Reproductive Medicine

Reproductive Medicine

Edited by **Chris Flagstad**

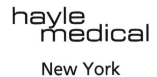

New York

Published by Hayle Medical,
30 West, 37th Street, Suite 612,
New York, NY 10018, USA
www.haylemedical.com

Reproductive Medicine
Edited by Chris Flagstad

International Standard Book Number: 978-1-63241-406-9 (Hardback)

Contents

Preface

In this highly competitive world people tend to delay their marriage and family planning decisions and therefore the demand for the advanced medicines and techniques in the field of reproductive medicine is constantly rising. This discipline helps to preserve and improve reproductive health of human beings and provides an option of having children at a particular time preferred by them. Its foundation lies in a combination of disciplines like molecular biology, biochemistry, anatomy, physiology, endocrinology and pathology. It mainly covers the issues related to family planning, birth control, puberty, sexual education, sexual dysfunction and infertility. This book is a vital tool for all researching or studying reproductive medicine as it gives incredible insights into emerging trends and concepts. The various advancements in this area are glanced at and their applications as well as ramifications are looked at in detail. Students, researchers, experts, medical experts and practitioners associated with reproductive medicine will benefit alike from this book.

This book has been the outcome of endless efforts put in by authors and researchers on various issues and topics within the field. The book is a comprehensive collection of significant researches that are addressed in a variety of chapters. It will surely enhance the knowledge of the field among readers across the globe.

It gives us an immense pleasure to thank our researchers and authors for their efforts to submit their piece of writing before the deadlines. Finally in the end, I would like to thank my family and colleagues who have been a great source of inspiration and support.

Editor

Randomized Comparison of Isosorbide Mononitrate and PGE2 Gel for Cervical Ripening at Term including High Risk Pregnancy

Kavita Agarwal,[1] Achla Batra,[1] Aruna Batra,[1] and Abha Aggarwal[2]

[1] *Department of Obstetrics & Gynaecology, Safdarjung Hospital, G-14, 92 Vrindavan Apartment, Gali No. 4, Krishna Nagar, Safdarjung Enclave, New Delhi 110029, India*
[2] *NIMS, Delhi 110029, India*

Correspondence should be addressed to Kavita Agarwal; drku93@gmail.com

Academic Editor: Robert Gaspar

Aims. Prostaglandin E2 is the most commonly used drug for cervical ripening prior to labour induction. However, there are concerns regarding uterine tachysystole and nonreassuring fetal heart (N-RFH). Isosorbide mononitrate (IMN) has been used successfully for cervical ripening. The present study was conducted to compare the two drugs for cervical ripening at term in hospital. *Methods.* Two hundred women with term pregnancies referred for induction of labour with Bishop score less than 6 were randomly allocated to receive either 40 mg IMN tablet vaginally ($n = 100$) or 0.5 mg PGE2 gel intracervically ($n = 100$). Adverse effects, progress, and outcomes of labour were assessed. *Results.* PGE2 group had significantly higher postripening mean Bishop score, shorter time from start of medication to vaginal delivery (13.37 ± 10.67 hours versus 30.78 ± 17.29 hours), and shorter labour-delivery interval compared to IMN group (4.53 ± 3.97 hours versus 7.34 ± 5.51 hours). However, PGE2 group also had significantly higher incidence of uterine tachysystole (15%) and N-RFH (11%) compared to none in IMN group, as well as higher caesarean section rate (27% versus 17%). *Conclusions.* Cervical ripening with IMN was less effective than PGE2 but resulted in fewer adverse effects and was safer especially in high risk pregnancies.

1. Introduction

Labour induction in unfavourable cervix is tedious and prolonged resulting in high incidence of failed induction and hence operative deliveries. Therefore, prostaglandin E2 (PGE2, dinoprostone gel) and PGE1 (misoprostol) are commonly used for success of labour induction and to reduce rate of caesarean section [1]. Prostaglandins are quite effective for cervical ripening [2] but have a high incidence of hyperstimulation and tachysystole which may compromise the fetus [3, 4]. An ideal cervical ripening agent should ripen cervix without stimulating uterine activity.

Nitric oxide (NO) donors such as isosorbide mononitrate (IMN) and glyceryl trinitrate (GTN) effectively induce cervical ripening without causing uterine contractions by rearranging cervical collagen and ground substance which softens the cervix [5–8].

The efficacy and safety of NO donors have been established in various studies [9–12] but there has been no Indian study to compare IMN with PGE2 gel for preinduction cervical ripening in term high risk pregnancies. With this background in mind, the present study was planned to compare the efficacy and safety of IMN with PGE2 gel for cervical ripening in term pregnancy in Indian population.

2. Methods

A prospective, randomized study was conducted from May 9, 2011, to April 8, 2012, at Safdarjung Hospital, New Delhi, India. The protocol was approved by the ethical committee of Safdarjung Hospital, Delhi, India.

Assuming that the percentages of women with a Bishop score less than 6 after 24 hours of the initiation of the IMN and PGE2 treatment would be 40% in the IMN group and

13% in the PGE2 group [13], it was determined that a sample size of 200 women, 100 in each group, would have 80% power to detect a 27% difference between the groups at $\alpha = 0.05$.

Study population comprised pregnant women >37 weeks hospitalised for induction of labour from outpatient department (O.P.D.) for either maternal or fetal indication. Low risk patients included postdated pregnancies (>42 weeks). High risk group included patients with hypertension, intrauterine growth restriction, cholestasis, or diabetes. All the participants had a singleton pregnancy with unfavourable cervix (Bishop score < 6), absence of uterine contractions, and intact membranes.

Exclusion criteria were fetal malpresentation, previous uterine incision, pregnancy with antepartum hemorrhage, severe anemia, heart disease or any contraindication to receive IMN or prostaglandins such as known allergy to drugs, bronchial asthma, hypotension, and palpitations.

Informed consent was obtained from all the participants. Simple randomization method was used. Patients were allocated to two groups by computer generated random numbers. The participants were enrolled by the first author and assigned to IMN and PGE2 group in accordance with the list of codes by the second author. This was a single blind trial as the participants did not know whether they were assigned to IMN or PGE2 group.

Baseline Bishop score of all the subjects was recorded. The participants were administered either 40 mg tablet of IMN (Monotrate; Sun pharmaceutical Industries, Mumbai, India) in posterior fornix which was repeated only once after 12 hours or three doses of 0.5 mg PGE2 gel (Cerviprime; Astra Zeneca Pharma India, Bangalore, India) intracervically given at 6 hours' interval.

The interval between 2 doses of vaginally administered IMN and its dosage was based on pharmacokinetics and serum profile data that revealed higher serum levels of vaginally administered 40 mg IMN tablet (337 μg/L) as compared to 144 μg/L with a 20 mg tablet. Cervical ripening was not improved by vaginal dose higher than 40 mg. The half-life is approximately 5 hours, the volume of distribution is 0.62 litre/kg, and systemic clearance is 115 mL/minute [14].

PGE2 is available as a 3 g endocervical gel containing 0.5 mg dinoprostone and can be repeated in 6 hours, not to exceed 1.5 mg in 24 hours. Half-life is 2.5 to 5 minutes. Onset of action is rapid and peaks in 30 to 45 minutes. T_{max} is 0.5 to 0.75 hours. C_{max} is approximately 484 pg/mL [15].

24 hours after first dose of IMN or PGE2, Bishop score was recorded and amniotomy done, if possible, irrespective of Bishop score. Labour was augmented by low dose oxytocin as per ACOG guidelines. Labour was immediately augmented by oxytocin if membranes ruptured spontaneously after IMN/PGE2 administration and further doses of drugs were withheld. Maternal and fetal condition and progress of labour were plotted on partogram.

Subjects who failed to achieve active phase of labour despite oxytocin stimulation for 6 hours were labelled as failed induction. Active labour was defined as at least 3 regular uterine contractions in 10 minutes, each lasting for at least 40 seconds with cervical dilatation of 3 cm or more.

The primary outcome variables were Bishop score at baseline and 24 hours after the first dose, initiation of treatment to vaginal delivery interval, and onset of active labour to vaginal delivery interval. Secondary outcome variables were subsequent need for oxytocin, operative delivery rates, and maternal side effects, that is, headache, hypotension, and complications such as hyperstimulation, tachysystole, and postpartum haemorrhage, and foetal outcome variables included abnormal foetal heart pattern, Apgar score at 1 and 5 minutes, and neonatal intensive care unit (NICU) admissions for Apgar ≤ 3 at 5 minutes of birth.

Statistical analysis was done using the following tests for comparison between IMN and PGE2 groups. Unpaired t-test was applied for age, gestational age, baseline Bishop score, Bishop score 24 hours after first dose, change in Bishop score, initiation of treatment to delivery interval, and labour delivery interval to see the difference between the two groups. Chi-square test has been applied for educational status, socioeconomic status, oxytocin requirement, caesarean section rate, headache, palpitation, tachysystole, hyperstimulation, postpartum haemorrhage, meconium stained liquor, nonreassuring foetal heart rate, Apgar score ≤ 3, and NICU admissions to see the association between two groups IMN and PGE2.

3. Results

A total of 200 women were recruited by computer generated random numbers, 100 to each IMN and PGE2 group (Figure 1), and simple randomization method was used. IMN group constituted 79% of women in low risk and 21% in high risk group. PGE2 group comprised 76% of patients in low risk and 24% in high risk group. Patients in low risk and high risk group were comparable in IMN and PGE2 groups. The maternal characteristics were similar in between the 2 groups (Tables 1 and 2). Most of the women were educated to more than middle school and belonged to lower middle class.

The mean Bishop score 24 hours after 1st dose of ripening agent was significantly higher in PGE2 group ($P = 0.006$). The mean change in modified Bishop score at 24 hours was 3.20 ± 1.61 for IMN and 3.87 ± 1.46 for PGE2 ($P = 0.002$; 95% CI, −1.09 to −0.24) (Table 3). The percentages of women with Bishop score < 6 at 24 hours of initiation of treatment were 35% in the IMN group and 12% in the PGE2 group ($P < 0.001$). Amniotomy was possible in all the patients. Oxytocin was required for 91% of participants in IMN group and 76% of participants in PGE2 group ($P = 0.004$). The mean time from treatment initiation to vaginal delivery was significantly shorter in PGE2 group (13.37 ± 10.67 hours) than in IMN group (30.78 ± 17.29 hours) with P value < 0.001 (95% CI, 12.98 to 20.99). Also, time from onset of labour to delivery interval was significantly shorter in PGE2 group ($P < 0.001$; 95% CI, 1.47 to 4.15) (Table 3).

Tachysystole was seen in a statistically significant number of patients in PGE2 group ($P < 0.001$) and 3 patients of PGE2 group had hyperstimulation whereas none of the participants in the IMN group had hyperstimulation or tachysystole (Table 4). There was no significant difference in the incidence of PPH in between the 2 groups.

TABLE 1: Maternal characteristics.

Variable	IMN N = 100	PGE2 N = 100	P value
Age (years)[a]	23.40 ± 2.391	23.57 ± 3.655	0.69
Gestational age (weeks)[a]	42.08 ± 1.066	41.99 ± 1.218	0.57
Parity			
Nulliparous[b]	54%	51%	0.671
Multiparous[b]	46%	49%	0.671
Baseline Bishop score[a] (pretreatment)	2.21 ± 1.241	2.20 ± 0.876	0.94

[a]Values are given as mean ± standard deviation.
[b]Values are given as percentage.

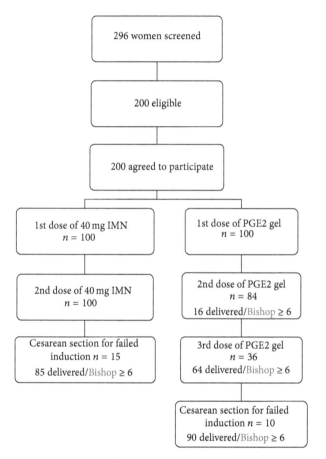

FIGURE 1: Flowchart of study participants.

TABLE 2: Indications for induction.

Indication	IMN N = 100	PGE2 N = 100
Low risk		
Postdated	79%	76%
High risk		
Hypertension	15%	18%
Intrauterine growth restriction	3%	2%
Cholestasis	3%	4%

initial treatment with IMN or PGE2 followed by artificial rupture of membranes and oxytocin, 15% of participants in IMN group and 10% in PGE2 group had caesarean section for failed induction. The most common indication for caesarean section in IMN group was for failed induction (88.2%) and in PGE2 group was for fetal distress. In PGE2 group, 40.7% of caesarean section were for fetal distress compared to none in the IMN group ($P < 0.001$).

The main side effects experienced in the IMN group were headache and palpitations; however, headache was not severe and none of the patients avoided the second dose of IMN. There were no changes in basic vital signs that required treatment in either group.

4. Discussion

IMN and PGE2 both are effective at cervical ripening but significant improvement in mean Bishop score and less number of women with Bishop score < 6 after 24 hours of initiation of treatment, higher change in Bishop score, less oxytocin requirement, and shorter initiation of treatment to delivery interval and labour delivery interval in PGE2 group support that PGE2 is more effective than IMN.

Chanrachakul et al. [10, 11] in 2 small trials compared IMN with prostaglandin E1 (PGE1) and nitric oxide (NO) donor glyceryl trinitrate (GTN) with PGE2 gel. Both trials demonstrated that 24 hours after initiation of treatment, increase in the median Bishop score was higher in prostaglandins group compared to NO donor. Osman et al. [13] also reported significantly higher change in modified Bishop score in PGE2 group ($P < 0.0001$) and percentages of

A statistically significant number of patients had nonreassuring foetal heart rate pattern in the PGE2 group compared to none in the IMN group ($P = 0.001$). Nonreassuring foetal heart rate (FHR) was found in 37.5% of women in high risk group compared to 2.6% in low risk group. Also, significant number of babies had Apgar ≤ 3 at 5 minutes ($P = 0.04$) and required NICU admission in PGE2 group. Apgar ≤ 3 at 5 minutes was seen only in high risk group (Table 5).

Caesarean delivery rate was more in PGE2 group compared to IMN group (27% versus 17%) but the difference was not statistically significant ($P = 0.22$) (Table 4). After

TABLE 3: Comparison of labour and delivery characteristics.

Variable	IMN $N = 100$	PGE2 $N = 100$	t value	P value	95% confidence interval	
					Lower	Upper
Bishop score at 24 hrs[a] (posttreatment)	5.41 ± 1.85	6.07 ± 1.52	-2.75	0.006	-1.13	-0.18
Change in Bishop score[a]	3.20 ± 1.61	3.87 ± 1.46	-3.07	0.002	-1.09	-0.24
Labour delivery interval (hours)[a]	7.34 ± 5.51	4.53 ± 3.97	4.13	<0.001	1.47	4.15
Initiation of treatment-delivery interval (hours)[a]	30.78 ± 17.29	13.37 ± 10.67	8.36	<0.001	12.98	20.99

[a]Values are given as mean ± standard deviation.

TABLE 4: Maternal and fetal outcome.

Variables	IMN $N = 100$	PGE2 $N = 100$	Chi-square value	P value
Headache	46%	0%		
Not requiring medication	40%	0%	50.0	<0.001
Requiring medication	6%	0%	6.18	0.013
Palpitation	12%	0%	12.76	<0.001
Tachysystole	0%	15%	16.21	<0.001
Hyperstimulation	0%	3%	3.05	0.08
Caesarean section	17%	27%	2.95	0.22
Postpartum hemorrhage	2%	3%	0.20	0.65
Nonreassuring FHR	0%	11%	11.64	0.001
Apgar $\leq$ 3 at 5 min (NICU admission)	0%	4%	4.08	0.04

TABLE 5: Fetal outcome.

Risk groups	IMN $N = 100$	PGE2 $N = 100$
Low risk		
Nonreassuring FHR	0%	2/76 (2.6%)
Apgar $\leq$ 3 at 5 min	0%	0%
High risk		
Nonreassuring FHR	0%	9/24 (37.5%)
Apgar $\leq$ 3 at 5 min	0%	4/24 (16.7%)

women with Bishop score < 6 requiring additional ripening agent 24 hours after initiation of treatment was found to be higher in the IMN group compared to PGE2 (40% versus 13%).

The oxytocin requirement was significantly less in PGE2 group ($P = 0.004$) compared to IMN group. Similarly, Chanrachakul et al. [10, 11] reported less oxytocin requirement in prostaglandins group compared to NO donors (75% in GTN versus 43% in PGE2 group, 92% in IMN versus 11% in PGE1 group).

In the present study, time from treatment initiation to delivery and labour delivery interval was significantly shorter in PGE2 group compared to IMN group ($P < 0.001$). Osman et al. [13] also found time from initiation of treatment to delivery interval significantly shorter in PGE2 group, 26.9 hours versus 39.7 hours in IMN group.

Tachysystole was seen in a significant number of patients in PGE2 group in the present study. There were 3 cases of hyperstimulation in PGE2 group and no case of hyperstimulation or tachysystole in IMN group. Chanrachakul et al. [10, 11] also found NO donors GTN and IMN to be less associated with uterine tachysystole compared to prostaglandins (0% in GTN versus 9% in PGE2 group, 0% in IMN versus 19% in PGE1 group). Hyperstimulation was found to be more associated with PGE1 group (0% in IMN versus 15% in PGE1 group). Sharma et al. [12] also reported hyperstimulation and tachysystole only in PGE1 (9% and 4.3%) and PGE2 groups (4.7% and 16.2%). Headache was reported in 48% of GTN subjects. In the present study, incidence of headache and palpitations was higher in IMN group compared to PGE2 group. Similar findings have also been reported in other previous studies [13, 16–18]. Headache and palpitations were more frequent with GTN and IMN group.

Statistically significant higher number of patients in the present study had nonreassuring foetal heart rate pattern in PGE2 group compared to none in IMN group. Similarly, Osman et al. [13] reported that 7% of patients had abnormal foetal heart rate patterns in PGE2 group compared to none in the IMN group.

The caesarean section rate was found to be higher in the PGE2 group than IMN (27% versus 17%) in the present study. Chanrachakul et al. [10, 11] in 2000 reported higher caesarean section rate in PGE2 group compared to IMN and GTN group (60% versus 40%).

To conclude, PGE2 is more effective than IMN for cervical ripening prior to induction of labour. However, it is associated with higher incidence of hyperstimulation, tachysystole, and nonreassuring foetal heart rate. There is only one study [13] in which IMN has been compared with PGE2 for cervical ripening at term pregnancy but they also have not categorised the results in high and low risk patients. In our study, we have compared the foetal outcome in low risk and high risk patients. Nonreassuring foetal heart rate in PGE2 group is higher in high risk group compared to low risk women. Apgar ≤ 3 at 5 minutes was seen only in high risk group in PGE2 group. Therefore, it may not be the ideal agent for cervical ripening especially in women with high risk pregnancy. IMN can be used safely in such cases.

Conflict of Interests

The authors declare that they have no conflict of interests regarding the publication of this paper.

References

[1] M. J. N. C. Keirse and H. J. De Koning Gans, "Randomized comparison of the effects of endocervical and vaginal prostaglandin E 2 gel in women with various degrees of cervical ripeness," *The American Journal of Obstetrics and Gynecology*, vol. 173, no. 6, pp. 1859–1864, 1995.

[2] M. J. N. C. Keirse, "Prostaglandins in preinduction cervical ripening: meta-analysis of worldwide clinical experience," *Journal of Reproductive Medicine for the Obstetrician and Gynecologist*, vol. 38, supplement 1, pp. 89–100, 1993.

[3] Y. Herabutya, P. O-Prasertsawat, and J. Pokpirom, "A comparison of intravaginal misoprostol and intracervical prostaglandin E2 gel for ripening of unfavorable cervix and labor induction," *Journal of Obstetrics and Gynaecology Research*, vol. 23, no. 4, pp. 369–374, 1997.

[4] D. A. Wing, M. M. Jones, A. Rahall, T. M. Goodwin, and R. H. Paul, "A comparison of misoprostol and prostaglandin E2 gel for preinduction cervical ripening and labor induction," *The American Journal of Obstetrics and Gynecology*, vol. 172, no. 6, pp. 1804–1810, 1995.

[5] W. Tschugguel, C. Schneeberger, H. Lass et al., "Human cervical ripening is associated with an increase in cervical inducible nitric oxide synthase expression," *Biology of Reproduction*, vol. 60, no. 6, pp. 1367–1372, 1999.

[6] M. A. Ledingham, A. J. Thomson, A. Young, L. M. Macara, I. A. Greer, and J. E. Norman, "Changes in the expression of nitric oxide synthase in the human uterine cervix during pregnancy and parturition," *Molecular Human Reproduction*, vol. 6, no. 11, pp. 1041–1048, 2000.

[7] M. Väisänen-Tommiska, M. Nuutila, K. Aittomäki, V. Hiilesmaa, and O. Ylikorkala, "Nitric oxide metabolites in cervical fluid during pregnancy: further evidence for the role of cervical nitric oxide in cervical ripening," *The American Journal of Obstetrics and Gynecology*, vol. 188, no. 3, pp. 779–785, 2003.

[8] K. Chwalisz, S. Shao-Qing, R. E. Garfield, and H. M. Beier, "Cervical ripening in guinea-pigs after a local application of nitric oxide," *Human Reproduction*, vol. 12, no. 10, pp. 2093–2101, 1997.

[9] B. Chanrachakul, Y. Herabutya, and P. Punyavachira, "Potential efficacy of nitric oxide for cervical ripening in pregnancy at term," *International Journal of Gynecology and Obstetrics*, vol. 71, no. 3, pp. 217–219, 2000.

[10] B. Chanrachakul, Y. Herabutya, and P. Punyavachira, "Randomized comparison of glyceryl trinitrate and prostaglandin E2 for cervical ripening at term," *Obstetrics and Gynecology*, vol. 96, no. 4, pp. 549–553, 2000.

[11] B. Chanrachakul, Y. Herabutya, and P. Punyavachira, "Randomized trial of isosorbide mononitrate versus misoprostol for cervical ripening at term," *International Journal of Gynecology and Obstetrics*, vol. 78, no. 2, pp. 139–145, 2002.

[12] Y. Sharma, S. Kumar, S. Mittal, R. Misra, and V. Dadhwal, "Evaluation of glyceryl trinitrate, misoprostol, and prostaglandin E 2 gel for preinduction cervical ripening in term pregnancy," *Journal of Obstetrics and Gynaecology Research*, vol. 31, no. 3, pp. 210–215, 2005.

[13] I. Osman, F. MacKenzie, J. Norrie, H. M. Murray, I. A. Greer, and J. E. Norman, "The "PRIM" study: a randomized comparison of prostaglandin E_2 gel with the nitric oxide donor isosorbide mononitrate for cervical ripening before the induction of labor at term," *American Journal of Obstetrics & Gynecology*, vol. 194, no. 4, pp. 1012–1021, 2006.

[14] C. D. Bates, A. E. Nicoll, A. B. Mullen, F. Mackenzie, A. J. Thomson, and J. E. Norman, "Serum profile of isosorbide mononitrate after vaginal administration in the third trimester," *BJOG*, vol. 110, no. 1, pp. 64–67, 2003.

[15] Dorland's Medical Dictionary for Health Consumers, 2007.

[16] S. S. Bollapragada, F. MacKenzie, J. D. Norrie et al., "Randomised placebo-controlled trial of outpatient (at home) cervical ripening with isosorbide mononitrate (IMN) prior to induction of labour—clinical trial with analyses of efficacy and acceptability. The IMOP Study," *BJOG*, vol. 116, no. 9, pp. 1185–1195, 2009.

[17] M. Bullarbo, M. E. Orrskog, B. Andersch, L. Granström, A. Norström, and E. Ekerhovd, "Outpatient vaginal administration of the nitric oxide donor isosorbide mononitrate for cervical ripening and labor induction postterm: a randomized controlled study," *American Journal of Obstetrics and Gynecology*, vol. 196, no. 1, pp. 50.e1–50.e5, 2007.

[18] S. M. Habib, S. S. Emam, and A. S. Saber, "Outpatient cervical ripening with nitric oxide donor isosorbide mononitrate prior to induction of labor," *International Journal of Gynecology and Obstetrics*, vol. 101, no. 1, pp. 57–61, 2008.

Impact of Exogenous Gonadotropin Stimulation on Circulatory and Follicular Fluid Cytokine Profiles

N. Ellissa Baskind,[1] Nicolas M. Orsi,[2] and Vinay Sharma[1]

[1] *The Leeds Centre for Reproductive Medicine, Leeds Teaching Hospitals NHS Trust, Seacroft Hospital, York Road, LS14 6UH Leeds, UK*
[2] *Women's Health Research Group, Leeds Institute of Cancer & Pathology, St James's University Hospital, Wellcome Trust Brenner Building, Beckett Street, LS9 7TF Leeds, UK*

Correspondence should be addressed to N. Ellissa Baskind; ellissa@doctors.org.uk

Academic Editor: Stefania A. Nottola

Background. The natural cycle is the prototype to which we aspire to emulate in assisted reproduction techniques. Increasing evidence is emerging that controlled ovarian hyperstimulation (COH) with exogenous gonadotropins may be detrimental to oogenesis, embryo quality, and endometrial receptivity. This research aimed at assessing the impact of COH on the intrafollicular milieu by comparing follicular fluid (FF) cytokine profiles during stimulated *in vitro* fertilization (IVF) and modified natural cycle (MNC) IVF. *Methods.* Ten women undergoing COH IVF and 10 matched women undergoing MNC IVF were recruited for this pilot study. 40 FF cytokine concentrations from individual follicles and plasma were measured by fluid-phase multiplex immunoassay. Demographic/cycle/cytokine data were compared and correlations between cytokines were computed. *Results.* No significant differences were found between COH and MNC groups for patient and cycle demographics, including outcome. Overall mean FF cytokine levels were higher in the MNC group for 29/40 cytokines, significantly so for leukaemia inhibitory factor and stromal cell-derived factor-1α. Furthermore, FF MNC cytokine correlations were significantly stronger than for COH data. *Conclusions.* These findings suggest that COH perturbs intrafollicular cytokine networks, in terms of both cytokine levels and their interrelationships. This may impact oocyte maturation/fertilization and embryo developmental competence.

1. Introduction

Controlled ovarian hyperstimulation (COH) with gonadotropins has improved success rates of *in vitro* fertilization (IVF) by increasing the number and opportunity for selection of embryos before transfer [1–3] as well as permitting the cryopreservation of supernumerary embryos for further fertility treatment [4, 5]. The basis of COH is to support the growth of multiple follicles to the preovulatory stage, a process achieved by bypassing physiological regulatory mechanisms. Urinary-derived or recombinant follicle stimulating hormone (FSH) is administered to increase serum concentrations above the threshold required for dominant follicle selection, thus enabling the entire cohort of recruited follicles to develop and attain preovulatory status [4]. Luteinising hormone (LH) is often coadministered although, following pituitary downregulation, this is not essential for follicular development as remnant basal LH levels are sufficient to stimulate the theca cells. Administration of a GnRH analogue (long protocol) or an antagonist (short protocol) that desensitizes the pituitary is primarily used to prevent premature LH surge as a consequence of supraphysiological serum oestradiol (E_2) levels which, if it occurs, can lead to premature luteinisation and/or ovulation.

With few exceptions [6], the last two decades have witnessed a mounting body of evidence indicating that ovarian stimulation has a detrimental effect on oogenesis, embryo quality, and endometrial receptivity [7–13]. More specifically, Sharma et al. [7] and Pellicer et al. [14] demonstrated that retrieval of >10 oocytes per woman adversely affected their quality based on oocyte/embryo morphology, fertilization, and implantation rates. More recently van der Gaast et al. [15] found 13 oocytes to be the optimum number retrieved in order to achieve a pregnancy using a long protocol, above which there was a fall in pregnancy rates. An extreme example of the negative impact of COH is the excessively high number of poor quality oocytes seen in ovarian hyperstimulation syndrome (OHSS), which is putatively attributable to detrimental supraphysiological E_2 levels [16]. These observations in humans are supported by a number of rodent studies that investigated the impact of exogenous gonadotropin stimulation on oocytes and demonstrated a delay in embryo development [17, 18]. It has been suggested that gonadotropin stimulation may affect oocyte maturation and the completion of meiosis, thus leading to an increased risk of having aneuploid oocytes and/or embryos [10, 19]. As such, *in vitro* maturation (IVM) has been proposed as an alternative strategy since it reduces exposure to exogenous gonadotropin stimulation, but the process itself introduces a host of other variables/complications (e.g., disruption of the meiotic spindle) that do not allow a fair comparison of these approaches to be made [20]. von Wolff et al. [21] recently demonstrated a varying endocrine follicular milieu together with the concentration of putative markers of oocyte quality, specifically anti-Müllerian hormone (AMH) between NC and COH FF, and suggest that this may be the cause for the lower oocyte quality following COH compared with naturally matured oocytes.

There has also been some concern that suppressed LH concentrations in the late follicular phase may be detrimental through downstream perturbations in follicular steroid synthesis. Consequently, stimulation protocols incorporating exogenous LH were developed, resulting in an increase in the percentage of diploid and good quality embryos obtained [22, 23]. By contrast, other investigators have reported a reduction in fertility and increased risk of miscarriage when incorporating exogenous LH into protocols [24, 25]. Such contradictory findings support the notion of a "LH window" below which E_2 production is inadequate and above which LH may begin premature luteinisation and be detrimental to follicular development [26]. von Wolff et al. [21] postulate that the reduced levels of intrafollicular AMH they demonstrated following COH compared with NC may be attributed to LH suppression, resulting initially in low follicular androgen concentrations, and subsequently to low AMH production which in turn may be responsible for lower oocyte quality.

Natural cycle IVF (NC-IVF) has been proposed as an alternative treatment for older women and poor responders [27]. Indeed, there has been a resurgence of interest in NC-IVF for all patients in recent years because it avoids COH and its potential sequelae. Moreover, this also supports the international drive to reduce multiple pregnancies rates with elective single embryo transfer and to minimise complications such as OHSS [28–30]. Pelinck et al. [1] conducted a systematic review of 1,800 natural IVF cycles reported between 1989 and 2000 and concluded that NC-IVF has a pregnancy rate of less than 10% per cycle. More recent reports concur, presenting a similar 15.2% live birth rate per initiated cycle in all reported unstimulated NCs in women <35 years ($n = 795$) in the United States (2006-2007) [31].

A compromise between these approaches has been described: mild ovarian stimulation IVF. This method incorporates the use of low dose gonadotropin stimulation together with a gonadotropin releasing hormone (GnRH) antagonist aimed at generating fewer than eight oocytes per cycle [32]. The term modified natural cycle IVF (MNC-IVF) is applied when drugs (e.g., human chorionic gonadotropin (hCG)) are used to induce final oocyte maturation whereby a GnRH antagonist is administered during a spontaneous cycle to reduce the risk of cancellation [33] and/or where luteal support is provided.

During folliculogenesis, follicular fluid (FF) composition exhibits dynamic changes as individual follicular cell types respond to gonadotropins by secreting different hormones and cytokines [34, 35]. As growth factors regulating all stages of folliculogenesis, cytokines have been shown to govern the development/function of somatic cells and the oocyte as well as the composition of FF [36–42]. Given that oocyte quality influences subsequent embryo viability [43], it has been suggested that the disruption in the balance of these intrafollicular mediators following COH may influence cycle outcome [44–52]. The correct regulation of cytokine networks is essential to support normal physiology and this central role is underscored by the fact that inflammatory/immune dysfunctions underpin many pathological reproductive conditions, resulting in both local and systemic changes in cytokine profiles [53–55].

Studies have measured individual FF cytokines throughout the menstrual cycle. For example, the levels of interleukin- (IL-) 8, a chemotactic and angiogenic cytokine essential to folliculogenesis, have been found to rise from the midfollicular to the late follicular phase. These levels are comparable to those found during a COH cycle [56], implying that granulosa cell (GC) and theca cell (TC) IL-8 secretion is a true physiological phenomenon associated with follicular growth/maturation rather than resulting from gonadotropin stimulation. *In vitro* enhancement of IL-8 secretion by cultured GCs and TCs was evident following exposure to IL-1α and IL-1β, but not tumour necrosis factor- (TNF-) α, suggesting that IL-8 is both gonadotropin and cytokine-induced and may thus be involved in the hormonally regulated stages of folliculogenesis and ovulation [57].

Although cytokines are readily detected in FF, the complexity of their network regulation makes their study in isolation difficult to interpret. In view of their biological properties (pleiotropism, synergy, antagonism, functional redundancy, and differential sensitivity) [58–60], cytokines should ideally be investigated in terms of their interrelationships as much as in terms of their absolute concentrations. Whilst a recent study by Bersinger et al. [61] failed to demonstrate a difference in 13 FF cytokines between women undergoing NC and COH IVF, no specific attention was paid towards the complex interrelations within the cytokine networks. To date, there has been a paucity of studies focusing on minimal stimulation regimens and MNCs, and comparisons of isolated cytokine concentrations (e.g., vascular endothelial growth factor (VEGF) in COH and NC-IVF) have been inconsistent [62, 63]. Exogenous gonadotropins may disrupt intrafollicular cytokine networks, in turn affecting oocyte developmental potential. Therefore, this pilot study aimed at examining the impact of gonadotropins on the intrafollicular cytokine milieu in MNC and following COH cycles.

2. Materials and Methods

2.1. Patient Recruitment and Sample Collection. From November 2008 to March 2009, ten women who required treatment with IVF/ICSI due to unexplained or male factor infertility aged 25–35 years with a body mass index (BMI) 19–30 were selected to undergo MNC-IVF/intracytoplasmic sperm injection (ICSI) at the Assisted Conception Unit, St James's University Hospital, Leeds, UK. These patients were matched with ten women undergoing COH-IVF/ICSI. Only nonsmokers and women who drank <6 units alcohol per week were included. They were required to be ovulatory (confirmed by transvaginal ultrasound scan (TVUSS), progesterone levels, or commercial LH surge kits within the preceding three months) and have a normal endocrine profile (early follicular phase FSH < 8.0 IU/L and E_2 50–200 pmol/L), a negative infection screen (including negative serum *Chlamydia* antigens), and normal pelvic anatomy confirmed by TVUSS and laparoscopy. Furthermore, they were required to have no risk factors for pelvic pathology (e.g., history of pelvic inflammatory disease, incomplete miscarriage, ectopic pregnancy, cervical dyskaryosis, and abdominal/pelvic/cervical surgery). Women with coexisting morbidity (e.g., autoimmune diseases, inflammatory conditions, and diabetes mellitus) and those taking regular medications were also excluded. The study protocol was approved by National Research Ethics Service, Leeds (East) Research Ethics Committee, and all participants provided written informed consent.

All women underwent a baseline TVUSS (ALOKA SSSD 1700) in the early follicular phase. In the MNC cohort, a TVUSS assessment was performed on alternate days from day 8 of the cycle, until the mean maximal diameter (MMD) measured in two planes (sagittal and transverse) of the dominant follicle measured ≥14 mm, after which they were performed daily. Women were asked to use urinary LH kits twice daily (06:00–08:00 and 18:00–20:00) in order to identify the onset of LH surge prior to spontaneous ovulation. An injection of 5,000 IU hCG (Pregnyl (Organon, Cambridge, UK)) was given when the MMD of the lead follicle measured ≥17 mm (17.0–18.1 mm). If the urinary LH kit was positive, ultrasound directed oocyte retrieval (UDOR) was performed the day after the surge was detected; otherwise it was planned for 36 h after hCG. For subsequent analysis, women who had a spontaneous LH surge and women who were administered exogenous hCG were grouped together as the MNC cohort. All women in the COH arm underwent the long protocol. Pituitary downregulation was attained using leuprorelin acetate SR 3.75 mg (Prostap (Wyeth, Maidenhead, Berkshire, UK)) administered on the first day of the menstrual cycle. COH was achieved with 225 IU human menopausal gonadotropin (HMG) daily (Menopur, Ferring, Slough, Berkshire, UK). As with the MNC-IVF/ICSI cycle, when one or more follicles had an MMD of ≥17 mm, 5,000 IU hCG (Pregnyl (Organon, Cambridge, UK)) was administered 36 h prior to UDOR.

All UDORs were performed between 09:00 and 11:00 to accommodate putative circadian variations in ovarian physiology. Whole blood was collected immediately before sedation in EDTA vacutainers. Dead space (containing 1.5 mL 0.9% sodium chloride solution) within the oocyte harvesting needle and tubing was constant/uniform throughout such that the first 1.5 mL aspirated was checked and discarded. Subsequent aspirate was considered to contain FF and, following oocyte assessment and retrieval, was subsequently labelled to ensure longitudinal tracking of the corresponding oocyte to its fate (for multifollicular cycles). Follicles were flushed up to four times with culture medium (Enhance HTF Culture Medium with HEPES; Conception Technologies, San Diego, California, USA) if no oocyte was obtained in the initial aspirate to minimise the risk of inadvertently aspirating a second follicle and collecting the oocyte from the previous one due to being contained within the dead space. All ultrasonically visible follicles were individually aspirated irrespective of their size. The aspiration pressure applied was uniform on all follicles (183–185 mm/Hg).

All samples were immediately stored on ice. Whole blood and FF samples were centrifuged (2,000 rpm at 4°C for 10 minutes) to isolate plasma and remove cell debris, respectively. All samples were frozen at −80°C within one hour of retrieval until required for analysis. In the MNC cohort, only the FF from the single dominant follicle was analysed. In the COH cohort, FF analysis was performed on the follicles yielding the oocytes that generated transferred embryos (since double ETs were performed in these cycles, the follicle selected for analysis was the one yielding the embryo with the highest morphological grading).

In both cycles, routine procedures for fertilization with IVF/ICSI were performed as previously described [64]. Embryo transfer (ET) was performed 84–90 h after hCG injection. A single ET was performed in the MNC cohort, whilst a double ET was performed in the COH cohort (as per ACU protocols at the time). All women in the MNC cohort who underwent an ET received 2,500 IU hCG (Pregnyl) on the day of ET and again 72 h later for luteal support. Women in the COH cohort who developed <15 follicles had an identical luteal support regimen, whereas those women with ≥15 follicles following COH were given daily intramuscular injection of 100 mg progesterone (Gestone, Nordic Pharma, Reading, Berkshire, UK), which was continued throughout the first trimester of pregnancy. Pregnancy tests were performed on first void urine 14 days after ET with a commercial urinary kit. A clinical pregnancy was defined as one demonstrating a gestational sac with a fetal pole and a fetal heart or an ectopic pregnancy by TVUSS at 6-7 weeks' gestation.

2.2. Fluid-Phase Multiplex Immunoassay. Cytokine levels in both FF and plasma were measured by fluid-phase cytometric multiplex immunoassay (Bio-Rad Laboratories, Hercules, CA, USA) (Bio-rad assays: Human Cytokine 27-plex Assay M50-0KCAF0Y; Human Cytokine 21-plex Assay MF0-005KMII) using a Luminex 100 cytometer (Luminex

Corporation, Austin, Texas, USA) equipped with BioPlex 4.0 Manager software (Bio-Rad Laboratories, Ltd., Hertfordshire, UK), as previously described [65]. Target cytokines included interleukin- (IL-) 1 receptor antagonist (ra), IL-2ra, IL-3, IL-6, IL-7, IL-8, IL-9, IL-10, IL-12 (p40), IL-12 (p70), IL-13, IL-15, IL-16, IL-18, leukaemia inhibitory factor (LIF), granulocyte macrophage-colony stimulating factor (GM-CSF), macrophage- (M-) CSF, granulocyte- (G-) CSF, stem cell factor (SCF), interferon- (IFN-) α, IFN-γ, IFN-γ inducible protein- (IP-10), TNF-α, TNF-β, TNF related apoptosis inducing ligand (TRAIL), VEGF, platelet derived growth factor (PDGF), basic fibroblast growth factor (b-FGF), nerve growth factor- (NGF-) β, stem cell growth factor- (SCGF-) β, growth regulated oncogene- (GRO-) α, macrophage inflammatory protein- (MIP-) 1β, monocyte chemoattractant protein- (MCP-) 1, MCP-3, eotaxin, regulated upon activation of normal T cell expressed and secreted (RANTES), stromal cell-derived factor- (SDF-) 1α, cutaneous T-cell attracting chemokine (CTACK), monokine induced by IFN-γ (MIG), and macrophage migration inhibitory factor (MIF).

2.3. Contamination and Standardisation. Oocyte retrieval frequently results in disruption of the intraovarian vasculature such that blood (macroscopic or microscopic) contaminates the FF retrieved [66]. Furthermore, although the needle and tubing were primed with normal saline at the commencement of aspiration of each ovary, in between subsequent follicular aspirations, protein-free flush medium formulated with gentamicin (enhanced HTF culture medium with HEPES; Conception Technologies, San Diego, California, USA) was used, with potential dilution of the FF [67]. Such contamination/dilution was accounted for in the FF cytokine analysis. This entailed cytokine, total protein (by Lowry assay, Bio-Rad), and von Willebrand factor (vWF; by enzyme-linked immunosorbent assay; R&D Systems, Abingdon, UK) measurement in both plasma and FF. Since vWF is a large plasma multimeric glycoprotein that does not pass through the basement membrane and is not produced by follicular cells, it enabled accurate quantification of FF blood (and therefore circulatory cytokine) contamination (present authors, manuscript under review). The dilutional effect of the flush medium was instead accounted for by standardising both FF and plasma (the latter to enable a valid comparison with the former) cytokine concentrations to total protein (pg cytokine/mg protein).

2.4. Statistical Analysis. Chi-squared, independent samples t-tests, or Mann-Whitney U tests were used to compare MNC and COH patient demographics, cycle details, FF, and plasma cytokines following tests for normal distribution by Shapiro-Wilk test (Stata/SE 11.1, Texas, USA). In order to address the interrelationships between multiple cytokines and the impact that COH has upon these, heat maps were generated using R 2.7.0 software (R Foundation for Statistical Computing, Vienna, Austria). Correlations between the different cytokines were determined for MNC and COH data using Kendall's tau as a measure of correlation (Stata/SE 11.1). Resulting P values were adjusted for multiple comparisons with Holm's correction ($P < 0.05$ was considered significant).

3. Results and Discussion

3.1. Participant, MNC, and COH Cycle Demographics. In the MNC cohort, one patient had a positive LH surge and therefore did not receive exogenous hCG. At the time of UDOR 12 hours after the positive surge, spontaneous ovulation had occurred such that no FF was retrieved and an oocyte was not obtained. This patient was therefore excluded from the study. No statistically significant differences were noted in patient demographics (age, BMI, baseline endocrine profile (FSH, LH, and E_2), and ethnicity), day of UDOR, follicular aspirate volume, oocyte maturity, and cycle outcome between the two groups (Table 1).

3.2. Follicular Fluid and Plasma Cytokines. Most FF cytokines (29 out of 40) were found to be at higher concentrations in the MNC group compared to the COH group (binomial test: $P < 0.001$). This relationship was statistically significant for LIF ($P < 0.01$) and SDF-1α ($P < 0.05$) (Figure 1). As with FF, the majority of circulatory cytokines in the MNC cohort were present at higher concentrations than in the COH group (Figure 2), a relationship which was significant for 12 of these: IL-2ra, IL-3, IL-12 (p40), LIF, M-CSF, IFN-α, TRAIL, NGF-β, GRO-α, MCP-3, RANTES, and SDF-1α ($P < 0.05$). Conversely, plasma IL-12 (p70) levels were present at significantly higher levels following COH ($P < 0.05$) (Figure 2).

Heat maps were generated following correlation analysis using Kendall's tau to demonstrate FF cytokine interrelationships (Figure 3). Significantly more pairs of cytokines exhibited strong correlations in the MNC data compared to the COH data (binomial test) ($P < 0.001$). Various relationship alterations were also noted; for example, LIF and TNF-α demonstrated a weak negative correlation in the MNC group (Kendall's tau: -0.08) compared with a strong positive correlation following COH (Kendall's tau: 0.46). When plasma:FF cytokine ratios were compared between the MNC and COH cohorts, no statistically significant differences were identified.

Gonadotropin use in COH has previously been recognised to perturb the intrauterine cytokine milieu. Significantly higher concentrations of various cytokines including IL-1β, IL-5, IL-10, IL-12, IL-17, TNF-α, and eotaxin have been recorded in endometrial secretions from stimulated cycles compared to NCs [68]. Similarly, in the ovary, it has been suggested that exogenous gonadotropins may influence the levels of cytokines such as IL-1β, IL-6, and TNF-α following earlier studies on FF [69]. More recently, de Los Santos et al. [70] demonstrated altered cumulus cell gene expression for leukocyte differentiation and T-cell activation and regulation following COH, which may in turn influence follicular cytokine profiles as highlighted by the present findings.

To the best of our knowledge, FF has not previously been analysed for such an extensive range of cytokines in NC/MNC and COH cycles. In the present pilot study, FF concentrations of 29 out of the 40 cytokines analysed were found to be higher in the MNC cohort, significantly so for LIF and SDF-1α. LIF is an embryotrophic cytokine whose secretion by GCs and stromal cells into FF has previously

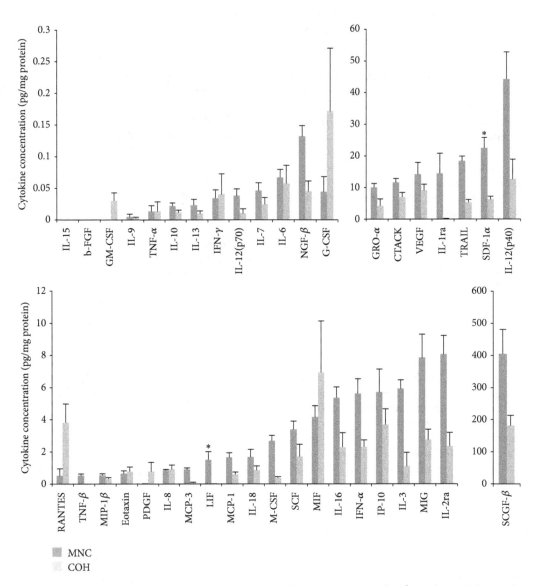

FIGURE 1: Mean (± SEM) FF cytokine concentrations in MNC (n = 9) and COH (n = 10) cycles (*significant difference from COH cycle; P < 0.05).

TABLE 1: Participant and cycle demographics in MNC and COH cycles.

	NC Cycle	COH Cycle	P-value
Age (years)	30.8 ± 0.72 (27–34)	31.9 ± 1.20 (24–35)	0.21
BMI (kg/m^2)	23.5 ± 0.86 (20.0–28.0)	24.0 ± 0.87 (20.0–30.0)	0.88
Baseline FSH (IU/L)	5.2 ± 0.40 (4.0–8.0)	6.0 ± 0.45 (3.9–7.9)	0.24
Baseline LH (IU/L)	5.2 ± 0.48 (2.6–7.1)	4.6 ± 0.55 (1.5–7.4)	0.44
Baseline E$_2$ (pmol/L)	115.2 ± 12.23 (73–162)	117.8 ± 18.14 (25–193)	0.92
Day of cycle for aspiration	14 ± 0.93 (10–20)	13.1 ± 0.34 (12–15)	0.35
Follicular volume (mL)	2.3 ± 0.40 (0.5–4.0)	3.0 ± 0.51 (1.0–6.5)	0.62
Mature oocyte (%)	70[a]	100[b]	0.06
Clinical pregnancy (%)	20[c]	30[c]	0.61

Mean ± SEM (range), unless otherwise specified. [a]One patient spontaneously ovulated, therefore 9 oocytes were retrieved; [b]Follicles yielding a mature oocyte which was subsequently transferred as an embryo were included in this cohort; [c]Clinical pregnancy rate calculated per embryos transferred [MNC: 7 embryos transferred; COH; 10 embryos transferred].

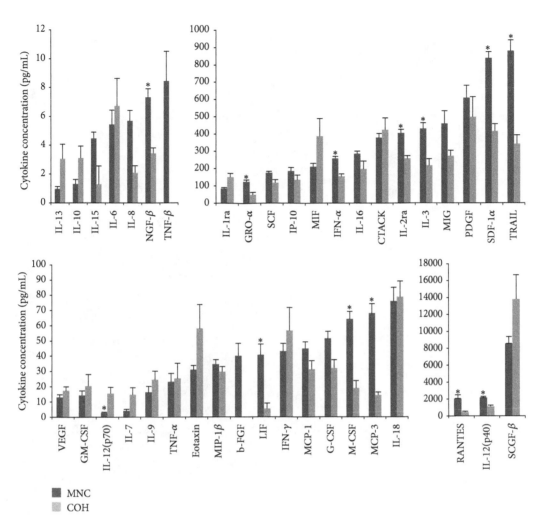

FIGURE 2: Mean (± SEM) plasma cytokine concentrations in MNC ($n = 9$) and COH ($n = 10$) cycles (*significant difference from COH cycle; $P < 0.05$).

been shown to be stimulated by hCG [71–73]. Since both the MNC and COH cohorts in this study received identical doses of exogenous hCG, the elevated levels of LIF in MNC FF may represent an enhanced response to hCG, whereas the likely perturbed cytokine response allied to COH may reflect a reduced sensitivity to hCG resulting in lower LIF concentrations. COH also appeared to perturb relationships between cytokines, highlighted by the relative changes in intrafollicular LIF and TNF-α (where the latter modulates ovarian stromal cell secretion of the former) [71]. The heat map displays a strong positive correlation between LIF and TNF-α in the MNC cohort whereas this relationship is weakened following COH. Interestingly, FF LIF concentrations have also been correlated with E_2 concentrations (possibly through its role in enhancing aromatase expression) which, in turn, relate to follicular maturity [74, 75]. Although a comparable causal association has not been identified to date in the ovary, 17-β oestradiol is known to induce LIF synthesis in bovine oviduct epithelial cells [76]. It is tempting to speculate that an analogous mechanism is at play in the ovary, where the supraphysiological E_2 levels associated with

COH may impair the induction of follicular LIF synthesis, with a consequent impact on the FF milieu and oocyte quality.

SDF-1α is a chemokine secreted by oocytes, which acts in a paracrine manner to prevent follicular activation, thereby controlling the entry of primordial follicles into the growing pool in NCs [77]. Furthermore, FF SDF-1α has previously been positively correlated with FF VEGF levels in COH cycles, where it is believed to play a proangiogenic role in supporting follicular growth [78]. Our findings corroborate this correlation in the COH group (Figure 3). By contrast, this relationship was much weaker in the MNC cohort, suggesting that it may thus in part be gonadotropin dependent.

Akin to what was noted for FF, plasma cytokine levels in the MNC group were higher than in COH cycles. The exception was circulatory IL-12 (p70), which was measured at significantly higher concentrations following COH. Furthermore, correlations between FF IL-12 (p70) and other cytokines were markedly altered following stimulation. In the MNC cohort, most FF cytokines were positively correlated with IL-12 (p70), whilst this relationship was reversed following COH. Conversely, IFN-γ and TNF-α were negatively

Natural cycle

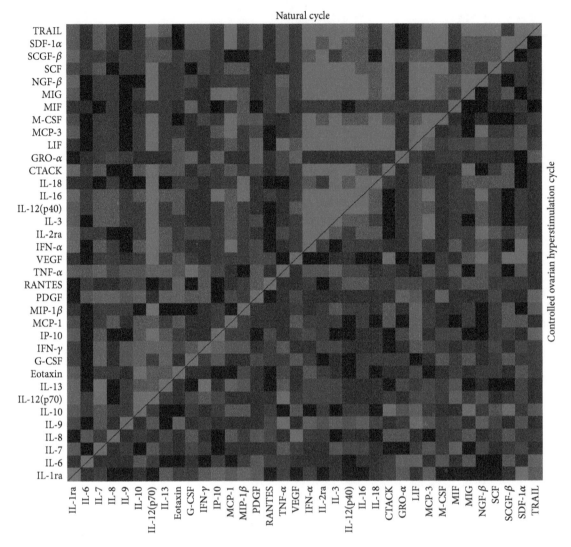

FIGURE 3: Heat maps demonstrating correlations between cytokines in periovulatory FF in MNC and COH cycles. Each square represents the correlation between specific cytokines: a red square represents a significantly positive correlation whilst a blue square represents a significantly negative correlation. A black square represents no significant relationship and the darker shades of red and blue represent weaker positive and negative correlations, respectively.

correlated with IL-12 (p70) in the MNC group and positively in the COH cohort. Interestingly, an intricate triumvirate relationship between these particular cytokines has been identified in the regulation of inflammatory responses. IL-12 (p70) induces IFN-γ production [79] and, in turn, IFN-γ markedly augments IL-12 (p70) production, thereby providing a key inflammatory amplifying mechanism [80]. By contrast, TNF-α is thought to inhibit IFN-γ-induced IL-12 (p70) production, as demonstrated by Hodge-Dufour et al. [81], whose TNF$^{+/+}$ mice exhibited a prompt inflammatory response which resolved spontaneously compared with a delayed, more vigorous, inflammatory response leading to death associated with elevated IL-12 levels in TNF$^{-/-}$ mice when injected with *Corynebacterium parvum*. Thus, TNF-α is thought to contribute to the resolution of IL-12- (p70-) driven inflammatory processes. In the MNC cohort, TNF-α was negatively correlated with both IL-12 (p70) and IFN-γ, thus

suggesting that, in the absence of stimulatory gonadotropins, TNF-α of follicular cell origin may play an analogous role via its capacity to regulate IL-12 (p70) production. A positive correlation between these FF cytokines in combination with significantly elevated systemic IL-12 (p70) levels suggests a disruption of this mechanism following COH. An analogous disruption in the ovary following COH could thus contribute to the detrimental sequelae of increased IL-12 (p70) and IFN-γ levels despite the observed compensatory rise in modulatory TNF-α levels.

Fluctuations in systemic white cell populations have been attributed to stimulation with exogenous gonadotropins such that the total number of circulatory leukocytes and neutrophils was increased on the day of hCG administration in COH compared to NCs [82]. Other studies have reported an increase in plasma white cell count and G-CSF, but not in M-CSF or IL-6, during COH [83]. Furthermore, various cytokines have been found to be elevated in FF following COH, including IL-1β, IL-6, and TNF-α [69]. The main difference between the present study and those cited is our administration of exogenous hCG in the MNC cohort. Both LH and hCG induce IL-1β and TNF-α, both of which subsequently upregulate GM-CSF expression [38]. Despite identical doses of hCG being used to trigger ovulation in both groups in the current study, GM-CSF in particular was measured at higher (although not statistically significant) levels following COH in both FF and plasma. Furthermore, following COH, there was a trend towards several other proinflammatory cytokines in both FF and plasma to be found at higher concentration, with IL-12 (p70) levels in particular being significantly higher in COH plasma samples. This provides further evidence that COH can induce both local and systemic inflammatory network deregulations featuring perturbations in cytokine interrelationships which, speculatively, may potentially also impact oocyte viability and treatment outcome. Unfortunately, the present pilot study was not powered to answer this particular question.

4. Conclusions

In conclusion, this investigation demonstrated that COH not only alters FF cytokine profiles compared to MNCs but also perturbs their circulatory levels and disrupts their interrelationships. Given their central role in orchestrating normal follicular physiology, these changes have the potential to adversely affect follicular function and compromise oocyte viability.

Conflict of Interests

The authors declare that there is no conflict of interests regarding the publication of this paper.

References

[1] M. J. Pelinck, A. Hoek, A. H. M. Simons, and M. J. Heineman, "Efficacy of natural cycle IVF: a review of the literature," *Human Reproduction Update*, vol. 8, no. 2, pp. 129–139, 2002.

[2] M. P. Rosen, S. Shen, A. T. Dobson, P. F. Rinaudo, C. E. McCulloch, and M. I. Cedars, "A quantitative assessment of follicle size on oocyte developmental competence," *Fertility and Sterility*, vol. 90, no. 3, pp. 684–690, 2008.

[3] S. X. Y. Wang, "The past, present, and future of embryo selection in *in vitro* fertilization: frontiers in reproduction conference," *The Yale Journal of Biology and Medicine*, vol. 84, no. 4, pp. 487–490, 2011.

[4] N. S. Macklon, R. L. Stouffer, L. C. Giudice, and B. C. J. M. Fauser, "The science behind 25 years of ovarian stimulation for *in vitro* fertilization," *Endocrine Reviews*, vol. 27, no. 2, pp. 170–207, 2006.

[5] J. P. Geraedts and L. Gianaroli, "Embryo selection and IVF," *Human Reproduction*, vol. 27, no. 9, pp. 2876–2877, 2012.

[6] E. H. Y. Ng, E. Y. L. Lau, W. S. B. Yeung, and P. C. Ho, "Oocyte and embryo quality in patients with excessive ovarian response during in vitro fertilization treatment," *Journal of Assisted Reproduction and Genetics*, vol. 20, no. 5, pp. 186–191, 2003.

[7] V. Sharma, J. Williams, W. Collins, A. Riddle, B. Mason, and M. Whitehead, "A comparison of treatments with exogenous FSH to promote folliculogenesis in patients with quiescent ovaries due to the continued administration of an LH-RH agonist," *Human Reproduction*, vol. 2, no. 7, pp. 553–556, 1987.

[8] V. Sharma, M. Whitehead, B. Mason et al., "Influence of superovulation on endometrial and embryonic development," *Fertility and Sterility*, vol. 53, no. 5, pp. 822–829, 1990.

[9] J. A. Horcajadas, A. Riesewijk, J. Polman et al., "Effect of controlled ovarian hyperstimulation in IVF on endometrial gene expression profiles," *Molecular Human Reproduction*, vol. 11, no. 3, pp. 195–205, 2005.

[10] E. B. Baart, E. Martini, M. J. Eijkemans et al., "Milder ovarian stimulation for *in-vitro* fertilization reduces aneuploidy in the human preimplantation embryo: a randomized controlled trial," *Human Reproduction*, vol. 22, no. 4, pp. 980–988, 2007.

[11] J. A. Horcajadas, P. Díaz-Gimeno, A. Pellicer, and C. Simón, "Uterine receptivity and the ramifications of ovarian stimulation on endometrial function," *Seminars in Reproductive Medicine*, vol. 25, no. 6, pp. 454–460, 2007.

[12] J. A. Horcajadas, P. Mínguez, J. Dopazo et al., "Controlled ovarian stimulation induces a functional genomic delay of the endometrium with potential clinical implications," *Journal of Clinical Endocrinology and Metabolism*, vol. 93, no. 11, pp. 4500–4510, 2008.

[13] M. A. Santos, E. W. Kuijk, and N. S. Macklon, "The impact of ovarian stimulation for IVF on the developing embryo," *Reproduction*, vol. 139, no. 1, pp. 23–34, 2010.

[14] A. Pellicer, A. Ruiz, R. M. Castellvi et al., "Is the retrieval of high numbers of oocytes desirable in patients treated with gonadotrophin-releasing hormone analogues (GnRHa) and gonadotrophins?" *Human Reproduction*, vol. 4, no. 5, pp. 536–540, 1989.

[15] M. H. van der Gaast, M. J. C. Eijkemans, J. B. van der Net et al., "Optimum number of oocytes for a successful first IVF treatment cycle," *Reproductive BioMedicine Online*, vol. 13, pp. 476–480, 2006.

[16] M. A. Aboulghar, A. M. Ramzy, R. T. Mansour, Y. M. Amin, and G. I. Serour, "Oocyte quality in patients with severe ovarian hyperstimulation syndrome," *Fertility and Sterility*, vol. 68, no. 6, pp. 1017–1021, 1997.

[17] G. Ertzeid and R. Storeng, "Adverse effects of gonadotrophin treatment on pre- and postimplantation development in mice," *Journal of Reproduction and Fertility*, vol. 96, no. 2, pp. 649–655, 1992.

[18] I. Van Der Auwera and T. D'Hooghe, "Superovulation of female mice delays embryonic and fetal development," *Human Reproduction*, vol. 16, no. 6, pp. 1237–1243, 2001.

[19] C. A. Hodges, A. Ilagan, D. Jennings, R. Keri, J. Nilson, and P. A. Hunt, "Experimental evidence that changes in oocyte growth influence meiotic chromosome segregation," *Human Reproduction*, vol. 17, no. 5, pp. 1171–1180, 2002.

[20] Y. Li, H.-L. Feng, Y.-J. Cao et al., "Confocal microscopic analysis of the spindle and chromosome configurations of human oocytes matured in vitro," *Fertility and Sterility*, vol. 85, no. 4, pp. 827–832, 2006.

[21] M. Von Wolff, Z. Kollmann, C. E. Flück et al., "Gonadotrophin stimulation for in vitro fertilization significantly alters the hormone milieu in follicular fluid: a comparative study between natural cycle IVF and conventional IVF," *Human Reproduction*, vol. 29, no. 5, pp. 1049–1057, 2014.

[22] A. N. Andersen, P. Devroey, and J.-C. Arce, "Clinical outcome following stimulation with highly purified hMG or recombinant FSH in patients undergoing IVF: a randomized assessor-blind controlled trial," *Human Reproduction*, vol. 21, no. 12, pp. 3217–3227, 2006.

[23] A. Weghofer, S. Munné, W. Brannath et al., "The impact of LH-containing gonadotropin stimulation on euploidy rates in preimplantation embryos: antagonist cycles," *Fertility and Sterility*, vol. 92, no. 3, pp. 937–942, 2009.

[24] L. Regan, E. J. Owen, and H. S. Jacobs, "Hypersecretion of luteinising hormone, infertility, and miscarriage," *The Lancet*, vol. 336, no. 8724, pp. 1141–1144, 1990.

[25] J. N. Hugues, J. Soussis, I. Calderon et al., "Does the addition of recombinant LH in WHO group II anovulatory women over-responding to FSH treatment reduce the number of developing follicles? A dose-finding study," *Human Reproduction*, vol. 20, no. 3, pp. 629–635, 2005.

[26] Z. Shoham, "The clinical therapeutic window for luteinizing hormone in controlled ovarian stimulation," *Fertility and Sterility*, vol. 77, no. 6, pp. 1170–1177, 2002.

[27] M. Schimberni, F. Morgia, J. Colabianchi et al., "Natural-cycle in vitro fertilization in poor responder patients: a survey of 500 consecutive cycles," *Fertility and Sterility*, vol. 92, no. 4, pp. 1297–1301, 2009.

[28] K.-G. Nygren, "Single embryo transfer: the role of natural cycle/minimal stimulation IVF in the future," *Reproductive BioMedicine Online*, vol. 14, no. 5, article 2841, 2007.

[29] R. Cutting, D. Morroll, S. Roberts, S. Pickering, and A. Rutherford, "Elective single embryo transfer: guidelines for practice British fertility society and association of clinical embryologists," *Human Fertility*, vol. 11, no. 3, pp. 131–146, 2008.

[30] Joint SOGC-CFAS, "Guidelines for the number of embryos to transfer following *in vitro* fertilization no. 182, September 2006," *International Journal of Gynecology & Obstetrics*, vol. 102, pp. 203–216, 2008.

[31] J. D. Gordon, M. Dimattina, A. Reh, A. Botes, G. Celia, and M. Payson, "Utilization and success rates of unstimulated in vitro fertilization in the United States: an analysis of the Society for Assisted Reproductive Technology database," *Fertility and Sterility*, vol. 100, no. 2, pp. 392–395, 2013.

[32] B. C. Fauser, G. Nargund, A. N. Andersen et al., "Mild ovarian stimulation for IVF: 10 years later," *Human Reproduction*, vol. 25, no. 11, pp. 2678–2684, 2010.

[33] G. Nargund, B. C. J. M. Fauser, N. Macklon, W. Ombelet, K. Nygren, and R. Frydman, "The ISMAAR proposal on terminology for ovarian stimulation for IVF," *Human Reproduction*, vol. 22, no. 11, pp. 2801–2804, 2007.

[34] W. M. Enien, S. El Sahwy, C. P. Harris, M. W. Seif, and M. Elstein, "Human chorionic gonadotrophin and steroid concentrations in follicular fluid: the relationship to oocyte maturity and fertilization rates in stimulated and natural in-vitro fertilization cycles," *Human Reproduction*, vol. 10, no. 11, pp. 2840–2844, 1995.

[35] M. J. De Los Santos, V. Garca-Lez, D. Beltrn-Torregrosa et al., "Hormonal and molecular characterization of follicular fluid, cumulus cells and oocytes from pre-ovulatory follicles in stimulated and unstimulated cycles," *Human Reproduction*, vol. 27, no. 6, pp. 1596–1605, 2012.

[36] D. Vinatier, C. Lefebvre-Maunoury, and C. Bernardi, "The ovaries, the immune system, cytokines: physiology," *Journal de Gynecologie Obstetrique et Biologie de la Reproduction*, vol. 22, no. 6, pp. 581–591, 1993.

[37] C. L. Best and J. A. Hill, "Interleukin-1α and -β modulation of luteinized human granulosa cell oestrogen and progesterone biosynthesis," *Human Reproduction*, vol. 10, no. 12, pp. 3206–3210, 1995.

[38] V. Machelon and D. Emilie, "Production of ovarian cytokines and their role in ovulation in the mammalian ovary," *European Cytokine Network*, vol. 8, no. 2, pp. 137–143, 1997.

[39] D. F. Albertini, C. M. H. Combelles, E. Benecchi, and M. J. Carabatsos, "Cellular basis for paracrine regulation of ovarian follicle development," *Reproduction*, vol. 121, no. 5, pp. 647–653, 2001.

[40] J. J. Eppig, "Oocyte control of ovarian follicular development and function in mammals," *Reproduction*, vol. 122, no. 6, pp. 829–838, 2001.

[41] M. K. Skinner, "Regulation of primordial follicle assembly and development," *Human Reproduction Update*, vol. 11, no. 5, pp. 461–471, 2005.

[42] S. Vujisić, S. Ž. Lepej, I. Emedi, R. Bauman, A. Remenar, and M. K. Tiljak, "Ovarian follicular concentration of IL-12, IL-15, IL-18 and p40 subunit of IL-12 and IL-23," *Human Reproduction*, vol. 21, no. 10, pp. 2650–2655, 2006.

[43] S. Vujisic and S. Zidovec, "Follicular immunology environment and the influence on in-vitro fertilization outcome," *Current Women's Health Reviews*, vol. 1, pp. 49–60, 2005.

[44] C. Mendoza, N. Cremades, E. Ruiz-Requena et al., "Relationship between fertilization results after intracytoplasmic sperm injection, and intrafollicular steroid, pituitary hormone and cytokine concentrations," *Human Reproduction*, vol. 14, no. 3, pp. 628–635, 1999.

[45] M. E. Hammadeh, A. K. Ertan, M. Baltes et al., "Immunoglobulins and cytokines level in follicular fluid in relation to etiology of infertility and their relevance to IVF outcome," *American Journal of Reproductive Immunology*, vol. 47, no. 2, pp. 82–90, 2002.

[46] C. Mendoza, E. Ruiz-Requena, E. Ortega et al., "Follicular fluid markers of oocyte developmental potential," *Human Reproduction*, vol. 17, no. 4, pp. 1017–1022, 2002.

[47] M. E. Hammadeh, C. Fischer-Hammadeh, A. S. Amer, P. Rosenbaum, and W. Schmidt, "Relationship between cytokine concentration in serum and preovulatory follicular fluid and in vitro fertilization/intracytoplasmic sperm injection outcome," *Chemical Immunology and Allergy*, vol. 88, pp. 80–97, 2005.

[48] M. Bedaiwy, A. Y. Shahin, A. M. AbulHassan et al., "Differential expression of follicular fluid cytokines: relationship to subsequent pregnancy in IVF cycles," *Reproductive BioMedicine Online*, vol. 15, no. 3, pp. 321–325, 2007.

[49] N. Lédée, R. Lombroso, L. Lombardelli et al., "Cytokines and chemokines in follicular fluids and potential of the corresponding embryo: the role of granulocyte colony-stimulating factor," *Human Reproduction*, vol. 23, no. 9, pp. 2001–2009, 2008.

[50] A. Revelli, L. D. Piane, S. Casano, E. Molinari, M. Massobrio, and P. Rinaudo, "Follicular fluid content and oocyte quality: from single biochemical markers to metabolomics," *Reproductive Biology and Endocrinology*, vol. 7, article 40, 2009.

[51] N. Lédée, M. Petitbarat, M. Rahmati et al., "New pre-conception immune biomarkers for clinical practice: interleukin-18, interleukin-15 and TWEAK on the endometrial side, G-CSF on the follicular side," *Journal of Reproductive Immunology*, vol. 88, no. 2, pp. 118–123, 2011.

[52] A. Sarapik, A. Velthut, K. Haller-Kikkatalo et al., "Follicular proinflammatory cytokines and chemokines as markers of IVF

success," *Clinical and Developmental Immunology*, vol. 2012, Article ID 606459, 10 pages, 2012.

[53] H. Hagberg, C. Mallard, and B. Jacobsson, "Role of cytokines in preterm labour and brain injury," *British Journal of Obstetrics and Gynaecology*, vol. 112, supplement 1, pp. 16–18, 2005.

[54] A. Agic, H. Xu, D. Finas, C. Banz, K. Diedrich, and D. Hornung, "Is endometriosis associated with systemic subclinical inflammation?" *Gynecologic and Obstetric Investigation*, vol. 62, no. 3, pp. 139–147, 2006.

[55] O. B. Christiansen, H. S. Nielsen, and A. M. Kolte, "Inflammation and miscarriage," *Seminars in Fetal and Neonatal Medicine*, vol. 11, no. 5, pp. 302–308, 2006.

[56] A. Arici, E. Oral, O. Bukulmez, S. Buradagunta, O. Engin, and D. L. Olive, "Interleukin-8 expression and modulation in human preovulatory follicles and ovarian cells," *Endocrinology*, vol. 137, no. 9, pp. 3762–3769, 1996.

[57] E. Runesson, K. Ivarsson, P. O. Janson, and M. Brännström, "Gonadotropin- and cytokin-regulated expression of the chemokine interleukin 8 in the human preovulatory follicle of the menstrual cycle," *Journal of Clinical Endocrinology and Metabolism*, vol. 85, no. 11, pp. 4387–4395, 2000.

[58] V. Baud and M. Karin, "Signal transduction by tumor necrosis factor and its relatives," *Trends in Cell Biology*, vol. 11, no. 9, pp. 372–377, 2001.

[59] R. P. Numerof and K. Asadullah, "Cytokine and anti-cytokine therapies for psoriasis and atopic dermatitis," *BioDrugs*, vol. 20, no. 2, pp. 93–103, 2006.

[60] S. Weiser, J. Miu, H. J. Ball, and N. H. Hunt, "Interferon-γ synergises with tumour necrosis factor and lymphotoxin-α to enhance the mRNA and protein expression of adhesion molecules in mouse brain endothelial cells," *Cytokine*, vol. 37, no. 1, pp. 84–91, 2007.

[61] N. A. Bersinger, Z. Kollmann, and M. von Wolff, "Serum but not follicular fluid cytokine levels are increased in stimulated versus natural cycle IVF: a multiplexed assay study," *Journal of Reproductive Immunology*, vol. 106, pp. 27–33, 2014.

[62] O. Tokuyama, Y. Nakamura, A. Muso, Y. Fujino, O. Ishiko, and S. Ogita, "Vascular endothelial growth factor concentrations in follicular fluid obtained from IVF-ET patients: a comparison of hMG, clomiphene citrate, and natural cycle," *Journal of Assisted Reproduction and Genetics*, vol. 19, no. 1, pp. 19–23, 2002.

[63] J. S. Cunha-Filho, N. Lemos, N. Stein, A. Laranjeira, and E. P. Passos, "Vascular endothelial growth factor and inhibin A in follicular fluid of infertile patients who underwent *in vitro* fertilization with a gonadotropin-releasing hormone antagonist," *Fertility and Sterility*, vol. 83, no. 4, pp. 902–907, 2005.

[64] C. McRae, N. E. Baskind, N. M. Orsi, V. Sharma, and J. Fisher, "Metabolic profiling of follicular fluid and plasma from natural cycle in vitro fertilization patients—a pilot study," *Fertility and Sterility*, vol. 98, no. 6, pp. 1449.e6–1457.e6, 2012.

[65] N. M. Orsi, N. Gopichandran, U. V. Ekbote, and J. J. Walker, "Murine serum cytokines throughout the estrous cycle, pregnancy and post partum period," *Animal Reproduction Science*, vol. 96, no. 1-2, pp. 54–65, 2006.

[66] P. F. Levay, C. Huyser, F. L. Fourie, and D. J. Rossouw, "The detection of blood contamination in human follicular fluid," *Journal of Assisted Reproduction and Genetics*, vol. 14, no. 4, pp. 212–217, 1997.

[67] C. Huyser, F. L. R. Fourie, and L. Wolmarans, "Spectrophotometric absorbance of follicular fluid: a selection criterion," *Journal of Assisted Reproduction and Genetics*, vol. 9, no. 6, pp. 539–544, 1992.

[68] C. M. Boomsma, A. Kavelaars, M. J. C. Eijkemans, B. C. J. M. Fauser, C. J. Heijnen, and N. S. MacKlon, "Ovarian stimulation for *in vitro* fertilization alters the intrauterine cytokine, chemokine, and growth factor milieu encountered by the embryo," *Fertility and Sterility*, vol. 94, no. 5, pp. 1764–1768, 2010.

[69] J. R. L. de Mola, J. M. Goldfarb, B. R. Hecht, G. P. Baumgardner, C. J. Babbo, and M. A. Friedlander, "Gonadotropins induce the release of interleukin-1β, interleukin-6 and tumor necrosis factor-α from the human preovulatory follicle," *American Journal of Reproductive Immunology*, vol. 39, no. 6, pp. 387–390, 1998.

[70] M. J. de Los Santos, V. Garca-Lez, D. Beltrn-Torregrosa et al., "Hormonal and molecular characterization of follicular fluid, cumulus cells and oocytes from pre-ovulatory follicles in stimulated and unstimulated cycles," *Human Reproduction*, vol. 27, no. 6, pp. 1596–1605, 2012.

[71] A. Arici, E. Oral, O. Bahtiyar, O. Engin, E. Seli, and E. E. Jones, "Leukaemia inhibitory factor expression in human follicular fluid and ovarian cells," *Human Reproduction*, vol. 12, no. 6, pp. 1233–1239, 1997.

[72] S. Coskun, M. Uzumcu, K. Jaroudi, J. M. G. Hollanders, R. S. Parhar, and S. T. Al-Sedairy, "Presence of leukemia inhibitory factor and interleukin-12 in human follicular fluid during follicular growth," *The American Journal of Reproductive Immunology*, vol. 40, no. 1, pp. 13–18, 1998.

[73] M. Jean, S. Mirallie, P. Barriere et al., "Leukaemia inhibitory factor expression in human follicular fluid," *Human Reproduction*, vol. 14, no. 2, article 571, 1999.

[74] Y. Zhao, J. E. Nichols, S. E. Bulun, C. R. Mendelson, and E. R. Simpson, "Aromatase P450 gene expression in human adipose tissue: role of a Jak/STAT pathway in regulation of the adipose-specific promoter," *The Journal of Biological Chemistry*, vol. 270, no. 27, pp. 16449–16457, 1995.

[75] O. Bukulmez and A. Arici, "Leukocytes in ovarian function," *Human Reproduction Update*, vol. 6, no. 1, pp. 1–15, 2000.

[76] K. C. Reinhart, R. K. Dubey, C. L. Mummery, M. Van Rooijen, P. J. Keller, and R. Marinella, "Synthesis and regulation of leukaemia inhibitory factor in cultured bovine oviduct cells by hormones," *Molecular Human Reproduction*, vol. 4, no. 3, pp. 301–308, 1998.

[77] J. E. Holt, A. Jackson, S. D. Roman, R. J. Aitken, P. Koopman, and E. A. McLaughlin, "CXCR4/SDF1 interaction inhibits the primordial to primary follicle transition in the neonatal mouse ovary," *Developmental Biology*, vol. 293, no. 2, pp. 449–460, 2006.

[78] A. Nishigaki, H. Okada, R. Okamoto et al., "Concentrations of stromal cell-derived factor-1 and vascular endothelial growth factor in relation to the diameter of human follicles," *Fertility and Sterility*, vol. 95, no. 2, pp. 742–746, 2011.

[79] T. Hamza, J. B. Barnett, and B. Li, "Interleukin 12 a key immunoregulatory cytokine in infection applications," *International Journal of Molecular Sciences*, vol. 11, no. 3, pp. 789–806, 2010.

[80] G. Trinchieri, "Interleukin-12: a proinflammatory cytokine with immunoregulatory functions that bridge innate resistance and antigen-specific adaptive immunity," *Annual Review of Immunology*, vol. 13, pp. 251–276, 1995.

[81] J. Hodge-Dufour, M. W. Marino, M. R. Horton et al., "Inhibition of interferon γ induced interleukin 12 production: a potential

mechanism for the anti-inflammatory activities of tumor necrosis factor," *Proceedings of the National Academy of Sciences of the United States of America*, vol. 95, no. 23, pp. 13806–13811, 1998.

[82] A. Giuliani, W. Schoell, J. Auner, and W. Urdl, "Controlled ovarian hyperstimulation in assisted reproduction: effect on the immune system," *Fertility and Sterility*, vol. 70, no. 5, pp. 831–815, 1998.

[83] A. Hoek, J. Schoemaker, and H. A. Drexhage, "Premature ovarian failure and ovarian autoimmunity," *Endocrine Reviews*, vol. 18, no. 1, pp. 107–134, 1997.

3

Comparison of Results of Cycles Treated with Modified Mild Protocol and Short Protocol for Ovarian Stimulation

F. Coelho,[1] L. F. Aguiar,[1] G. S. P. Cunha,[1] N. Cardinot,[1] and E. Lucena[2]

[1] Centro de Infertilidade e Medicina Fetal do Norte Fluminense, Hospital Escola Álvaro Alvim, Rua Barão da Lagoa Dourada, 409-2° pavimento, Centro, 28035-210 Campos dos Goytacazes, RJ, Brazil
[2] Centro Colombiano de Fertilidad y Esterilidad (CECOLFES) S.A.S., Calle 102 No. 14A-15, 56769 Bogota, Colombia

Correspondence should be addressed to F. Coelho; coelhoaf@ig.com.br

Academic Editor: Dimitris Loutradis

The ovarian stimulation has been applied in order to increase the number of oocytes to compensate for the poor results of in vitro fertilization, allowing the selection of one or more embryos to be transferred. Our aim is to compare the results obtained in IVF/ICSI cycles using the short protocol for controlled ovarian stimulation to the results from the modified mild protocol used in our department. A total of 240 cycles were conducted from January 2010 to December 2011. When comparing both protocols, it could be observed that there was a significant difference in the quantity of gonadotropins doses in the mild protocol and in the short protocol. No significant difference was observed regarding pregnancy rates per cycle, 22% and 26.2%, in short and mild protocols, respectively. The protocols of controlled ovarian stimulation are often associated with high risk of complications such as ovarian hyperstimulation syndrome, excessive emotional stress, high rates of treatment dropouts, and abdominal discomfort. With the data obtained in this study, one can conclude that there are less risks and complications for the patient when using the mild stimulation protocol. It was also observed that in this group there was a slightly higher rate.

1. Introduction

Ovarian stimulation is a fundamental part of the technologies involving assisted reproduction. For over 30 years, ovarian stimulation has been applied in order to increase the number of oocytes to compensate for the inefficiency of the in vitro fertilization procedure (IVF), allowing the selection of one or more embryos to be transferred [1–3]. For many years the concept of number generosity of ovules was associated with the also generous number of embryos and directly related to the reproductive treatments prognosis.

In parallel, the number of eggs recruited and the consequent number of resulting embryos contributed to increase the number of multiple pregnancies and the incidence of ovarian hyperstimulation syndrome (OHSS). However, the pregnancy rate did not rise as expected [4].

Likewise, previous studies indicate that the successful embryo implantation depends on an optimal communication between good quality embryos and a receptive endometrium [5]. In IVF the main reason for these poor results of implantation may be the endometrium quality which is affected during the pharmacological treatment (ovarian stimulation and hormone replacement) that is evidenced when comparing both implantation and pregnancy rates among natural cycles and IVF [6].

Recently, a stimulation protocol called mild stimulation protocol has been proposed in order to make the treatment the closest to natural as possible, using low doses of gonadotropins to obtain the success rate similar to the "conventional" stimulus and with fewer side effects to the patients.

This study aims to compare the results obtained in IVF/ICSI cycles using the "short" controlled ovarian stimulation protocol with the results of mild modified protocol used in our department.

2. Material and Method

This study was conducted at the Department of Human Reproduction of the Álvaro Alvim Teaching Hospital, in Campos dos Goytacazes, Rio de Janeiro. A total of 160 cycles using the "short" controlled ovarian stimulation protocol and 80 cycles using the mild modified protocol were conducted from January 2010 to December 2011.

In the 80 cycles in which the mild modified protocol for ovarian stimulation was used, 2 tablets of 50 mg clomiphene citrate (Clomid or Indux) were administered daily during a 5-day period associated with urinary gonadotropin 75 IU (Menopur) for 6 days and the pituitary blocking was performed using indomethacin (50 mg Inducid) three times a day for 5 days when a 15-centimeter ovarian follicle was formed. For follicles luteinization a 0.02 mL dose of 0.1 mg leuprolide acetate (Lupron) was administered taking advantage of the endogenous LH when a 17-centimeter or larger ovarian follicle was formed.

From the puncture day on, 3 tablets of 200 mg progesterone (Utrogestan) were administered in a daily basis during a 14-day period, in order to support the luteal phase and provide initial support in case of pregnancy.

In the 160 cycles in which the "short" protocol for ovarian stimulation was used, 0.02-milliliter doses of 0.1 mg leuprolide acetate (Lupron) were administered from the first or second day of the menstrual cycle on, and the ovarian stimulation was initiated on the third day of the cycle using 75 IU/day of recombinant gonadotropins 450 IU/mL (Gonal-F) for 9 days. In addition, 1 daily ampoule of 75 IU urinary gonadotropin (Menopur) was administered during a 10-day period. One ampoule of 250 mg recombinant (r-hCG) chorionic gonadotropin alpha hCG (Ovidrel) was also used. The use of 2 mg estradiol valerate (Primogyna) was initiated when two 17-centimeter ovarian follicles were formed, then it was carried on making use of 2 tablets daily for 16 days until the pregnancy test.

In both groups the needle puncture-aspiration was performed 36 hours after the leuprolide acetate administration, using a 17G COOK needle under a 120 mmHg aspiration pressure, guided by a 7.5 MHz (ALOKA 500-JAPAN) transvaginal ultrasound probe, while the patient was sedated with 10 mg/mL 1% Propofol (Fresofol).

For most patients, the embryo transfer was performed on day 3; however, 12 patients had embryo transfer on day 2 and 10 other patients had embryo transfer on day 5. The embryo quality was monitored daily until the transfer day.

The transfer was performed using SURE-PRO ULTRATM WALLACE transfer catheter coupled to a 1 mL TERUMO syringe and a disposable speculum. The number of preembryos transferred to the uterine cavity followed the Brazilian Resolution of the Federal Council of Medicine (CFM 1957/10) concerning the number of embryos to be transferred where the following determinations are made: (a) up to two embryos for women up to 35 years old; (b) up to three embryos for women between 36 and 39 years old; (c) up to four embryos for 40-year-old women and older.

The statistical analysis consisted of the means and standard errors of the variables for each treatment (short protocol

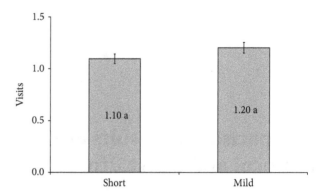

FIGURE 1: Number of visits to service for monitoring the follicular growth. Means followed by the same letter do not differ significantly through the t-test at a 5% probability.

and mild protocol) presentation, as well as the comparison of the means through the t-test and of the frequencies through the chi-square test. A 5% significance level was adopted being the analysis performed in the application Statistical and Genetic Analyzes Systems (SAEG, version 9.1).

3. Results

During the 23-month study period, a total of 240 cycles were performed in our service with patients with a mean age of 34.5. The cycles were divided into two groups: one containing 160 patients stimulated with the "short" protocol for ovarian stimulation and the other one containing 80 patients stimulated with the mild protocol. There was no significant difference between the two groups regarding the number of visits to the service for monitoring the follicular growth (Figure 1). The number of days of stimulation (Figure 2) and the number of gonadotropins doses used (Figure 3) were both significantly lower in the group of patients stimulated with the mild protocol.

The number of retrieved oocytes (6.24 versus 4.42) was statistically similar in both groups. Analyzing the retrieved oocytes (Figure 4(a)) no significant difference was found in the number of retrieved oocytes in germinal vesicle (GV) (Figure 4(b)) and in immature oocytes (MI) (Figure 4(c)). A significant difference was observed in the quantity of mature oocytes (MII) (5.37 versus 3.39) (Figure 4(d)) and in the quantity of degenerated oocytes (0.12 versus 0,62) (Figure 4(e)). No statistical significance was observed regarding the fertilization rate (Figure 5(b)), even though there was a significant difference in the fertilized ovules quantity (Figure 5(a)). A significant difference was observed in the average number of embryos transferred per cycle (2.34 versus 1.92) (Figure 5(c)). However, no significant difference was noticed regarding the pregnancy rate (Figure 5(d)) between the two groups.

4. Discussion

Controlled ovarian stimulation is a key step in assisted reproduction. The concern for oocyte maturation is constant since the end of last century [7].

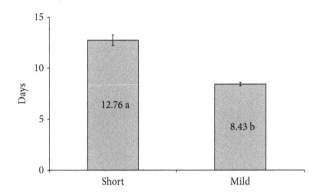

FIGURE 2: Number of days of stimulation. Means followed by different letters differ significantly through the t-test at a 5% probability.

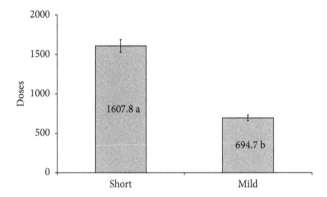

FIGURE 3: Doses of gonadotropins. Means followed by different letters differ significantly through the t-test at a 5% probability.

The development of ovarian stimulation protocols used in conjunction with use of the agonist and antagonist and HCG favored the development of ovarian stimulation protocols. However, success rates have lagged the development of drugs and other stimulus protocols [8].

The conventional GnRH agonist stimulation protocol, resulting in pituitary and ovarian desensitization with the GnRH antagonist stimulation allows the endogenous FSH cycle to occur [9]. Therefore, the cyclic follicular recruitment and gonadotropin-dependent follicles recruited in early stages of growth may continue unimpaired [10, 11].

15, 50, 54, observed that the ovarian stimulation and simultaneous high levels of estradiol were shown to have a negative impact on the potential development of the embryo and its implantation.

The FSH and HCG promote recruitment and maturation of ovules that normally deteriorate in physiological cycles resulting in availability of ova of dubious quality.

This variation of oocyte quality directly affects the embryo quality, a matter of great concern today.

Thus, the increased availability of eggs without the parallel rise of the expected results motivated the transfer of a high number of embryos to compensate for the low success rate. This attempt to offset considerably increased the rate of multiple pregnancy in assisted reproductive technology

cycles. This combination, in addition to observed outcomes, resulted in considerable increase in the costs of assisted reproduction treatments and expenditures for perinatal care in such a way that the past 3-4 decades single embryo transfer is a reality and a possibility for mild stimulation.

The purpose of this study was to evaluate the results obtained in IVF/ICSI cycles using the "short" controlled ovarian stimulation protocol with the results of mild modified protocol. The mild modified stimulation protocol we use in our service is a simple and more physiological protocol, which takes advantage of the physiological variations of endogenous gonadotropins, requiring a smaller number of visits for ovarian control and, therefore, reducing any potential risk of medical complications for patients. Ovarian hyperstimulation syndrome (OHSS) corresponds to 1% of complications in assisted reproduction treatments and an important complication of controlled ovarian stimulus [12]. Besides, the SHO controlled ovarian stimulation protocols are often associated with high risk of excessive emotional stress [13] and high rates of treatment dropouts and abdominal discomfort [14]. Moreover, protocols medication used for stimulation is complex, expensive, require weeks of daily injections, and frequent [12].

The mild protocol did not show any complications related to severe ovarian stimulation besides the complaints already related to it as discomfort and abdominal pain. Likewise, there was a reduction in the number of medical visits for ovarian control and consequently, a significant reduction in the cost of treatments. As a result of these observed benefits, the use of LLINs protocols contributed to greater adhesion of patients to treatment proposals. Furthermore, it contributed to the reduction of cases of multiple pregnancies and the need for freezing of surplus embryos; thereby our observations agree with the observations from [5].

Conventional ovarian stimulation may affect mechanisms involved in maintaining accurate chromosome segregation and this is associated with increased incidence of morphological and chromosomal abnormalities [8, 15–18].

Moreover, the mild protocol also relates the best quality embryos and the lowest rate of embryonic aneuploidy when compared to conventional stimulation [19].

Indomethacin can play an important role to overcome a major obstacle in IVF cycles. Furthermore, the safety profile and low cost of this medication make their use attractive.

Indomethacin, an anti-inflammatory nonsteroidal drug, when added to the treatment protocol may prevent ovulation [20]. It inhibits prostaglandin production, especially through the inhibition of cyclooxygenase, the enzyme that catalyzes prostaglandin synthesis and is an essential mediator of ovulation and implantation and also essential to the rupture of the follicle and ovulation. It has been demonstrated that indomethacin administered before ovulation prevents rupture of the follicle, with no apparent lasting effects on the menstrual cycle or FSH, LH, estradiol, and progesterone [13, 21] concern that justified the pituitary suppression with agonist and antagonist [8].

The work in [21] showed that indomethacin administered at the time of positive urinary LH might retard follicular

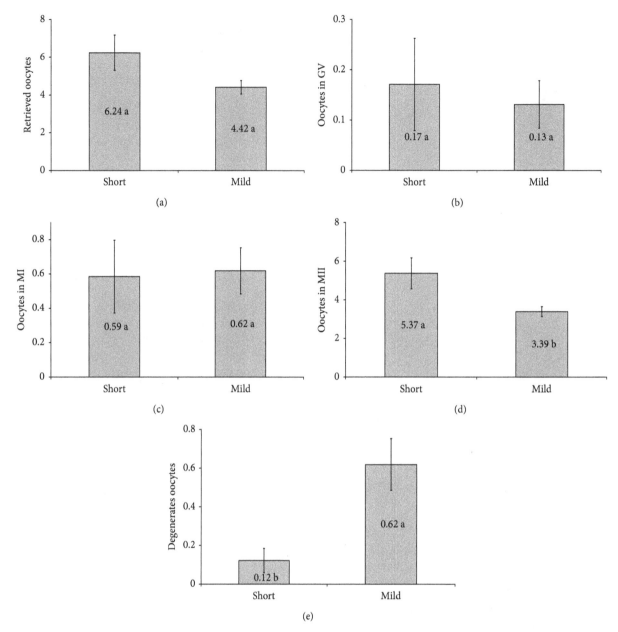

FIGURE 4: Average number of oocytes per cycle: (a) average of oocytes retrieved, (b) stage of oocytes retrieved at the germinal vesicle (GV), (c) retrieved oocytes in metaphase I (MI), (d) in metaphase II oocytes retrieved (MII), and (e) degenerates oocytes. Means followed by the same letter do not differ significantly by t-test at 5% probability.

rupture, with an associated reduction in blood flow intrafollicular but without apparent effect on hormone or menstrual status. The mechanism of action of indomethacin, therefore, is probably inhibition of "inflammation" associated with follicular rupture.

The work in [22] contends that indomethacin did not interfere with the effectiveness of assisted reproduction cycles and does not interfere with canceled cycles and, therefore, improves the effectiveness of IVF cycles. The work in [22] also stated that the rate of oocyte retrieval and transfer by procedure were not significantly affected by the use of indomethacin demonstrating that it has no deleterious effects

to the embryonic development, and the clinical pregnancy rate per cycle was increased.

In our study we observed that with the use of mild protocol there was a reduction in the number of oocytes retrieved and a greater synchronization of follicles reducing the number of immature oocytes, the number of preembryos transferred and cryopreserved without reducing the overall rates of success treatment IVF confirming the findings of [3]. The observed relationship between low numbers of oocytes and the possibility of success in assisted reproduction cycles after mild stimulation suggests that when some oocytes are obtained, they are likely to represent a homogeneous group

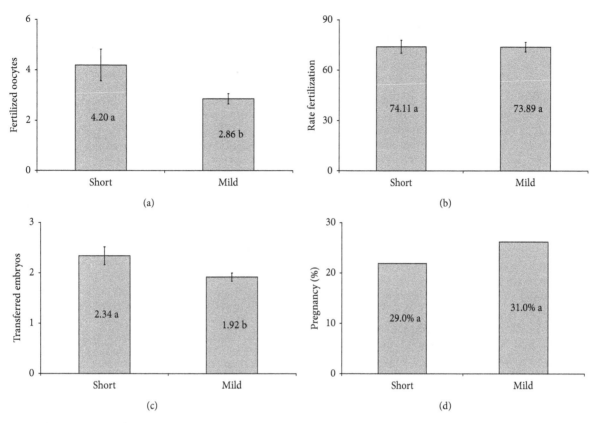

FIGURE 5: Fertilization rates and pregnancy: (a) average oocytes fertilized, (b) fertilization rate, (c) average number of embryos transferred, and (d) the pregnancy rate. Means followed by the same letter do not differ significantly by t-test at 5% probability.

of good quality oocytes. This could be the result of the interference with the subtle natural selection of good quality oocytes or minimized exposure of growing follicles to the potentially negative effects of ovarian stimulation.

However, a possible reduction in pregnancy rate was described. This reduction can be confirmed by less comorbidity of mild Protocol for greater comfort, increased safety, reduced likelihood of ovarian hyperstimulation associated with significant reduction of treatment costs and promoting a high rate of adherence to treatment, and the possibility of execution of successive cycles with reduction or pregnancy rate stability, without compromising the rate of drinking at home [2, 18, 23–30].

However, increasing the effectiveness of procedures for IVF and the global trend to limit the number of embryos transferred reduced the need for large amounts of oocytes. The observed relationship between low numbers of oocytes and a high chance of achieving an ongoing pregnancy after mild stimulation suggests that when some oocytes are obtained, they are likely to represent a homogeneous group of good quality oocytes.

When ovarian mild stimulation is combined with a policy of single embryo transfer, the costs associated with pregnancy complications were reduced [29]. The results of this study showed that the use of LLINs modified protocol does not compromise fertilization rates and pregnancy rates if compared to the use of the "short" stimulation protocol. However,

the number of days of stimulation, the financial cost, the complications, and the number of doses of gonadotropins used were significantly shorter.

A decrease in the pregnancy rate in patients with a more pronounced ovarian response to stimulation using mild may be associated with the occurrence of premature LH rises [1]. The occurrence of premature LH elevation has a negative impact on the possibility of achieving an ongoing pregnancy [16].

The trigger ovulation, hCG, which is thought to have an effect of "proestablishment" is becoming a prime target in the search for substances with a negative role in endometrial receptivity [10, 31].

Studies that have examined the fate of oocytes demonstrated that prolonged exposure to hCG in the proliferative phase adversely affects the pregnancy rate [32].

Likewise, the "natural" ovulation determined by monitoring the LH surge results in higher implantation rates and ongoing pregnancy in normoovulatory women versus those in which ovulation is triggered with hCG IUI and frozen embryo transfers [33].

The implantation is a highly complex process that requires close synchronization between the development of the embryo and the endometrium [34].

Moreover, the endometrium could respond to embryonic signals such as hCG, to facilitate preparation for implantation.

The supporting evidence regarding a possible adverse effect of supraphysiological levels of steroids in endometrial receptivity [4, 9], corpus luteum function [14, 35], oocyte, and embryo quality [36] indicates that the response of limited ovarian stimulation may have a beneficial effect on the potential of implantation.

In assisted reproduction treatment one of the main reasons for the poor results in the implantation of the endometrium is the quality that is affected during pharmacological treatment (ovarian stimulation and hormone replacement) that is emphasized when comparing the rates of implantation and pregnancy rates between natural cycles and FIV [37]. According to [34, 38] increased progesterone during the late follicular phase has been considered a negative factor for clinical outcomes. The mechanism that may be attached to this observation can be the fact that high serum levels of progesterone on the day of hCG administration induce both the advanced endometrial maturation and the differential expression of endometrium genes, which may be related to the deployment failure [39–41].

The work in [9] noted that considering the concentrations of estradiol isolated was independent to the number of oocytes retrieved. Implantation rates and pregnancy were significantly reduced when estradiol concentrations were elevated.

In our reality, a developing country, the main barrier to access for couples to acquire assisted reproduction treatments, is the financial cost involved, because there is no coverage for public assistance. Thus, only a small privileged fraction of the population has access to these treatments.

Thus the mild protocol we use in our service associated with the blockade of ovulation with indomethacin and its triggering with GnRH agonist substantially reduces the cost of treatment and possible complications expenditures when compared to the SHO. The use of LLINs as trigger associated with using the endogenous LH agonist, as no pituitary suppression, eliminates the risk of OHSS. Besides, the use of low doses of gonadotropin and no use of hCG often associated with the pathophysiology of OHSS. Thus the financial expenses related complications by any hospital admissions are also eliminated. All this makes for easy access for couples who generally would be limited by the financial cost of treatment.

Likewise, when the programs of assisted reproduction are associated with a single embryo transfer, it reduces the rate of multiple pregnancies and subsequent expenses with neonatal intensive treatment systems.

In conclusion, mild protocol did not interfere with treatment outcomes, achieving greater compliance and cost reduction and it acts as an important gateway to assisted reproductive treatments in developing countries and may be an option for models of public assistance to infertility in these countries.

Conflict of Interests

The authors declare that there is no conflict of interests regarding the publication of this paper.

References

[1] G. Borm and B. Mannaerts, "Treatment with gonadotrophin-releasing hormone antagonist ganirelix in women undergoing ovarian stimulation with recombinant follicle stimulating hormone is effective, safe and convenient: results of a controlled, randomized, multicentre trial," *Human Reproduction*, vol. 15, pp. 1490–1498, 2000.

[2] E. F. Branigan and M. A. Estes, "Minimal stimulation IVF using clomiphene citrate and oral contraceptive pill pretreatment for LH suppression," *Fertility and Sterility*, vol. 73, no. 3, pp. 587–590, 2000.

[3] B. C. Fauser, P. Devroey, S. S. Yen et al., "Minimal ovarian stimulation for IVF: appraisal of potential benefits and drawbacks," *Human Reproduction*, vol. 14, no. 11, pp. 2681–2686, 1999.

[4] P. Devroey, C. Bourgain, N. S. Macklon, and B. C. J. M. Fauser, "Reproductive biology and IVF: ovarian stimulation and endometrial receptivity," *Trends in Endocrinology and Metabolism*, vol. 15, no. 2, pp. 84–90, 2004.

[5] R. H. Reindollar and M. B. Goldman, "Gonadotropin therapy: a 20th century relic," *Fertility and Sterility*, vol. 97, no. 4, pp. 813–818, 2012.

[6] S. D. Keay, N. H. Liversedge, R. S. Mathur, and J. M. Jenkins, "Assisted conception following poor ovarian response to gonadotrophin stimulation," *British Journal of Obstetrics and Gynaecology*, vol. 104, no. 5, pp. 521–527, 1997.

[7] C. A. Gemzell, P. Roos, and F. E. Loeffler, "Follicle stimulating hormone extracted from human pituitary," in *Progress in Infertility*, S. J. Behrman and R. W. Kistner, Eds., pp. 479–493, Little, Brown and Company, Boston, Mass, USA, 1975.

[8] R. Roberts, A. Iatropoulou, D. Ciantar et al., "Follicle-stimulating hormone affects metaphase I chromosome alignment and increases aneuploidy in mouse oocytes matured in vitro," *Biology of Reproduction*, vol. 72, no. 1, pp. 107–118, 2005.

[9] C. Simon, F. Cano, D. Valbuena, J. Remohi, and A. Pellicer, "Clinical evidence for a detrimental effect on uterine receptivity of high serum oestradiol concentrations in high and normal responder patients," *Human Reproduction*, vol. 10, no. 9, pp. 2432–2437, 1995.

[10] B. C. J. M. Fauser and A. M. Van Heusden, "Manipulation of human ovarian function: Physiological concepts and clinical consequences," *Endocrine Reviews*, vol. 18, no. 1, pp. 71–106, 1997.

[11] E. A. McGee and A. J. W. Hsueh, "Initial and cyclic recruitment of ovarian follicles," *Endocrine Reviews*, vol. 21, no. 2, pp. 200–214, 2000.

[12] M. J. Pelinck, N. E. A. Vogel, A. Hoek et al., "Cumulative pregnancy rates after three cycles of minimal stimulation IVF and results according to subfertility diagnosis: a multicentre cohort study," *Human Reproduction*, vol. 21, no. 9, pp. 2375–2383, 2006.

[13] K. E. Hester, M. J. K. Harper, and D. M. Duffy, "Oral administration of the cyclooxygenase-2 (COX-2) inhibitor meloxicam blocks ovulation in non-human primates when administered to simulate emergency contraception," *Human Reproduction*, vol. 25, no. 2, pp. 360–367, 2010.

[14] B. C. J. M. Fauser and P. Devroey, "Reproductive biology and IVF: ovarian stimulation and luteal phase consequences," *Trends in Endocrinology and Metabolism*, vol. 14, no. 5, pp. 236–242, 2003.

[15] J. J. Eppig, M. J. O'Brien, F. L. Pendola, and S. Watanabe, "Factors affecting the developmental competence of mouse oocytes grown in vitro: follicle-stimulating hormone and insulin," *Biology of Reproduction*, vol. 59, no. 6, pp. 1445–1453, 1998.

[16] P. Humaidan, L. Bungum, M. Bungum, and C. Y. Andersen, "Ovarian response and pregnancy outcome related to mid-follicular LH levels in women undergoing assisted reproduction with GnRH agonist down-regulation and recombinant FSH stimulation," *Human Reproduction*, vol. 17, no. 8, pp. 2016–2021, 2002.

[17] S. Munné, C. Magli, A. Adler et al., "Treatment-related chromosome abnormalities in human embryos," *Human Reproduction*, vol. 12, no. 4, pp. 780–784, 1997.

[18] J. Van Blerkom and P. Davis, "Differential effects of repeated ovarian stimulation on cytoplasmic and spindle organization in metaphase II mouse oocytes matured *in vivo* and *in vitro*," *Human Reproduction*, vol. 16, no. 4, pp. 757–764, 2001.

[19] T. Haaf, A. Hahn, A. Lambrecht et al., "A high oocyte yield for intracytoplasmic sperm injection treatment is associated with an increased chromosome error rate," *Fertility and Sterility*, vol. 91, no. 3, pp. 733–738, 2009.

[20] T. M. Rijken-Zijlstra, M. L. Haadsma, C. Hammer et al., "Effectiveness of indometacin to prevent ovulation in modified natural-cycle IVF: a randomized controlled trial," *Reproductive BioMedicine Online*, vol. 27, pp. 297–304, 2013.

[21] S. Athanasiou, T. H. Bourne, A. Khalid et al., "Effects of indomethacin on follicular structure, vascularity, and function over the periovulatory period in women," *Fertil. Steril*, vol. 65, pp. 556–560, 1996.

[22] I. J. Kadoch, M. Al-Khaduri, S. J. Phillips et al., "Spontaneous ovulation rate before oocyte retrieval in modified natural cycle IVF with and without indomethacin," *Reproductive BioMedicine*, vol. 16, no. 2, pp. 245–249, 2008.

[23] E. B. Baart, E. Martini, M. J. Eijkemans et al., "Milder ovarian stimulation for in-vitro fertilization reduces aneuploidy in the human preimplantation embryo: a randomized controlled trial," *Human Reproduction*, vol. 22, no. 4, pp. 980–988, 2007.

[24] K. Diedrich and R. Felberbaum, "New approaches to ovarian stimulation," *Human Reproduction*, vol. 13, supplement 3, pp. 1–13, 1998.

[25] M. G. Katz-Jaffe, A. O. Trounson, and D. S. Cram, "Chromosome 21 mosaic human preimplantation embryos predominantly arise from diploid conceptions," *Fertility and Sterility*, vol. 84, no. 3, pp. 634–643, 2005.

[26] G. Nargund and R. Frydman, "Towards a more physiological approach to IVF," *Reproductive BioMedicine Online*, vol. 14, no. 5, pp. 550–552, 2007.

[27] F. Olivennes and R. Frydman, "Friendly IVF: the way of the future?" *Human Reproduction*, vol. 13, no. 5, pp. 1121–1124, 1998.

[28] F. Olivennes, "GnRH antagonists: do they open new pathways to safer treatment in assisted reproductive techniques?" *Reproductive Biomedicine Online*, vol. 5, supplement 1, pp. 20–25, 2002.

[29] G. Pennings and W. Ombelet, "Coming soon to your clinic: patient-friendly ART," *Human Reproduction*, vol. 22, no. 8, pp. 2075–2079, 2007.

[30] F. M. Ubaldi, L. Rienzi, E. Baroni et al., "Hopes and facts about mild ovarian stimulation," *Reproductive BioMedicine Online*, vol. 14, no. 6, pp. 675–681, 2007.

[31] D. Kyrou, E. M. Kolibianakis, H. M. Fatemi et al., "Spontaneous triggering of ovulation versus HCG administration in patients undergoing IUI: a prospective randomized study," *Reproductive BioMedicine Online*, vol. 25, no. 3, pp. 278–283, 2012.

[32] N. Prapas, A. Tavaniotou, Y. Panagiotidis et al., "Low-dose human chorionic gonadotropin during the proliferative phase may adversely affect endometrial receptivity in oocyte recipients," *Gynecological Endocrinology*, vol. 25, no. 1, pp. 53–59, 2009.

[33] B. S. Shapiro, S. T. Daneshmand, F. C. Garner, M. Aguirre, C. Hudson, and S. Thomas, "Evidence of impaired endometrial receptivity after ovarian stimulation for in vitro fertilization: a prospective randomized trial comparing fresh and frozen-thawed embryo transfer in normal responders," *Fertility and Sterility*, vol. 96, no. 2, pp. 344–348, 2011.

[34] A. Bermejo, C. Iglesias, M. Ruiz-Alonso et al., "The impact of using the combined oral contraceptive pill for cycle scheduling on gene expression related to endometrial receptivity," *Human Reproduction*, vol. 29, no. 6, pp. 1271–1278, 2014.

[35] N. G. M. Beckers, P. Platteau, M. J. Eijkemans et al., "The early luteal phase administration of estrogen and progesterone does not induce premature luteolysis in normo-ovulatory women," *European Journal of Endocrinology*, vol. 155, no. 2, pp. 355–363, 2006.

[36] D. Valbuena, J. Martin, J. L. De Pablo, J. Remohí, A. Pellicer, and C. Simón, "Increasing levels of estradiol are deleterious to embryonic implantation because they directly affect the embryo," *Fertility and Sterility*, vol. 76, no. 5, pp. 962–968, 2001.

[37] R. J. Paulson, M. V. Sauer, and R. A. Lobo, "Embryo implantation after human in vitro fertilization: importance of endometrial receptivity," *Fertility and Sterility*, vol. 53, no. 5, pp. 870–874, 1990.

[38] E. G. Papanikolaou, G. Pados, G. Grimbizis et al., "GnRH-agonist versus GnRH-antagonist IVF cycles: Is the reproductive outcome affected by the incidence of progesterone elevation on the day of HCG triggering? A randomized prospective study," *Human Reproduction*, vol. 27, no. 6, pp. 1822–1828, 2012.

[39] A. M. Elnashar, "Progesterone rise on the day of HCG administration (premature luteinization) in IVF: an overdue update," *Journal of Assisted Reproduction and Genetics*, vol. 27, no. 4, pp. 149–155, 2010.

[40] W. Schoolcraft, E. Sinton, T. Schlenker, D. Huynh, F. Hamilton, and D. R. Meldrum, "Lower pregnancy rate with premature luteinization during pituitary suppression with leuprolide acetate," *Fertility and Sterility*, vol. 55, no. 3, pp. 563–566, 1991.

[41] K. M. Silverberg, W. N. Burns, D. L. Olive, R. M. Riehl, and R. S. Schenken, "Serum progesterone levels predict success of in vitro fertilization/embryo transfer in patients stimulated with leuprolide acetate and human menopausal gonadotropins," *Journal of Clinical Endocrinology and Metabolism*, vol. 73, no. 4, pp. 797–803, 1991.

4

Family Planning Knowledge, Attitudes, and Practices among Married Men and Women in Rural Areas of Pakistan: Findings from a Qualitative Need Assessment Study

Ghulam Mustafa,[1] Syed Khurram Azmat,[1,2] Waqas Hameed,[1] Safdar Ali,[1] Muhammad Ishaque,[1] Wajahat Hussain,[1] Aftab Ahmed,[1] and Erik Munroe[3]

[1]Marie Stopes Society, Research, Monitoring and Evaluation, Technical Services Department, 21-C, Commercial Area, Old Sunset Boulevard, DHA-II, Karachi, Sindh 75500, Pakistan
[2]Department of Urogynecology, Faculty of Medicine and Health Sciences, University of Gent, Sint-Pietersnieuwstraat 25, 9000 Gent, Belgium
[3]Marie Stopes International, Research, Monitoring and Evaluation Department, 1 Conway Street, Fitzroy Square, London W1T 6LP, UK

Correspondence should be addressed to Syed Khurram Azmat; syedkhurram.azmat@ugent.be

Academic Editor: Hind A. Beydoun

This paper presents the findings of a qualitative assessment aimed at exploring knowledge, attitudes, and practices regarding family planning and factors that influence the need for and use of modern contraceptives. A descriptive exploratory study was conducted with married women and men aged between 15 and 40. Overall, 24 focus group discussions were conducted with male and female participants in three provinces of Pakistan. The findings reveal that the majority knew about some modern contraceptive methods, but the overall contraceptive use was very low. Knowledge and use of any contraceptive method were particularly low. Reasons for not using family planning and modern contraception included incomplete family size, negative perceptions, in-laws' disapproval, religious concerns, side-effects, and lack of access to quality services. The majority preferred private facilities over the government health facilities as the later were cited as derided. The study concluded the need for qualified female healthcare providers, especially for long term family planning services at health facilities instead of camps arranged occasionally. Addressing issues around access, affordability, availability, and sociocultural barriers about modern contraception as well as involving men will help to meet the needs and ensure that the women and couples fulfill their childbearing and reproductive health goals.

1. Background

Despite being the sixth most populous country on the planet with the population exceeding 184 million, Pakistan is facing a huge challenge of poverty where 61% of its population is living below US$2 a day [1, 2]. About 45% of its population has limited access to health services both public and private, especially in rural areas where 65% of its population resides [2]. The country lags far behind on almost all development indicators, particularly with regard to maternal and child health [3]. It has been estimated that approximately 28,000 women die annually in Pakistan due to preventable pregnancy-related complications [2]. In 2008, Pakistan was included amongst the six countries that contributed to more than 50% of maternal deaths happening worldwide [3].

Maternal and neonatal health are strongly interlinked. Around 33% of neonates in Pakistan die due to maternal infections and other problems related to pregnancy and delivery [4]. The level of health among Pakistani women is alarmingly poor and contributes to both maternal and child morbidity and mortality. Some estimates from recent studies suggest that the lifetime risk of maternal death for Pakistani women is one in 93 [5]. Only half of the deliveries in Pakistan take place in the presence of skilled health provider and rural and less educated women are less likely to revive skilled delivery care [2]. Not only maternal mortality is high in Pakistan but there is a substantial rural-urban differential in maternal mortality (319 versus 175 per 100,000, resp.) [2]. Antenatal care coverage is far from optimal; 27% of pregnant women in Pakistan still receive no antenatal care and 40% do not receive postnatal care after delivery [2].

In addition to maternal health, newborn health and survival are another priority area for improvement. The Pakistan Demographic and Health Survey (PDHS) 2006-7 indicates that the neonatal mortality rate (NMR) has remained virtually unchanged over the past 15 years. It highlighted regional disparities also in this regard [6]. For example, the 10-year NMR is much higher in Punjab (58 per 1,000) and Sindh (53 per 1,000) than in NWFP and Baluchistan (41 and 30 per 1,000, resp.).

Modern FP methods, which have been documented to be highly effective means of improving maternal health by preventing unintended pregnancies in order to ensure healthy timing and spacing of births, only account for 26% of FP use in Pakistan. Moreover, the overall levels of FP use in rural areas continue to remain very low (around 31%), compared to 45% in urban areas. Similarly, women from the poorest households and those with no education have the lowest CPR [2].

Furthermore, the PDHS 2012-13 documents a significant unmet need for contraception at 20% [2]. According to an estimate, 890,000 induced abortions occur annually in Pakistan whereby one in seven pregnancies is terminated by induced abortion often performed in clandestine conditions [7] and abortion being used as means to control fertility and an outcome of failed contraception [7]. Out of the total fertility rate (TFR) of 3.8 in Pakistan, one birth is unwanted [2]. There are a number of structural and sociocultural issues that pose a challenge to improving maternal and newborn health (MNH) status in Pakistan. Lack of money, transportation, denial of family permission, or/and distance from health facility are some of the critical problems the majority of women face in Pakistan [2].

The average distance to a reproductive health facility in rural areas is larger than that to urban areas which makes access to services for rural women without transportation or funds extremely difficult [2]. It is also noteworthy that despite the large government infrastructure of primary, secondary, and tertiary care facilities in many areas throughout the country, as well as a Lady Health Worker (LHW) program, more than 70% of the population seeks healthcare through the private sector [6].

In addition, the dynamics of decision-making between a husband and wife also create barriers to access. Several studies have examined the influence of social and cultural factors on contraceptive use in Pakistan [8]. These studies have emphasized the influence of the mother-in-law and the husband on family planning decision-making [9, 10] and have highlighted the importance of communication between spouses regarding the use of contraception [11, 12]. Despite the huge benefits, family planning is one of the most difficult and least discussed topics, particularly amongst males in a conservative and patriarchal society where men have the final decision-making power regarding most issues, including reproductive health. Nevertheless, there have been some efforts to target men through either advocacy or behavioral change interventions, but very little have been achieved.

Healthy timing and spacing of pregnancy (HTSP) is a family planning intervention to help women and couples delay, time, space, or limit their pregnancies to achieve the healthiest outcomes for women, newborns, infants, and children regardless of the total number of children [13]. It has been documented that perinatal outcomes and child survival can be improved mainly by lengthening interpregnancy intervals [14, 15]. Over one million maternal deaths were averted between 1990 and 2005 because the fertility rate in developing countries has declined and by reducing high parity births family planning contributed to reducing the maternal mortality ratio [16]. On the contrary, birth to pregnancy intervals of less than 18 months are associated with risk of low birth weight, preterm birth, small size for gestational age, and stillbirth [17]. Despite the increased awareness and acknowledgement of birth spacing in improving maternal and child health outcomes, there is little evidence on effective, scalable, and sustainable programs for birth spacing in developing countries like Pakistan, particularly in rural areas. Moreover, there is a need to package evidence in creative ways to support program and policy decision-making at multiple levels: from community to policy arenas of Pakistan [18].

"Evidence for Innovating to Save Lives" was a 36-month operations' research initiative, implemented by Marie Stopes Society (MSS) from 2010 to 2013 aiming to promote birth spacing and modern contraceptive uptake in poor segments of population of Pakistan (http://mariestopespk.org/raf/research-project/). The overall goal of the project was to improve MNH through healthy timing and spacing of pregnancies in rural and underserved areas of Sindh, Punjab, and Khyber Pakhtunkhwa (KPK) provinces of Pakistan. Before the implementation of the project, MSS conducted a qualitative need assessment study with the potential target population, including men and women, in proposed project areas. The study aimed to explore knowledge, attitudes, and practices concerning family planning and birth spacing; perceptions about quality of care; health seeking behavior; community need assessment; and barriers and facilitators that influence contraceptive uptake. This paper presents the findings of the need assessment study.

2. Study Design and Methodology

Using the descriptive exploratory design, the need assessment study employed Focus Group Discussions (FGDs) technique for data collection. Overall, twenty-four FGDs were conducted, 8 FGDs with males and 16 FGDs with females. The FGDs took place in 2 districts of Sindh, 3 districts of Punjab, and 3 districts of Khyber Pakhtunkhwa provinces of Pakistan (refer to Table 1).

2.1. Inclusion/Exclusion Criteria and Recruitment. The participants for the FGDs were selected randomly from the household who were fathers and mothers having at least one

TABLE 1: Area- and participant-wise data collection details of the study participants.

Province	District	Male		Female	
		Number of FGDs	Age group (in years)	Number of FGDs	Age group (in years)
Sindh	Nawabshah	1	18–24	2	(15–18) (19–23)
	Naushahro Feroze	1	26–39	2	(24–30) (15–18)
Lower Punjab	Bahawalpur	1	18–24	2	(19–23) (24–30)
	Khanewal	1	26–39	2	(15–18) (19–23)
	Pakpattan	1	18–24	2	(24–30) (15–18)
Khyber Pakhtunkhwa	Haripur	1	26–39	2	(19–23) (24–30)
	Mansehra	1	25–30	2	(18–24) (19–23)
	Abbottabad	1	26–39	2	(24–30) (18–24)

child less than 2 years and no child above 2 years; having total household income of about 6000 Rupees per month (US 60$); and residing in houses classified as Kacha (made of clay) or Semi-Pakka (made of clay and some concrete). Using a specially designed screening/recruitment questionnaire which was made in line with the preset criteria of the target participants, the researchers visited households in the villages in person and identified the potential participants and recruited the eligible participants for the FGDs with their informed consent. The households were selected on the basis of their placement within the 2-3-kilometer catchment areas of the nearest reproductive health services delivery outlet. Local community health workers, from public and private sectors, contributed to the identification of potential households and only the ones meeting the set criteria (all as mentioned above) were invited to participate in the FGDs.

2.2. Target Population and Sampling. The study targeted young and newly married men and women with no child older than two years as this is the reproductive age group mainly identified in Pakistan Demographic Health Survey (DHS) 2006-7 and 2012-13 lacking contraceptive exposure [2, 6]. The participants of FGDs were in an age group of 18–40 years (male) and 15–30 years (female); refer to Table 1. All the participants had at least one child less than 2 years of age. One FGD with males and two FGDs with females were conducted in each of the eight project districts (making a total of 8 groups for males and 16 for females); refer to Table 1 for details.

2.3. Study Sites. The study was carried out in 8 villages of the 8 rural districts of Sindh, Punjab, and Khyber Pakhtunkhwa provinces in Pakistan (refer to Table 1 for details). As the study was conducted in remote rural villages of the study districts, arrangements were made to conduct FGDs at places which had easy access to participants and where they felt comfortable, for example, autaq/baithak (community hall style places for male participants), schools, and/or homes for females.

2.4. Research Instrument and Data Collection. FGD guides were designed and developed by the MSS research team in English and were translated into the national language

Urdu after pretesting in order to accommodate professional and cultural validation. The interviews were conducted in participants' native language and the data were collected by qualified researchers comprised of male and female moderators. The moderators facilitating the FGDs were university graduates trained and experienced in social science research techniques and were fluent in local languages. Additional training on family planning and reproductive health concepts and qualitative methods of data collection was also provided to the moderators. The FGDs were carried out separately with male and female participants using separate guidelines due to cultural and local area sensitivities. Each FGD group consisted of 6 to 8 participants. As a standard procedure, male moderators conducted FGDs with males, whereas female moderators conducted FGDs with female groups. Each FGD was audiotape-recorded and, in addition to audiotape recording, field and observational notes were also taken by research assistants.

2.5. Data Analysis. Audio-recording of the FGDs was transcribed word to word/verbatim and translated from Urdu/local language into English by the researcher fluent in both languages. These transcripts were used for detailed analysis. Using the thematic analysis approach, the researchers read and reread all of the transcripts several times to be familiar with the data and to identify predetermined and emerging themes from the data. Along with the manual analysis technique employed in the initial phase of data analysis, the data was also coded and thematically analyzed using QSR NVIVO 8 software for Windows. The codes were further refined, combined, and categorized to develop additional codes for a detailed analysis.

2.6. Ethical Considerations. The ethical approval for the project was provided by Program Oversight Committee (POC) of Research and Advocacy Fund (RAF) and National Bioethics Committee (NBC) of Pakistan (Ref. number 4-87/10/NBC-43/RDC/). Further, all of the study participants were briefed about the purpose of the study and their right to refuse to answer any question or withdraw from the FGDs at any time. They were informed that there was no "right" or "wrong" answer and they were requested to express their opinions and thoughts freely. They were informed that their

TABLE 2: Identified themes and subthemes.

Themes	Subthemes
Sociodemographic profile	Socioeconomic status
	Household structure
	Family size
Reproductive history	Approximate age at marriage
	Number of pregnancies and any history or experience of miscarriages or pregnancy termination
	Number of children
	Desired family size
Health seeking behavior	General health service seeking behavior
	Health service seeking behavior regarding family planning/reproductive health
Knowledge, attitudes, perceptions, and practices about family planning and modern contraceptive methods	Type of contraceptive methods known including modern contractive methods
	Perceptions about safety/effectiveness of contraceptive methods
	Knowledge, attitudes, perceptions, and practices regarding family planning and contraceptive methods
Sources of knowledge	Interpersonal including friends and relatives
	Mass media including radio, TV and cable, and newspaper
Current contraceptive practices	Modern contraceptive methods
	The preferred method
	Reasons of use, nonuse, and discontinuation
Decision-making regarding contraceptive use	Decision-making dynamics about family planning and spousal communication
Barriers on family planning and contraceptive use	Religious barriers
	Lack of knowledge
	Fear of side-effects
	Social stigma and social pressure
	Husband/in-laws' disapproval
	Lack of access
	Lack of affordability

names or any identification leading to them will be kept strictly confidential and that their names will not appear in any report or publication resulting from this study. They were further informed that the audio-recordings and hard copies of the transcripts will be kept under lock and key and subsequently destroyed in due time. Before the start of FGDs, verbal and informed consent was also taken from the study participants.

3. Findings

The following themes and subthemes (refer to Table 2) were identified and used for thematic analysis of data. The detailed findings will follow this table of themes.

3.1. Sociodemographic Characteristics and Reproductive History. The majority of the participants, including men and women, belonged to a very low socioeconomic status (SES) with average monthly income around 6000 PKR (1 USD$ = 89 PKR). Mostly, they were living in a large joint family setup, especially in Sindh and Khyber Pakhtunkhwa. Females from

KPK said, *"we live together with our in laws. Including the mother-in-law, father in law, sister-in-law, brother-in-law, his wife and children; we are all around 15 people living together."* The majority of male and female participants had entered into marriage at an early age, especially females at a very young age ranging between 15 and 24 years and males between 20 and 30 years.

3.2. Pregnancy-Related Problems. There were some complications in last pregnancy and miscarriages experienced by participants in all regions. A female from KPK said, *"my first pregnancy resulted in a miscarriage at 5th month; I lifted something heavy and got a miscarriage,"* while a female from Punjab shared a quite different reason for her miscarriage and said, *"I had lost a child after 6 months of pregnancy, my uterus was weak, the doctor advised spacing to strengthen the uterus and now I have a child after almost two years."* Participants from Sindh having miscarriage were quite uncertain to find any reason. A female from Sindh said, *"I lost a child when I was 40 days pregnant, there was no reason. I was just sitting at home and miscarried."*

However, many women in KPK and Sindh opted for induced abortion to end their pregnancies often in a potentially harmful way. In some cases women even have to rely on Dais (traditional birth attendants) or visit private hospitals outside their village for an abortion owing to poverty as they either do not want to have a female child or they do not want more children. A female from Sindh said, *"they go to a private hospital for this, everything can be done there, and they get themselves aborted and cleaned there in secrecy."* Another female from Sindh said, *"yes, there are women who find it difficult to raise children, so they waste the fetus."*

3.3. Health Service Seeking Behavior

3.3.1. General Health Service Seeking Behavior. There was lack of basic health facilities in respective rural areas/villages of Sindh, Punjab, and Khyber Pakhtunkhwa. It was found that the majority of men and women prefer to go to private hospitals/clinics if they could afford owing to the perceived availability of various facilities. A male from Punjab said, *"Private hospitals have all kinds of facilities; they have every machine, ultrasound, blood tests and ambulance."* The majority of men and women in those rural areas heavily relied on quacks for many healthcare needs which include dispensers and compounders in most cases, who were engaged in private practice in their respective villages. Despite the awareness that these were not qualified doctors, they visited them for lack of a choice available to them. A female from KPK said, *"there is only one doctor available in our area. He does not have an MBBS degree. He is a local practitioner."*

3.3.2. Health Service Seeking Behavior regarding Family Planning/Reproductive Health. Absence of FP/RH across the regions was prevailing in the same intensity. The majority of men and women have to travel outside in case of emergency which in a way affect the choice of availing FP methods. A male from Sindh said, *"there is no such facility in our village to provide services on birth-spacing or birth related complication. We have to go to the main city Sakrand which is 14–16 kilometers away from our village."*

The majority of men and women in Sindh and Punjab were satisfied with the role of LHWs as they provide information and services at doorsteps with concerns over the IUCD procedure performed by them. A male from Sindh said, *"LHWs provide information and contraceptive methods. We listen to their advice carefully and trust them altogether. But we don't trust the operation that they do because it is done in the camp which is set up for only 2-3 days."*

In contrast, majority of women in KPK were not satisfied as LHWs in their area barely provided services at the doorstep. In addition, LHWs charge their late visit at night in case of emergency and they provide pills and injections to their relatives and neighbors only. A female from KPK said, *"Lady Health Workers get medicines from the government and they distribute them among their relatives."*

3.4. Knowledge of and Perceptions about Family Planning and Modern Contraception.

The men and women across the regions were familiar with different family planning methods, especially modern contraception except vasectomy. Among traditional methods, the majority of participants had little knowledge and were indifferent toward breast feeding as a natural way to avoid pregnancy. A male from Sindh said, *"We have heard that some women breast feed their children and don't get pregnant whereas in some cases women breast feed their children and from the second month they start getting their menses."*

The majority of participants across the regions were assured that FP is essential for the health of the mother and child and welfare of the family. A female from KPK said, *"Because there is one earner and many dependents, if we plan a family only then can you survive on one source of earning."* A male from Sindh said, *"if there are fewer children then we can raise them properly; providing better facilities, food, education, etc. to them."*

Moreover, it is interesting to note that indifferent approaches to FP/birth spacing still strongly prevail in rural areas of Pakistan. The majority of men in Sindh and KPK still seemed resistant to accept the use of FP/birth spacing and did not seem much in favor of family planning for financial and religious reasons. A male from Sindh said, *"if one has limited resources then only he should do FP, but once he is in a position to afford then he should put a stop to FP, this is the right approach, but those who go for tubal ligation that is not the right way which is against the religion."* However, it is alarming to note that some married adolescent women in Sindh and Punjab were intending to use contraception only when they complete their family size having 5-6 children. This attitude was prevailing mainly among the young men and women of these regions (19–23 years of age). A female from Sindh said, *"We don't want to do family planning, we are very young, once we will have 5 to 6 children then only we will think, some females do want to have less children but males wants them to produce more children."*

3.5. Sources of Knowledge regarding Family Planning and Modern Contraception.

The majority of men and women identified word of mouth as the main and most reliable and immediate source of information across the region. A female from Sindh said, *"We live in one village, so if anybody finds out any information they share it with each other."* In addition, women with previous experience of contraceptive use and television were mentioned as important sources of information. A female from Punjab said, *"we find out about pills and injection from TV."* Another female from KPK said, *"We have heard about different contraceptive methods from people around us who had used these methods."*

3.6. Current Contraceptive Use and Behavior.

The majority of men and women across all regions were not using any family planning method mainly because they wanted more children, had negative perceptions about family planning, or had concerns about side-effects and due to lack of access to information and services. A female from Punjab said, *"My cousin did family planning and after that she couldn't have children. She used the method of IUCD for spacing between children. But suddenly both of her children died and after that she cannot get pregnant.*"

In contrast, there were only few who used modern methods as these ensured better health of the mother and child. A female from KPK said, "*We did plan and tried that we should not have another child because our first child was too young; therefore we wanted to have another child once our first child was grown enough; so we used condoms.*" Method-wise, condoms were mostly preferred by men. To quote a female from Punjab, "*The idea of using a condom was my husband's; he had asked the doctor and decided.*" The majority of women perceived IUCD and tubal ligation relatively safer compared to pills and injections. A female from Sindh said, "*my neighbor told me to have IUCD inserted for five years. It is safe and I can decide when to remove it whenever I want.*"

3.7. Decision-Making regarding Contraceptive Use. Discussions about decision-making regarding family planning and modern contraception yielded that husband and in-laws mainly influence how, when, and whether to practice family planning and use contraception. A female from Sindh said, "*my mother-in-law and father-in-law say that I should have as many children as I can.*"

Despite that, there did exist some mutual understanding and communication found between few spouses in some areas across the regions. A female from Punjab informed that "*It is a mutual decision; the husband tells us to take advice from the doctor because she has a better understanding.*"

3.8. Barriers towards Family Planning and Modern Contraception. Findings of the study confirmed few barriers identified in previous studies. Nevertheless, findings provided some new insight into the perception that impedes the use of family planning/birth spacing.

3.8.1. Religious Barriers. The majority of men across the region do not practice FP/birth spacing owing to religious reasons. Quoting various religious injunctions and traditions, they discussed that bearing many children is advocated by Islam and is also beneficial for growth of Muslim Ummah (the Muslim brotherhood). A male from KPK said, "*we don't do family planning because of our religion; The Prophet (PBUH) had said that one should marry a woman whose family has more children.*" Similarly, a female from Punjab described it thus: "*The religion prohibits it because the prophet said that the more children a woman bears the more my Ummah (Muslim brotherhood) will grow.*"

3.8.2. Lack of Knowledge and Fear of Side-Effects. Across all regions, the majority of participants, especially women, associated different types of side-effects with different contraceptive methods, for example, dangerous for fertility, black spots and hair growing on face, and impotency and lack of knowledge. A male from Punjab said, "*People do not practice family planning mainly because they do not know how, when and what to do use,*" whereas a female from Punjab said that "*People don't use methods because of fear; someone woman I*

know got herself injected, and for a whole month she bled and became weak as a result."

3.8.3. Social Stigma and Pressure. It is important to note that the majority of young married males and females do not practice FP owing to various social stigmas. Social pressure to bear more children is identified as a barrier towards family planning as parents with more children are seen with more respect. A male from Sindh said, "*people here feel very shy telling anybody at home or anywhere else that he is going for family planning services with his wife. They either laugh at you or scorn you.*" A female from KPK said, "*People say if there are more children they will prove helpful in the future; and they will bring honor to the family name.*"

3.8.4. Husband/In-Laws Disapproval. Females do not practice family planning without their husbands and mothers-in-law approval. This is the most pivotal restriction to cope within Pakistan which is at times linked with sociocultural and health issues. A female from Sindh said, "*My husband does not allow me; he wants me to keep having children; some men say that spacing leads to illness and if a woman keeps having children then she is healthy.*"

3.8.5. Restrictions on Female Mobility. It is interesting to note that stringent restrictions on female mobility emerged as a major barrier across the regions. Females are not allowed to step out alone without the permission of their husbands or mothers-in-law. Women going alone even for medical help are thought to bring dishonor to the family. A female from KPK said that "*we cannot go freely or alone to get family planning services. We need permission from our husband or mother-in-law.*"

3.8.6. Lack of Access and Affordability to FP/RH Services. There were persistent problems of accessibility, affordability, and unavailability of the doctors prevailing in the rural/village areas of Pakistan. A male from Punjab said that "*The men and women in this area want to practice family planning but it is not within their reach; it is hard for them to reach family planning centers in other cities which are far away from our residence.*" It is interesting to note that affordability issue was mainly highlighted by the females as they mentioned that their husbands were earning limited incomes and they were dependent on their husband's income. A female from Sindh said, "*My husband's salary is spent in running the expenses of the household, so we cannot spend money on these things. Also there is no Centre here and to go to Sakrand you need to arrange conveyance and that requires extra expenditure.*"

In addition, the majority of men and women highlighted the importance of having female doctor in their respective areas as they were not comfortable to discuss gynecological or reproductive health issues with the male doctors due to various sociocultural boundaries. A female from Punjab said that "*There is no female doctor here; we need one because currently we have to travel to the city to see female doctor. It is difficult to consult a male doctor on reproductive health issues.*"

4. Discussion

Almost all of the participants had entered into marriage very early with women entering into marriage relatively earlier than men, which is similar to national figures that report that on average women enter into marriage at the age of 18. Both men and women reported that the ideal number of children they would like to have in a family is four comprising boys and girls with greater emphasis on boys. In line with findings of the PDHS 2012-13, males were reported as wanting more children than females [2]. Spouse (husband) involvement appears to be a key factor in deciding to take a family planning method and it is also equally important with regard to the number of children a couple will have [16]. Joint decision-making (both spouses) is rarely seen with regard to the number of children or the taking-up of an FP method.

As shown by previous research evidence [6], men and women, depending on the ability to afford, preferred to go to private health facilities as these were perceived to have sufficient and responsive staff, were well equipped, and provided quality services. Government health facilities, most of the participants claimed, either were dysfunctional or lacked staff/services and were discriminatory in provision of services where prompt and quality services were only provided to well-off people.

Most of the participants had knowledge of at least one modern contraceptive method with condom being the most commonly known method which is also concurrent with the findings of Pakistan DHS 2012-13 [2]. However, in contrast to the present national data [2], long acting Intrauterine Device (IUD) was the most commonly known method after condom and female sterilization and was considered safer and having fewer side-effects by women in comparison to short term methods including injectable and pills. It is interesting to note that word of mouth is the most common source of information for both men and women in these rural communities which is also supported by previous research findings [19].

Both positive and negative perceptions about FP were recorded during the discussions. On the positive side, both male and female participants stated that increased awareness and financial pressure were the two main factors making couples keep their family sizes smaller. Besides, lack of awareness and sociocultural pressures (including in-laws' pressure on females and peers' on males) and shyness negatively affected perceptions about family planning and discouraged family planning uptake.

Regarding current or ever use of contraception, only a few participants, either male or female, reported positively. The dominant reason for not using contraceptives included desire for more children. Hence, being qualitative in nature, this study was not able to measure the real "unmet need for contraception"; instead the study tried to capture the perceived need for contraceptive services which seem to be very low in the target communities due to the desire of having more children expressed by the majority of the participants. Therefore, there is no real need for contraception. Likewise, the participants were mostly young and newly married and no participant had more than two children which led to such

low perceived need for contraception. This is also concurrent with Pakistan DHS 2012-13 results which demonstrate that contraceptive use increases with age and the number of children and reaches optimal level when the couples have achieved their desired number of children [2]. However, the study findings also draw attention to other factors like lack of awareness about the range of family planning methods, absence of health facilities providing quality family planning services, inability to afford the quality services in remote cities, and sociocultural issues like peer-pressure, restrictions on female mobility, and in-laws' disapproval. These findings are also in agreement with previous research studies [6]. Fear of side-effects also emerged as an important impediment to contraceptive use which is also a recurrent theme in many studies conducted in developing countries including Pakistan, India, Bangladesh, and Ethiopia [19–22]. In addition, religious concerns were also cited by some participants as a reason for not using contraception which was also reported as important factor impeding contraceptive adoption by previous national DHS surveys [2, 6]. Some other studies have also highlighted religions as an important factor influencing an individual's decision to adopt contraception [23].

Nevertheless, the study findings need to be treated cautiously to avoid overgeneralization due to some limitations mainly arising from the study design. First of all, this is a qualitative study and is conducted with a limited number of people and may not represent the views of the whole population in the targeted communities. Secondly, the study documented the opinions of the married men and women who mostly were newly married, had no more than two children, and belonged to lower socioeconomic status and thus their opinions may vary from the opinions of men and women with different sociodemographic characteristics.

5. Conclusion and Recommendations

The study provides insights into the local contexts related to family planning knowledge, attitudes, perceptions, and practices and also highlights the need for contraceptives, especially for long acting and reversible contraceptives. In the wake of changing attitudes towards family planning and desired family size, more women and couples will be seeking family planning services. Addressing obstacles such as access, affordability, and availability will help meet these needs and ensure that women and couples can meet their childbearing and reproductive health goals. In addition, a very low perceived need for contraception was found amongst the respondents wanting more children expressed almost equally by male and female respondents.

The study also identified the need for qualified and trained female healthcare providers, especially for long term family planning services, including IUD, at well-established health facilities instead of camps setup occasionally. Both male and female participants were of the opinion that a female professional (ideally a doctor) should be made available in their areas to which people can have a quick and easy access. The men also emphasized that a male with training and adequate knowledge in family planning should be made available in their communities to inform men about the benefits of family planning and birth spacing.

In addition, the study findings reveal that mostly men and women do not use contraception either because they are newly married or because they have few children. Despite this, many young women and men expressed their intention to use contraception, though late in married life, depending on the quality and availability of the services. Well-targeted behavior change and communication campaigns can change the attitudes regarding birth spacing practices. These behavior change campaigns should encourage both men and women to adopt healthy birth spacing practices from the start or during the early period of marriage instead of letting them wait for completing their desired family size and then starting with contraception as is the current practice.

Moreover, the study also identified strong need for involving men in healthcare programs designed to improve women's and newborns' health as they mostly influence decision-making at the household level and this will also result in active male participation and community ownership. Young, especially first time, fathers need support and empowerment. Encouraging communication between wife and husband about family planning and birth spacing should also be part of such campaigns to promote mutual decision-making between wife and husband and make husbands responsible partners in family planning/birth spacing decisions and ease the burden of decision-making on women.

Furthermore, family planning and birth spacing interventions need to focus on alleviating fears about side-effects among men and women through effective counseling and providing adequate information to both men and women about method-related side-effects and how to manage them. In addition, involving community leaders, religious clerics, and health workers in awareness raising campaigns can help address sociocultural and religious concerns.

Conflict of Interests

The authors declare that there is no conflict of interests regarding the publication of this paper.

References

[1] Population Reference Bureau, "World Population Data Sheet," 2013, http://www.prb.org/Publications/Datasheets/2012/world-population-data-sheet.aspx.

[2] National Institute of Population Studies (NIPS) and ICF International, *Pakistan Demographic and Health Survey 2012-13*, National Institute of Population Studies (NIPS), Islamabad, Pakistan; ICF International, Calverton, Md, USA, 2013.

[3] UNDP, *The Real Wealth of the Nations: Pathways to Human Development*, 2014.

[4] Z. Bhutta, G. Darmstadt, E. Ramson, A. Starrs, and A. Inker, "Basing newborn and maternal health policies on evidence," Tech. Rep., JHPIEGO, 2013.

[5] D. Anthony, *The State of the World's Children 2011: Adolescence: An Age of Opportunity*, United Nations Children's Fund (UNICEF), New York, NY, USA, 2011.

[6] National Institute of Population Studies (NIPS) and Macro International, *Pakistan Demographic and Health Survey 2006-07*, National Institute of Population Studies (NIPS), Macro International, Islamabad, Pakistan, 2006.

[7] Z. A. Sathar, S. Singh, and F. F. Fikree, "Estimating the incidence of abortion in Pakistan," *Studies in Family Planning*, vol. 38, no. 1, pp. 11–22, 2007.

[8] I. Sirageldin, D. Norris, and J. G. Hardee, "Family planning in Pakistan: an analysis of some factors constraining use," *Studies in Family Planning*, vol. 7, no. 5, pp. 144–154, 1976.

[9] O. Pasha, F. F. Fikree, and S. Vermund, "Determinants of unmet need for family planning in squatter settlements in Karachi, Pakistan," *Asia-Pacific Population Journal*, vol. 16, no. 2, pp. 93–108, 2001.

[10] M. M. Kadir, F. Fikree, A. Khan, and F. Sajan, "Do mothers-in-law matter? Family dynamics and fertility decision-making in urban squatter settlements of Karachi, Pakistan," *Journal of Biosocial Science*, vol. 35, no. 4, pp. 545–558, 2003.

[11] R. M. Salem, J. Bemstein, T. M. Sullivan, and R. Lamde, *Communication for Better Health. Population Reports*, Johns Hopkins Bloomberg School of Public Health, Baltimore, Md, USA, 2008.

[12] N. Mahmood and K. Ringheim, "Factors affecting contraceptive use in Pakistan," *The Pakistan Development Review*, vol. 35, no. 1, pp. 1–22, 1996.

[13] C. Marston, *Report of WHO Technical Consultation on Birth Spacing*, World Health Organization, Geneva, Switzerland, 2005.

[14] J. Cleland, S. Bernstein, A. Ezeh, A. Faundes, A. Glasier, and J. Innis, "Family planning: the unfinished agenda," *The Lancet*, vol. 368, no. 9549, pp. 1810–1827, 2006.

[15] J. Cleland, A. Conde-Agudelo, H. Peterson, J. Ross, and A. Tsui, "Contraception and health," *The Lancet*, vol. 380, no. 9837, pp. 149–156, 2012.

[16] J. Stover and J. Ross, "How increased contraceptive use has reduced maternal mortality," *Maternal and Child Health Journal*, vol. 14, no. 5, pp. 687–695, 2010.

[17] B.-P. Zhu, "Effect of interpregnancy interval on birth outcomes: Findings from three recent US studies," *International Journal of Gynecology and Obstetrics*, vol. 89, no. 1, pp. S25–S33, 2005.

[18] B. T. Shaikh, "Unmet need for family planning in Pakistan-PDHS 2006-7: it's time to re-examine déjà vu," *Open Access Journal of Contraception*, vol. 1, pp. 113–118, 2010.

[19] S. K. Azmat and G. Mustafa, "Barriers and perceptions regarding different contraceptives and family planning practices amongst men and women of reproductive age in rural Pakistan: a qualitative study," *Pakistan Journal of Public Health*, vol. 2, no. 1, pp. 17–23, 2012.

[20] R. Neeti, D. K. Tanjea, K. Ravneet, and G. K. Ingle, "Factors affecting contraception among women in a minority community in Delhi: a qualitative study," *Health and Population: Perspectives and Issues*, vol. 33, pp. 10–15, 2014.

[21] H. Nuruzzaman, "Unmet need for contraceptive: the case of married adolescent women in Bangladesh," *International Journal of Current Research*, vol. 9, pp. 29–35, 2010.

[22] T. Tilahun, G. Coene, S. Luchters et al., "Family planning knowledge, attitude and practice among married couples in jimma zone, ethiopia," *PLoS ONE*, vol. 8, no. 4, Article ID e61335, 2013.

[23] M. H. Bernhart and M. M. Uddin, "Islam and family planning acceptance in Bangladesh," *Studies in Family Planning*, vol. 21, no. 5, pp. 287–292, 1990.

5

Comparison of IVF Outcomes between Minimal Stimulation and High-Dose Stimulation for Patients with Poor Ovarian Reserve

Tal Lazer,[1,2] Shir Dar,[1,2] Ekaterina Shlush,[1,2] Basheer S. Al Kudmani,[1,2] Kevin Quach,[1] Agata Sojecki,[1] Karen Glass,[1,2,3] Prati Sharma,[1,2,3] Ari Baratz,[1,2,3] and Clifford L. Librach[1,2,3]

[1] CReATe Fertility Centre, 790 Bay Street, Suite 1100, Toronto, ON, Canada M5G 1N8
[2] Department of Obstetrics & Gynecology, University of Toronto, Toronto, ON, Canada M5S 2J7
[3] Division of Reproductive Endocrinology and Infertility, Department of Obstetrics and Gynecology, Women's College Hospital, Toronto, ON, Canada M5S 1B2

Correspondence should be addressed to Clifford L. Librach; drlibrach@createivf.com

Academic Editor: Hind A. Beydoun

We examined whether treatment with minimum-dose stimulation (MS) protocol enhances clinical pregnancy rates compared to high-dose stimulation (HS) protocol. A retrospective cohort study was performed comparing IVF and pregnancy outcomes between MS and HS gonadotropin-antagonist protocol for patients with poor ovarian reserve (POR). Inclusion criteria included patients with an anti-Müllerian hormone (AMH) ≤8 pmol/L and/or antral follicle count (AFC) ≤5 on days 2-3 of the cycle. Patients from 2008 exclusively had a HS protocol treatment, while patients in 2010 had treatment with a MS protocol exclusively. The MS protocol involved letrozole at 2.5 mg over 5 days, starting from day 2, overlapping with gonadotropins, starting from the third day of letrozole at 150 units daily. GnRH antagonist was introduced once one or more follicles reached 14 mm or larger. The HS group received gonadotropins (≥300 IU/day) throughout their antagonist cycle. Clinical pregnancy rate was significantly higher in the MS protocol compared to the HS protocol ($P = 0.007$). Furthermore, the live birth rate was significantly higher in the MS group compare to the HS group ($P = 0.034$). In conclusion, the MS IVF protocol is less expensive (lower gonadotropin dosage) and resulted in a higher clinical pregnancy rate and live birth rate than a HS protocol for poor responders.

1. Introduction

Patients with poor ovarian response (POR) are both challenging to treat and represent a large proportion of patients presenting with infertility [1, 2]. Patients with POR, who are often of advanced maternal age, have a high cycle cancellation rate, higher miscarriage rate, and significantly reduced live birth rate per cycle. To date, there is no universally accepted definition for POR. These patients generally have one or more of the following characteristics: advanced maternal age, low AMH levels, high FSH in the early follicular phase (~day 3) (≥10 mIU/mL), low early follicular phase antral follicle count (AFC) (3–7) [3, 4], low number of mature retrieved oocytes (<4) after superovulation with a moderate to high-dose protocol, low peak E2 levels (<3300 pmol/L), and prior cycle cancellation(s) due to poor response [5–7]. The European Society of Human Reproduction and Embryology (ESHRE) attempted to standardize the definition of POR in 2010 and this resulted in a consensus definition called the Bologna criteria. At least two of the following three features must be present: (1) advanced maternal age (≥40 years) or any other risk factors for POR, (2) a previous POR (≤3 oocytes) with a conventional stimulation protocol, and/or (3) an abnormal ovarian reserve test (AFC < 5–7 follicles or AMH < 0.5–1.1 ng/mL) (REF).

The management of POR is highly controversial as well. There is still no consensus regarding the "ideal" protocol and so far no one treatment protocol has proven to be superior for this group. The majority of the strategies aim to recruit a higher number of follicles either by increasing the dose of gonadotropins, decreasing the dose of GnRH analogs, suppressing an early rise in FSH with "estrogen priming," or optimizing the endogenous FSH flare effect [1]. In addition, adjunctive growth hormone is advocated by some studies [1, 7] while aromatase inhibitors have also been suggested in other studies [8].

Letrozole is a potent and highly specific nonsteroidal third generation aromatase inhibitor, originally approved for use in postmenopausal women with hormone receptor positive breast cancer to suppress estrogen production [9]. It inhibits the aromatase enzyme resulting in decreased estradiol synthesis. Letrozole is increasingly being utilized for ovulation induction in infertility. By decreasing early follicular phase estrogen synthesis, there is a decrease in estradiol-mediated negative feedback at the hypothalamus, with a resultant increase in endogenous gonadotropin secretion. Healey et al. [10] demonstrated that the addition of letrozole to gonadotropins increases the number of preovulatory follicles without having a negative impact on pregnancy rate. In addition, letrozole was found to cause an increase in intraovarian androgen levels which in turn increases FSH receptor expression on follicular granulosa cells [11]. Thus, letrozole may improve the ovarian response to FSH in poor responders [11].

In our study, we compared a standard high-dose gonadotropin-antagonist (HS) protocol for poor responders to a minimal stimulation (MS) protocol involving letrozole overlapping with a low dose of gonadotropins, for poor responders. Our hypothesis was that using a MS protocol with letrozole might enhance clinical pregnancy rates over a HS protocol.

2. Materials and Methods

2.1. Patients. This is a retrospective cohort study using data from IVF cycles in patients with poor ovarian reserve, carried out at the CReATe Fertility Centre in Toronto, Canada. The inclusion criteria included patients with poor ovarian reserve as defined by the Bologna criteria [12]. Due to predicted poor outcome, cycles where only a single dominant follicle developed were cancelled and excluded.

In 2008 we were performing exclusively HS protocols on these patients. There were a total of 71 IVF cycles that met these criteria during that year. During 2009, after some early positive reports on MS, we began using a MS protocol in an attempt to improve pregnancy rates in this poor prognosis population. Based on our early observations of higher success with this protocol, by 2010 we transitioned to using, almost exclusively, the MS protocol for this group of patients. There were a total of 70 cycles that met these criteria during 2010. Therefore, we compared our 2008 cycles to 2010 in order to avoid selection bias. All cycles included for each group represented their first IVF attempt. This study was approved by the University of Toronto Research Ethics Committee (REB Approval number 28824).

2.2. Treatment Protocol. All patients had an initial transvaginal ultrasound examination to measure the uterine lining and perform an antral follicle count on day 2 of the cycle. Baseline blood levels of estradiol, FSH, LH, and progesterone were also

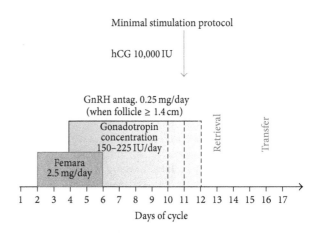

FIGURE 1: Treatment scheme for the minimal stimulation protocol.

measured at the same visit. The MS protocol consisted of low dose letrozole (Femara; Novartis, Dorval, Quebec, Canada) 2.5 mg PO over 5 days, starting from cycle day 2 (Figure 1). On day 4 of the cycle (day 3 of the letrozole treatment) overlapping low dose gonadotropins, menopur (Ferring Inc., Toronto, ON, Canada) was initiated. The initial gonadotropin dose was 150 IU per day. After 3 days on menopur, the patient was reviewed for standard ultrasound and blood hormone monitoring and the dose was titrated according to the initial response. Depending on the response, the gonadotropin dose was either maintained or increased up to 225 IU, but not higher. When one or more follicles reached 14 mm in size, gonadotropin releasing hormone (GnRH) antagonist, cetrotide (EMD Serono, Darmstadt, Germany) 0.25 mg, was introduced to avoid a premature LH surge. Human chorionic gonadotropin (hCG) (PPC, Richmond Hill, ON, Canada) 10000 IU was administered for final maturation when at least 1 or 2 follicles reached 18 mm or above. Cycles where there was a single dominant follicle were cancelled. Oocyte retrieval was performed approximately 36 hours after the hCG injection. Intracytoplasmic sperm injection (ICSI) was performed in almost all cases in order to optimize fertilization for the small number of oocytes. The control group received high levels of gonadotropins (≥300 IU/day) starting from day 2 of their cycle and throughout their short antagonist cycle. Antagonist initiation, hCG administration timing, and oocyte retrieval timing were the same as those for the MS protocol.

Embryo transfer was performed on day 3 under ultrasound guidance. Luteal support was with either intramuscular administration progesterone in ethyl oleate oil (2 cc of 50 mg/mL) (compounded by our local pharmacist (R.B.)) or progesterone suppositories 100 mg qid (compounded by our local pharmacist (R.B.)), started on the day of retrieval. Serum βhCG levels were tested starting 2 weeks after embryo transfer, and then serially, if positive, followed by a transvaginal ultrasound examination between 6 and 7 weeks of gestation. Clinical pregnancy was defined for this study as the presence of a gestational sac, with or without fetal cardiac activity.

Data were expressed as mean ± standard deviation. The student's t-test and χ^2 testing were used for data comparisons adjusting variables using a 95% confidence interval. A *P* value less than 0.05 was considered statistically significant. SPSS version 15.0 (SPSS Inc. Chicago, IL, USA) was used for data analysis.

3. Results

A total of 141 cycles ($n = 70$ for 2010 and $n = 71$ for 2008) met the inclusion criteria. Patients' demographic and clinical data are shown in Table 1. There was no significant difference between the MS and HS groups with respect to age (39.1 ± 3.8 versus 39.0 ± 3.9, resp.). The E2 level on the day of hCG administration (MS 1580.8 ± 1141.2 versus HS 5575 ± 3295.1 pmol/L, $P < 0.001$) and the total units gonadotropins administered during the stimulation protocol (MS 1332.9 ± 435.7 versus HS 5575.2 ± 1945 IU, $P < 0.001$) were significantly higher in the HS group. There was no significant difference in the number of oocytes retrieved with the MS versus HS protocol (2.9 ± 1.5 versus 3.5 ± 1.5 resp., $P > 0.05$). Cancelled cycles due to the formation of a single dominant follicle represented 5% of cycles started in each group (NS). There was no significant difference in the number of fertilized eggs (2PN) between the two protocols (1.5 ± 1.1 versus 1.5 ± 1.2 resp., $P > 0.05$), and no significant difference in the number of embryos transferred per cycle for the MS versus the HS protocols (1.8 ± 0.7 versus 1.4 ± 1.2 resp., $P > 0.05$) was found. Clinical pregnancy rate was significantly higher in the MS versus HS protocols (22/70, 31.4% versus 9/78, 12.7%, resp., $P < 0.05$). The live birth rate was significantly higher in the MS group compared to the HS group (15/70, 21.4% versus 5/71 7.0%, resp., $P < 0.05$).

A power analysis was conducted for a chi-square of the two groups. We assumed a significance level of 0.05 and a power level of 0.80. At an "n" of 79 for group 1 (2008) and a proportion of 0.14, the largest and smallest detectable proportions for group 2 (2010) are 0.35 and 0.0097, respectively.

4. Discussion

Treating patients with poor ovarian response remains one of the biggest challenges in reproductive medicine. It is usually a problem of advanced reproductive age patients [13]; however previous ovarian surgery [14], pelvic infections [15], and environmental factors or genetic factors may be associated with it in younger patients as well [16]. The objective of this study was to compare IVF laboratory results, clinical pregnancy rate, and live birth rate from a MS protocol using a combination of letrozole (aromatase inhibitor) and low dose gonadotropins versus a HS protocol. We found that our MS protocol resulted in a significantly higher clinical pregnancy rate and live birth rate.

There is no consistent definition for a "poor responder" in the literature and so it is difficult to compare studies and reach consensus on treatment effects. The ESHRE consensus, otherwise known as the Bologna criteria, establishes a guideline for poor ovarian reserve. However, this guideline is not universally accepted. Poor responders often present with a

shortened follicular phase, which decreases the time available for follicular recruitment. In addition, lower FSH receptor expression levels in granulosa cells may also be found in this group of patients [17]. In order to overcome the shorter follicular phase and create a longer window of opportunity for follicular recruitment, we hypothesized that the introduction of an aromatase inhibitor may be beneficial, through decreasing estrogen levels and prolonging the action of FSH. In addition, a letrozole-mediated increase in intraovarian androgen concentration may improve ovarian responsiveness to exogenous gonadotropins in poor responders. Hillier [18] was the first to introduce the idea of androgens as a treatment to promote gonadotropin responsiveness in granulosa cells. Weil et al. [19] suggested that androgen treatment may promote follicular growth and estrogen biosynthesis. Androgens are also known to stimulate IGF-1 and IGF-1 receptor gene expression which are known to promote follicular steroidogenesis [1, 17].

Letrozole is a potent, low cost, and highly specific non-steroidal aromatase inhibitor administered orally. It inhibits the aromatase enzyme by competitively binding to the heme domain of the enzyme's cytochrome P450 subunit, resulting in a blockade of androgen conversion into estrogens with a subsequent increase in intraovarian androgens [17]. Garcia-Velasco et al. [17] in a prospective pilot study were able to demonstrate that aromatase inhibition with letrozole at the beginning of ovarian stimulation significantly increases intraovarian androgen concentrations. They showed that follicular fluid levels of testosterone and androstenedione are significantly elevated in women given letrozole during ovarian stimulation for IVF. Other investigators have advocated the use of androgen supplementation, such as DHEA [20], but this is controversial. It is hypothesized that androgens or aromatase inhibitors may play a role in preantral and antral follicular development and may therefore improve ovarian responsiveness.

MS usually refers to stimulation protocols that yield a maximum of five oocytes [5]. This concept was first introduced by Corfman et al. [21]. Their MS protocol involved using CC 100 mg orally on days 3–7 of the cycle, followed by a single injection of 150 IU of IM hMG on cycle day 9. Although the number of retrieved oocytes was statistically lower using a MS protocol, this variability did not correlate to a statistically significant difference in pregnancy rate [21]. Subsequently, many papers introduced a variety of different protocols termed "minimal stimulation," which combined CC or letrozole with low levels of gonadotropins.

Although there is no conclusive data regarding the optimal doses for letrozole in reproductive medicine, letrozole at doses of 1–5 mg/day inhibits aromatase activity by 97–99% [11, 17]. Most published studies have involved a once-daily dose of 2.5–5 mg for 5 days [22]. A randomized study comparing 2.5 and 5 mg of letrozole in women with unexplained infertility suggested that a higher dose of letrozole might be associated with the development of more follicles in patients with normal ovarian reserve. However, higher doses of letrozole were found to cause persistent inhibition of aromatase and lower estrogen levels for endometrial growth at ovulation [11]. In our protocol, we chose to use the lower dose of

TABLE 1: Data comparison of minimal stimulation and high-dose stimulation protocols for low responders. Not significant results are denoted by NS.

	Minimum stimulation	High stimulation	P value
Number of patients	70	71	
Age (yr)	39.4 ± 3.2	39.2 ± 4.0	NS
Peak estradiol (pmol/L)	1580.8 ± 1141.2	5279.4 ± 3295.1	$P < 0.001$
Gonadotropin total dose (IU)	1332.9 ± 435.7	5575.2 ± 1945.0	$P < 0.001$
Antral follicle count	3.7 ± 1.0	4.5 ± 0.7	$P < 0.001$
Number of oocytes retrieved	2.9 ± 1.5	3.5 ± 1.5	NS
Number of fertilized oocytes	1.5 ± 1.1	1.5 ± 1.2	NS
Cancellation rate	3/71 (4.2%)	4/79 (5.0%)	NS
Number of embryos transferred	1.8 ± 0.7	1.4 ± 1.2	NS
Clinical pregnancy rate/cycle	22/70 (31.4%)	9/71 (12.7%)	$P < 0.05$
Live birth rate	15/70 (21.4%)	5/71 (7.0%)	$P < 0.05$

letrozole (2.5 mg), to avoid oversuppression and it was our group's clinical impression that this dose was more effective for patients with poor ovarian reserve. However, a RCT for the poor responder population would be required to test this hypothesis.

Conversely, we hypothesize that higher levels of gonadotropins, as well as the resultant very high levels of estrogen, may negatively impact the growing follicles, oocytes, and the endometrium, thus reducing the chances of a successful pregnancy for poor responders.

Mohsen and El Din [23] showed no difference in clinical pregnancy rates in poor responders when comparing a GnRHa microflare protocol to a letrozole antagonist protocol; however the days of stimulation and total dose of gonadotropins were significantly lower in the letrozole group. Yarali et al. [9] also studied a microdose GnRH agonist protocol versus a letrozole antagonist protocol in poor responders. They used a lower dose of gonadotropins and there was a shorter duration of treatment for the letrozole antagonist group, but again there was no difference in pregnancy rate. As a result, the minimal stimulation protocol tended to be easier to tolerate for patients and the cost of medication was greatly reduced.

Strengths: our fertility practices changed during the two years of the study from using one stimulation protocol (HS) to using another stimulation (MS) protocol in the poor ovarian reserve, poor responder population. The HS and MS protocols were used exclusively in 2008 and 2010, respectively. Thus, there was no bias towards choosing one protocol over the other in studied time periods.

Weaknesses: since we were comparing two groups, from two years apart (2008 and 2010), it is possible that the increase in pregnancy rate we observed was due to unrelated improvements in our embryology laboratory between these two years. To address this possibility, we compared pregnancy rates in normal and high responders and in egg donation cycles between these two years and there were no significant differences. In our clinic, egg donors had a pregnancy success rate of 53.6% and 52.5% in 2008 and 2010, respectively ($P > 0.05$). Normal responders of all ages had an overall pregnancy success rate of 35.3% and 32.8% in 2008 and 2010, respectively

($P > 0.05$). In 2008 and 2010, high responders had a pregnancy success rate of 41.4% and 38.6%, respectively ($P < 0.05$). Since one protocol being compared involved letrozole and the other did not, we cannot be certain that our results were not related to the use of letrozole rather than high versus low dose gonadotropins. Since this is a retrospective cohort study, in order to address this issue and confirm our overall findings, an adequately powered, prospective randomized controlled trial would be required. In addition, to determine if our findings are due to the lower dose of gonadotropins or the use of letrozole in this protocol, one would require a 3-armed prospective trial.

In conclusion, the MS protocol was less expensive (in terms of total gonadotropins used) and improved both clinical pregnancy and live birth rates, compared to the HS protocol. Based on our results, a prospective randomized controlled trial is warranted in order to confirm these findings.

Conflict of Interests

The authors declare that there is no conflict of interests regarding the publication of this paper.

References

[1] D. Kyrou, E. M. Kolibianakis, C. A. Venetis, E. G. Papanikolaou, J. Bontis, and B. C. Tarlatzis, "How to improve the probability of pregnancy in poor responders undergoing in vitro fertilization: a systematic review and meta-analysis," Fertility and Sterility, vol. 91, no. 3, pp. 749–766, 2009.

[2] B. Vollenhoven, T. Osianlis, and J. Catt, "Is there an ideal stimulation regimen for IVF for poor responders and does it change with age?" Journal of Assisted Reproduction and Genetics, vol. 25, no. 11-12, pp. 523–529, 2008.

[3] E. R. Klinkert, F. J. M. Broekmans, C. W. N. Looman, J. D. F. Habbema, and E. R. te Velde, "Expected poor responders on the basis of an antral follicle count do not benefit from a higher starting dose of gonadotrophins in IVF treatment: a randomized controlled trial," Human Reproduction, vol. 20, no. 3, pp. 611–615, 2005.

[4] M. F. Mutlu, M. Erdem, A. Erdem et al., "Antral follicle count determines poor ovarian response better than anti-müllerian hormone but age is the only predictor for live birth in in vitro fertilization cycles," *Journal of Assisted Reproduction & Genetics*, vol. 30, no. 5, pp. 657–665, 2013.

[5] S. M. Zarek and S. J. Muasher, "Mild/minimal stimulation for in vitro fertilization: an old idea that needs to be revisited," *Fertility & Sterility*, vol. 95, no. 8, pp. 2449–2455, 2011.

[6] E. R. Klinkert, F. J. M. Broekmans, C. W. N. Looman, and E. R. Te Velde, "A poor response in the first in vitro fertilization cycle is not necessarily related to a poor prognosis in subsequent cycles," *Fertility and Sterility*, vol. 81, no. 5, pp. 1247–1253, 2004.

[7] E. S. Surrey and W. B. Schoolcraft, "Evaluating strategies for improving ovarian response of the poor responder undergoing assisted reproductive techniques," *Fertility and Sterility*, vol. 73, no. 4, pp. 667–676, 2000.

[8] M. F. M. Mitwally and R. F. Casper, "Use of an aromatase inhibitor for induction of ovulation in patients with an inadequate response to clomiphene citrate," *Fertility and Sterility*, vol. 75, no. 2, pp. 305–309, 2001.

[9] H. Yarali, I. Esinler, M. Polat, G. Bozdag, and B. Tiras, "Antagonist/letrozole protocol in poor ovarian responders for intracytoplasmic sperm injection: a comparative study with the microdose flare-up protocol," *Fertility & Sterility*, vol. 92, no. 1, pp. 231–235, 2009.

[10] S. Healey, S. L. Tan, T. Tulandi, and M. M. Biljan, "Effects of letrozole on superovulation with gonadotropins in women undergoing intrauterine insemination," *Fertility and Sterility*, vol. 80, no. 6, pp. 1325–1329, 2003.

[11] R. F. Casper and M. F. M. Mitwally, "Use of the aromatase inhibitor letrozole for ovulation induction in women with polycystic ovarian syndrome," *Clinical Obstetrics and Gynecology*, vol. 54, no. 4, pp. 685–695, 2011.

[12] A. P. Ferraretti, A. La Marca, B. C. J. M. Fauser, B. Tarlatzis, G. Nargund, and L. Gianaroli, "ESHRE consensus on the definition of 'poor response, to ovarian stimulation for in vitro fertilization: the Bologna criteria," *Human Reproduction*, vol. 26, no. 7, pp. 1616–1624, 2011.

[13] V. A. Akande, C. F. Fleming, L. P. Hunt, S. D. Keay, and J. M. Jenkins, "Biological versus chronological ageing of oocytes, distinguishable by raised FSH levels in relation to the success of IVF treatment," *Human Reproduction*, vol. 17, no. 8, pp. 2003–2008, 2002.

[14] G. Nargund, W. C. Cheng, and J. Parsons, "The impact of ovarian cystectomy on ovarian response to stimulation during in-vitro fertilization cycles," *Human Reproduction*, vol. 11, no. 1, pp. 81–83, 1996.

[15] S. D. Keay, N. H. Liversedge, and J. M. Jenkins, "Could ovarian infection impair ovarian response to gonadotrophin stimulation?" *British Journal of Obstetrics & Gynaecology*, vol. 105, no. 3, pp. 252–254, 1998.

[16] D. Nikolaou and A. Templeton, "Early ovarian ageing: a hypothesis: detection and clinical relevance," *Human Reproduction*, vol. 18, no. 6, pp. 1137–1139, 2003.

[17] J. A. Garcia-Velasco, L. Moreno, A. Pacheco et al., "The aromatase inhibitor letrozole increases the concentration of intraovarian androgens and improves in vitro fertilization outcome in low responder patients: a pilot study," *Fertility and Sterility*, vol. 84, no. 1, pp. 82–87, 2005.

[18] S. G. Hillier, "Current concepts of the roles of follicle stimulating hormone and luteinizing hormone in folliculogenesis," *Human Reproduction*, vol. 9, no. 2, pp. 188–191, 1994.

[19] S. Weil, K. Vendola, J. Zhou, and C. A. Bondy, "Androgen and follicle-stimulating hormone interactions in primate ovarian follicle development," *Journal of Clinical Endocrinology and Metabolism*, vol. 84, no. 8, pp. 2951–2956, 1999.

[20] N. Gleicher and D. H. Barad, "Dehydroepiandrosterone (DHEA) supplementation in diminished ovarian reserve (DOR)," *Reproductive Biology and Endocrinology*, vol. 9, article 67, 2011.

[21] R. S. Corfman, M. P. Milad, T. L. Bellavance, S. J. Ory, L. D. Erickson, and G. D. Ball, "A novel ovarian stimulation protocol for use with the assisted reproductive technologies," *Fertility and Sterility*, vol. 60, no. 5, pp. 864–870, 1993.

[22] H. Al-Fozan, M. Al-Khadouri, S. L. Tan, and T. Tulandi, "A randomized trial of letrozole versus clomiphene citrate in women undergoing superovulation," *Fertility and Sterility*, vol. 82, no. 6, pp. 1561–1563, 2004.

[23] I. A. Mohsen and R. E. El Din, "Minimal stimulation protocol using letrozole versus microdose flare up GnRH agonist protocol in women with poor ovarian response undergoing ICSI," *Gynecological Endocrinology*, vol. 29, no. 2, pp. 105–108, 2013.

6

A Comparative Study of Prevalence of RTI/STI Symptoms and Treatment Seeking Behaviour among the Married Women in Urban and Rural Areas of Delhi

Anjana Verma, Jitendra Kumar Meena, and Bratati Banerjee

Department of Community Medicine, Maulana Azad Medical College, New Delhi 110002, India

Correspondence should be addressed to Anjana Verma; anjanaverma504@gmail.com

Academic Editor: Hind A. Beydoun

Background. In developing countries, women are at high risk for several reproductive health problems especially RTI/STIs. Since all RTIs/ STIs are preventable and most of them are curable, it is pertinent to study the determinants of the health seeking behaviour. *Objectives.* To compare the prevalence and treatment seeking behaviour about RTI/STI symptoms among the married women of reproductive age group (18–45 years) living in urban and rural area of Delhi. *Methods.* A cross-sectional study was done among the married women of reproductive age group residing in Pooth Khurd, a village in North West district of Delhi, and Delhi Gate, an urban locality situated in central Delhi. *Results.* In this study, the prevalence of RTI/STI symptoms was found to be similar in both urban (42.3%) and rural area (42%). In urban area, 73% sought treatment, while in rural area only 45.6% sought treatment. Prevalence of the symptoms was found to be higher among the study subjects who were not using any contraceptive method, had history of abortion, and were with lower educational status, in both urban and rural areas. Treatment seeking behaviour was significantly higher among the educated women, contraceptive users, and older age group women in both rural and urban area.

1. Introduction

Some 340 million new cases of curable sexually transmitted infections (STIs) occur every year. The figure does not include HIV or other viral STIs like hepatitis B, genital herpes, and genital warts, which are not curable. The most common of the curable STIs are gonorrhea, syphilis, chlamydia, and trichomoniasis. Sexually transmitted infections constitute a significant health burden and increase the risks of transmission of HIV [1]. Reproductive tract infection (RTI) is a global health problem among women, living in South East Asian Region (SEAR) countries. Studies have found the prevalence of RTI in India, Bangladesh, Egypt, and Kenya is in the range of 52–90 per cent. More than a million women and infants die of the complications of RTI every year [2]. Reproductive tract infections (RTIs) are caused by organisms normally present in the reproductive tract or introduced from the outside during sexual contact or medical procedures. These different but overlapping categories of RTI are called endogenous, sexually transmitted infections (STIs), and iatrogenic, reflecting how they are acquired and spread [3].

The prevalence of self-reported RTI symptoms among Indian women has been found to be 11–18% in nationally representative studies [4, 5] and 40–57% in various other studies [6–8], while the prevalence of laboratory-diagnosed RTIs has ranged from 28% to 38% [9, 10]. According to studies that have explored women's patterns of seeking treatment for RTI symptoms, between one-third and two-thirds of symptomatic women did not seek treatment [6, 8–10].

2. Materials and Methods

2.1. Study Design. It is a community based cross-sectional study.

2.2. Study Area. The study area is Pooth Khurd, a village in North West district of Delhi, and Darya Ganj, urban locality in central Delhi.

2.3. Study Population. Married women of reproductive age group residing in Pooth Khurd and Darya Ganj area of Delhi are the study population.

2.4. Study Period. The study was carried out from January 2012 to May 2013.

2.5. Sample Size Calculation. Taking the prevalence of RTI symptoms among married women (15–44 years) as 37% (RCH-II survey), with relative error of 20%, and taking nonresponse rate of 10%, total sample size is calculated to be 215, each in rural and urban area.

2.6. Methodology. Sampling was done using the simple random sampling technique. A sample of 215 women was selected using the random number table from the list of eligible couples noted in the registers at health centres serving these areas. In case the subject was not found eligible for the study (residing in the area for less than 6 months), then the woman listed next in the eligible couple register was selected. Investigation was carried out by the investigator, who was pursuing the postgraduation in community medicine in the duration of study period, by paying house to house visits. During the house visits, investigator introduced herself to the eligible women, explained the purpose and procedure of the study, and ensured complete confidentiality of their responses. In this study, the mean age of the study subjects was 31.3 years in urban and 28.4 years in rural area. Most of the study subjects were between the age of 26 and 35 years in both urban and rural area.

2.7. Study Tools. A predesigned, pretested, and semistructured questionnaire was used to take the interview of eligible women. The questionnaire had both open and closed ended questions. Questionnaire included following parts:

(A) questions to assess sociodemographic profile of the subject, identification data, namely, age, address, religion, occupation, socioeconomic status, and so forth;

(B) questions about the menstrual history of the women;

(C) questions about the obstetric history;

(D) questions to assess the knowledge regarding RTIs and history of occurrence of any RTI symptom in the past 3 months;

(E) questions to assess the treatment seeking behaviour for RTI symptoms.

2.8. Ethical Issues. The aims, objectives, and procedure of the study were explained to all the women. Informed consent was taken from all the participants. Complete confidentiality regarding patient information was maintained through all the stages of the study.

2.9. Statistical Tests. Data was analysed using SPSS version 17. Percentage and proportions were calculated for prevalence of the symptoms and treatment seeking behaviour. Chi square

TABLE 1: Sociodemographic characteristics of the study subjects of urban and rural area ($n = 215$).

Characteristics	Urban n (%)	Rural n (%)
Age		
18–25	54 (25)	60 (28)
26–35	110 (51)	103 (48)
36–45	51 (24)	52 (24)
Educational status		
Illiterate	52 (24.2)	63 (29.2)
Primary	13 (6)	15 (7)
Middle	45 (21)	43 (20)
High school	43 (20)	41 (19.1)
Secondary	35 (16.3)	34 (15.8)
Graduate	20 (9.3)	15 (7)
Postgraduate	7 (3.2)	4 (1.9)
Occupation		
Housewife	200 (93)	198 (92.1)
Unskilled worker	4 (1.8)	6 (2.8)
Semiskilled worker	3 (1.4)	4 (1.9)
Skilled worker	2 (1)	3 (1.4)
Shopkeeper/clerical	3 (1.4)	2 (0.9)
Semiprofessional	3 (1.4)	2 (0.9)
Monthly per capita income		
Up to 1000	70 (32.6)	77 (35.8)
1001–2000	50 (23.3)	52 (24.2)
2001 or more	95 (44.1)	86 (40)

and Fisher Exact test were used as tests of significance in univariate analysis. A P value of less than 0.05 was considered significant.

3. Results

In this study, the prevalence of RTI/STI symptoms was found to be similar in both urban (42.3%) and rural area (42%). In urban area, 73% sought treatment, while in rural area only 45.6% sought treatment. Table 1 shows the sociodemographic characteristics of the respondents.

Table 2 shows various obstetric and behavioural characteristics of the respondents. 39% of study subjects in urban area and 37.2% in rural area had history of abortion. Out of these, induced abortions comprised 81% in urban and 79% in rural area. Most of the women in both urban and rural area were using sanitary pad as method of menstrual hygiene. 76% of study subjects in urban and 51.6% in rural area were using some method of contraception. Condom was the most common method of contraception followed by tubectomy in both urban and rural area.

When asked about the knowledge of RTI/STI symptoms, 50.2% of respondents in urban and 41.8% in rural area were aware about the presence of discharge as an indication for infection. Only 20% of respondents in urban and 10%

TABLE 2: Obstetric and behavioural characteristics of the study subjects ($N = 215$).

Characteristics	Urban n (%)	Rural n (%)
Parity		
0	2 (1)	23 (10.7)
1-2	101 (47)	138 (64.2)
3-4	107 (50)	50 (23.2)
>4	5 (2)	4 (1.9)
History of abortions		
Yes	84 (39)	80 (37.2)
No	131 (61)	135 (62.8)
Last abortion, how many years back		
≤1 year	12 (14.3)	8 (10)
>1 year	72 (85.7)	72 (90)
Type of abortion		
Spontaneous	16 (19)	17 (21)
Induced	68 (81)	63 (79)
Menstrual hygiene practices		
Ordinary cloth	54 (25)	69 (32.1)
Sanitary pad	129 (60)	111 (51.6)
Both sanitary pad and cloth	32 (15)	35 (16.3)
Usage of contraceptive methods		
Yes	163 (76)	111 (51.6)
No	52 (24)	104 (48.4)
Methods of contraception		
None	52 (24)	61 (28)
Pills	19 (9)	10 (4.7)
Condom	95 (44.2)	90 (42)
IUCD	6 (2.8)	20 (9.3)
Safe period	1 (0.5)	0
Withdrawal	10 (4.7)	0
Tubectomy	32 (14.8)	34 (16)

TABLE 3: Knowledge and prevalence of RTI/STI among study subjects.

Characteristic	Urban n (%)	Rural n (%)
Knowledge of symptoms*		
Discharge	108 (50.2)	90 (41.8)
Dyspareunia	4 (2)	2 (1)
Dysuria	9 (4)	4 (2)
Lower abdominal pain	43 (20)	22 (10)
Infertility	2 (1)	2 (1)
Burning micturition	9 (4)	6 (3)
Genital ulcer	2 (1)	2 (1)
How does one get the disease?		
Poor genital hygiene	54 (25.1)	80 (37)
Infected sexual partner	75 (34.9)	43 (20)
Do not know	86 (40)	92 (42.8)
History of symptoms experienced		
Yes	91 (42.3)	90 (42)
No	124 (57.7)	125 (58)
History of symptoms experienced*		
Discharge	32 (35)	70 (77.8)
Lower backache	57 (63)	46 (51.1)
Lower abdominal pain	45 (49)	23 (25.6)
Itching over vulva	15 (7)	5 (5.6)
Dyspareunia	0 (0)	2 (2.2)
Infertility	2 (2)	4 (4.4)
Genital ulcer	2 (2)	2 (2.2)
Burning micturition	18 (20)	10 (11.1)

*Mutually not exclusive.

in rural area had heard of lower abdominal pain as a symptom of RTI/STI. Very few respondents knew about other symptoms of RTI/STI such as dyspareunia, dysuria, burning micturition, infertility, and genital ulcer. When participants were asked about the possible ways of contracting the disease, 34.9% of women living in urban area and 20% of rural women replied that disease can be acquired from infected partner. Poor genital hygiene was reported to be the cause of RTI/STI symptoms by 25% of urban respondents and 37% of rural women. In this study the prevalence of RTI/STI symptoms was found to be similar in both urban (42.3%) and rural area (42%). Vaginal discharge (77.8%) was reported as the most common symptom by the rural women followed by lower backache (51%) and lower abdominal pain (25.6%), whereas in urban area lower backache (63%) was the most common symptom followed by lower abdominal pain (49%) and vaginal discharge (35%) (Table 3).

Table 4 shows that, out of the 91 symptomatic women in urban area, 66 (73%) sought treatment, 46 (70%) consulted private practitioner, and 20 (30%) went to a government hospital. 92% of the treatment seeking women were compliant to the treatment. In rural area, out of the 90 symptomatic women, 41 (45.6%) sought treatment, 21 (51%) consulted private practitioner, and 20 (49%) went to a government hospital. 90% of the treatment seeking women were compliant to the treatment in rural area.

Table 5 shows the prevalence of RTI/STI symptoms in relation to some sociodemographic, obstetric, and behavioural factors in urban and rural Delhi. Based on the presence of one or more symptoms, the prevalence of RTI/STI symptoms was found to be 42.3% in urban area. It was highest in the 18 to 25 years of age group than other age groups; however the difference was not statistically significant. The prevalence of RTI/STI symptoms was found to be highest among the illiterate respondents (54%) and decreases significantly with increasing level of education (P value = 0.03). There was no significant difference in the prevalence of symptoms due to occupation, per capita income, menstrual hygiene practices, and parity.

TABLE 4: Treatment seeking behaviour of the respondents.

Characteristic	Urban n (%)	Rural n (%)
Treatment seeking symptomatic women	66 (73)	41 (45.6)
Government hospital	20 (30)	20 (49)
Private practitioner	46 (70)	21 (51)
Compliance to the treatment among women	61 (92)	37 (90)

TABLE 5: Prevalence of symptoms suggestive of RTI/STI in relation to sociodemographic, obstetric, and behavioural factors in urban and rural area.

Characteristics	Urban			Rural		
	Symptoms present n (%)	Total n (%)	P value	Symptoms present n (%)	Total n (%)	P value
Age						
18–25	29 (54)	54 (25)		32 (53.3)	60 (28)	
26–35	53 (48)	110 (51)	0.710	48 (46.6)	103 (48)	0.622
36–45	9 (17.6)	51 (24)		10 (19.2)	52 (24)	
Education						
Illiterate	28 (54)	52 (24)		27 (43)	63 (29.3)	
Up to high school	40 (40)	101 (47)	**0.032**	45 (45.5)	99 (46)	**0.046**
Post-high school	23 (37.1)	62 (29)		18 (34)	53 (24.7)	
Occupation						
Working	6 (40)	15 (7.5)	0.970	7 (41.2)	17 (7.9)	0.952
Housewife	85 (42.5)	200 (93)		83 (42)	198 (92.1)	
Monthly income per capita						
Up to 1000	30 (42.8)	70 (32.6)		28 (36)	77 (35.8)	
1001–2000	21 (42)	50 (23.3)	0.124	28 (54)	52 (24.2)	0.121
2001 or more	40 (42)	95 (44.1)		34 (40)	86 (40)	
Menstrual hygiene practices						
Ordinary cloth	23 (42)	54 (25)		32 (46.4)	69 (32.1)	
Sanitary pad	58 (45)	129 (60)	0.198	48 (43.2)	111 (51.6)	0.201
Both sanitary pad and cloth	10 (31.25)	32 (15)		10 (28.6)	35 (16.3)	
Parity						
0	0 (0)	2 (1)		4 (17.4)	23 (10.7)	
1-2	43 (42.6)	101 (47)	0.124	60 (43.4)	138 (64.2)	**0.009**
3-4	45 (42)	107 (50)		24 (48)	50 (23.3)	
>4	3 (60)	5 (2)		2 (50)	4 (1.8)	
Contraceptive usage						
Yes	63 (38.6)	163 (76)	**0.021**	39 (35.1)	111 (51.6)	**0.029**
No	28 (54)	52 (24)		51 (49)	104 (48.4)	
Gynaecological risk factors						
Abortion	47 (56)	84 (39)		43 (54)	80 (37.2)	
CuT	0 (0)	6 (2.8)	**0.04**	6 (30)	20 (9.3)	**0.004**
Nil	44 (35)	125 (58.2)		41 (35.7)	115 (53.5)	

Contraceptive users had lesser prevalence (38.6%) of RTI/STI symptoms as compared to nonusers (54%) and the difference was statistically significant (P value = 0.021). The prevalence was highest (56%) in those who had history of abortion and (35%) in those with none of the risk factors of abortion or inserted IUCD (P value = 0.04).

In rural Delhi, the prevalence of RTI/STI symptoms was 42.3%. It was highest in the 18 to 25 years of age group than other age groups; however the difference was not statistically significant. The prevalence of RTI/STI symptoms was found to be highest among the respondents who were educated up to high school (45%) and was lowest among the respondents who were post-high school educated (P value = 0.046). There was no significant difference in the prevalence of symptoms due to occupation, per capita income, and menstrual hygiene practices. The prevalence of symptoms was found to be significantly associated with parity (P value = 0.009). Contraceptive users were found to have lesser prevalence (35.1%) of RTI/STI symptoms than nonusers (49%) and the difference was statistically significant (P value = 0.029). The prevalence

TABLE 6: Treatment seeking behaviour in relation to some sociodemographic, obstetric, and behavioural factors in urban and rural area.

Characteristics	Urban ($n = 91$)			Rural ($n = 90$)		
	Sought treatment n (%)	Total symptomatic respondents n (%)	P value	Sought treatment n (%)	Total symptomatic respondents n (%)	P value
Age						
18–25	19 (65)	29 (32)		6 (18.8)	32 (36)	
26–35	40 (75)	53 (58)	**0.001**	28 (58.3)	48 (53)	0.000
36–45	7 (78)	9 (10)		7 (70)	10 (11)	
Education						
Illiterate	16 (59.3)	27 (30)		10 (37)	27 (30)	
Up to high school	35 (78)	45 (50)	**0.003**	22 (48.9)	45 (50)	**0.04**
Post-high school	15 (83.3)	18 (20)		9 (50)	18 (20)	
Occupation						
Working	4 (67)	6 (7)	0.120	5 (71)	7 (8)	**0.04**
Housewife	62 (73)	85 (93)		35 (42)	83 (92)	
Monthly income per capita						
Up to 1000	21 (70)	30 (33)		11 (40)	28 (31)	
1001–2000	14 (67)	21 (23)	0.085	12 (43)	28 (31)	0.074
2001 or more	31 (78)	40 (44)		16 (47)	34 (38)	
Contraception usage						
Yes	50 (79.4)	63 (69)	**0.001**	21 (53.8)	39 (43)	**0.041**
No	16 (57.1)	28 (31)		20 (39.2)	51 (57)	

was highest (54%) in those who had history of abortion and (30%) in those with CuT insertion (P value = 0.04).

Table 6 shows the treatment seeking behaviour of the symptomatic women in relation to some sociodemographic, obstetric, and behavioural factors in urban and rural Delhi. In urban area, it was found that treatment seeking behaviour increased with age (P value = 0.001) and education status (P value = 0.003) of the study subjects. Contraceptive users had higher percentage of treatment seeking behaviour as compared to the nonusers with a significant P value of 0.001. Treatment seeking behaviour was higher among the women with higher per capita income, but this difference was not statistically significant. Similarly, in rural Delhi (Table 6), treatment seeking behaviour was found to be associated significantly with higher age (P value = 0.001), higher education (P value = 0.003), and contraceptive usage (P value = 0.001). However, treatment seeking behaviour was also found to be associated with the occupational status of the women. Working women had higher percentage of seeking treatment as compared to housewives with statistically significant difference (P value = 0.04).

4. Discussion

4.1. Prevalence of RTI/STI Symptoms. In this study the prevalence of RTI/STI symptoms was found to be similar in both rural (42%) and urban (42.3%) area of Delhi. This is higher than that reported in RCH-II survey (2002–04), according to which the prevalence of RTI/STI symptoms was 39.3% in

rural and 33.6% in urban women [11]. In a study conducted by Kosambiya et al. in Surat, the prevalence of RTI/STIs was higher in urban (69%) than rural area (53%). The higher prevalence among urban population was attributed to greater proportion of migratory population residing in urban areas of Surat [12].

Vaginal discharge (77%) was reported as the most common symptom by the rural women followed by lower backache (51%) and lower abdominal pain (25.6%), whereas in urban area lower backache (63%) was the most common symptom followed by lower abdominal pain (495) and vaginal discharge (36%).

4.2. Knowledge about RTI. When asked about the knowledge of RTI/STI symptoms, 50.2% of respondents in urban and 41.8% in rural area were aware about the presence of discharge as an indication for infection. 20% of respondents in urban and 10% in rural area had heard of lower abdominal pain as a symptom of RTI/STI. This is much higher than reported in another study done by Kosambiya et al. in Surat, in which only 14% of the respondents were aware about the presence of discharge as an indication of infection and 9% knew lower abdominal pain as the symptom of RTI [12]. Very few respondents knew about other symptoms of RTI/STI such as dyspareunia, dysuria, burning micturition, infertility, and genital ulcer. When participants were asked about the possible ways of contracting the disease, 34.9% of women living in urban area and 20% of rural women replied that disease is acquired from infected partner. This finding is similar to that reported in Surat, in which 22% of rural and 41% of urban area replied infected partner is the source of infection [12]. Unhygienic conditions were reported to be the cause of RTI/STI symptoms by 37% of rural women and 25% of urban respondents.

4.3. Factors Associated with RTI Symptoms. The prevalence of RTI/STI symptoms was found to be associated with education in both urban and rural areas, which decreased significantly with increasing level of education (P value < 0.05). This finding is comparable to a study carried out in Rajasthan by Bansal et al. in which RTI was highly prevalent among illiterates (62.5%) as compared to literates (48.3%). Number of RTI cases decreased with an increase in educational status, showing a direct relationship between the two [13]. The prevalence of symptoms was found to be significantly associated with parity (P value = 0.009) in rural area. The prevalence of symptoms was found to be lowest among the nulliparous and highest among the women with parity of four or more. This finding is comparable to a study done by Rani et al. in Gorakhpur, which revealed that overall prevalence of RTIs was maximum (42.0%) in women who were having five or more children and minimum (34.2%) in women who had one or no child. This difference was statistically significant (P value = 0.01) [14]. Similar finding was reported in a study done in Ludhiana by Philip et al. in which it was found that the prevalence of the symptoms increased with parity, with the prevalence being lowest (7.7%) in the nulliparous and highest (25.0%) in the multiparous with parity >4. The prevalence was 16.8% in those with parity 1-2 and 18.3% in those with parity 3-4 [15].

Contraceptive users were found to have lesser prevalence of RTI/STI symptoms than nonusers and the difference was statistically significant (P value = 0.021) in both urban and rural areas. The prevalence was highest in those who had history of abortion in both urban and rural areas. Similar findings were reported by Rani et al. [14] and Philip et al. [15], in which prevalence was highest among the study subjects who had history of abortion. This can be attributed to the fact that operative procedures make women more prone to ascending infections.

There was no significant difference in the prevalence of symptoms due to occupation, per capita income, and menstrual hygiene practices.

4.4. Treatment Seeking Behaviour. In the present study, out of the 91 symptomatic women in urban area, 66 (73%) sought treatment, 46 (70%) consulted private practitioner, and 20 (30%) went to a government hospital, while 25 (27%) did not seek any treatment. This proportion is much higher than reported by a study done in Ludhiana by Philip et al., in which the majority (64.4%) of the respondents with symptoms did not seek any treatment. The preferred source of treatment was a private practitioner, followed by "desi" medicines [15]. This can be attributed to the differences in education status and

health awareness among the study subjects living in Delhi and Ludhiana.

In rural area, out of the 90 symptomatic women, 41 (45.6%) sought treatment, 21 (50%) consulted private practitioner, and 20 (49%) went to a government hospital, while 49 (54.4%) did not seek any treatment. This proportion is higher than reported in a study done by Aggarwal et al. in a rural area of Dehradun, in which 36.4 per cent of the respondents responded that they would like to visit an STD specialist and 19.3 per cent expressed that they would consult an MBBS doctor. 5.7 per cent of the symptomatic women still wanted to be treated by quacks and 4.5 per cent wanted to take treatment from other traditional healers [16]. In a study done by Ravi and Kulasekaran in rural area of Tamil Nadu it was revealed that 80.7% of the women sought treatment [17]. This is much higher than found in present study. This difference can be because of the differences in sociodemographic characteristics of the populations.

In urban area, out of 91 symptomatic women, 66 (73%) sought treatment, 46 (70%) consulted private practitioner, and 20 (30%) went to a government hospital. 92% of the treatment seeking women were compliant to the treatment. Easy accessibility to the private practitioners can be the possible reason for the preference of private practitioner for seeking treatment. In rural area, out of the 90 symptomatic women, 41 (45.6%) sought treatment, 21 (50%) consulted private practitioner, and 20 (49%) went to a government hospital. This finding is similar to other studies, in which the majority of women had consulted private providers, suggesting that a preference for these providers persists despite the numerous initiatives undertaken by the Indian government to improve access to sexual and reproductive health services in the public sector [8, 9, 18–20].

4.5. Factors Associated with Treatment Seeking Behaviour. In present study, treatment seeking behaviour increased with educational status of the study subjects in both urban and rural area. This finding is similar to that reported in a study done by Ravi and Kulasekaran in Tamil Nadu, in which overwhelming proportion of women received treatment of STIs who completed secondary education (85.7%) compared to those who completed primary education (70.0%) and illiterates (66.7%) [17]. Similarly in other studies, schooling was associated with treatment seeking behaviour of the study subjects [10, 18], from formal providers, likely because young women with more schooling had more information about protective actions and the resources to adopt them than did others [18].

In our study treatment seeking behaviour was found to be associated with older age as compared to younger women. This finding differs from study done by Ravi and Kulasekaran in Tamil Nadu, in which it was observed that younger women were much more likely to receive treatment for their STIs than the older women [17]. This can be explained because of the differences in sociodemographic profile and level of health awareness among the women of these two states. In our study older age group women were found to have better treatment seeking behaviour than younger women. This can be attributed to the fact that younger women do not have decision making power regarding seeking health services as compared to older age group women, because of various traditional cultural beliefs and attitudes of the people living in this area.

In present study, working women had better treatment seeking behaviour than nonworking women in rural area. This finding is comparable to that found in a study done by Sabarwal and Santhya in which the greater proportion of the working women sought treatment as compared to the nonworking women [18].

In present study, the contraceptive users had higher percentage of treatment seeking behaviour as compared to the nonusers, likely because contraceptive users had more information and awareness about health care services, due to regular visits to the health centre and communication with health workers.

5. Conclusion

In this study, it was found that the prevalence of RTI/STI symptoms is high in both urban (42.3%) and rural (42%) areas. Prevalence of the symptoms was found to be higher among the study subjects who were not using any contraceptive method, had history of abortion, and were with lower educational status, in both urban and rural areas. In rural area, in addition to above factors, prevalence of symptoms was found to be significantly associated with parity. The treatment seeking behaviour is better in urban area (73%), as compared to rural area (45.6%). However, in both areas, women preferred private practitioner for seeking treatment compared to government facilities, because of the long waiting time and unavailability of medicines in government health facilities. Treatment seeking behaviour was significantly higher among the educated women, contraceptive users, and older age group women in both rural and urban area.

There is a need to educate women about the symptoms of RTI/STI, their prevention, and the importance of timely treatment in both urban and rural areas. The availability of the RTI/STI treatment kits should be ensured in all the primary health centres to increase the usage of the government services.

Conflict of Interests

The authors declare that there is no conflict of interests regarding the publication of this paper.

References

[1] UNFPA, *Top Level Push to Tackle Priorities in Sexual and Reproductive Health*, United Nations Population Fund, New York, NY, USA, 2006.

[2] UNFPA, *Common Reproductive Tract Infections*, No. 9, 1999.

[3] WHO, *Sexually Transmitted and Other Reproductive Tract Infections: Integrating STI/RTI Care for Reproductive Health*, 2005.

[4] International Institute for Population Sciences (IIPS), *District Level Household and Facility Survey (DLHS-3), 2007-08*, IIPS, Mumbai, India, 2010.

[5] IIPS and Macro International, *National Family Health Survey (NFHS-3), 2005-06: India*, vol. 1, IIPS, Mumbai, India, 2007.

[6] M. N. Bhanderi and S. Kannan, "Untreated reproductive morbidities among ever married women of slums of Rajkot City, Gujarat: the role of class, distance, provider attitudes, and perceived quality of care," *Journal of Urban Health*, vol. 87, no. 2, pp. 254–263, 2010.

[7] S. Sudha, S. Morrison, and L. Zhu, "Violence against women, symptom reporting, and treatment for reproductive tract infections in Kerala State, Southern India," *Health Care for Women International*, vol. 28, no. 3, pp. 268–284, 2007.

[8] M. Rani and S. Bonu, "Rural Indian women's care-seeking behavior and choice of provider for gynecological symptoms," *Studies in Family Planning*, vol. 34, no. 3, pp. 173–185, 2003.

[9] J. H. Prasad, S. Abraham, K. M. Kurz et al., "Reproductive tract infections among young married women in Tamil Nadu, India," *International Family Planning Perspectives*, vol. 31, no. 2, pp. 73–82, 2005.

[10] V. Patel, H. A. Weiss, D. Mabey et al., "The burden and determinants of reproductive tract infections in India: a population based study of women in Goa, India," *Sexually Transmitted Infections*, vol. 82, no. 3, pp. 243–249, 2006.

[11] G. S. Desai and R. M. Patel, "Incidence of reproductive tract infections and sexually transmitted diseases in India: levels and differentials," *Journal of Family Welfare*, vol. 57, no. 2, pp. 48–59, 2011.

[12] J. K. Kosambiya, V. K. Desai, P. Bhardwaj, and T. Chakraborty, "RTI/STI prevalence among urban and rural women of Surat: a community-based study," *Indian Journal of Sexually Transmitted Diseases & AIDS*, vol. 30, no. 2, pp. 89–93, 2009.

[13] K. M. Bansal, K. Singh, and S. Bhatnagar, "Prevalence of lower RTI among married females in the reproductive age group (15–45)," *Health and Population: Perspectives and Issues*, vol. 24, no. 3, pp. 157–163, 2001.

[14] V. Rani, S. Seth, P. Jian, C. M. Singh, S. Kumar, and N. P. Singh, "Prevalence of reproductive tract infections in married women in association with their past reproductive behaviour in district Gorakhpur," *Indian Journal of Preventive & Social Medicine*, vol. 40, no. 3, pp. 199–202, 2009.

[15] P. S. Philip, A. I. Benjamin, and P. Sengupta, "Prevalence of symptoms suggestive of reproductive tract infections/sexually transmitted infections in women in an urban area of Ludhiana," *Indian Journal of Sexually Transmitted Diseases*, vol. 34, no. 2, pp. 83–88, 2013.

[16] P. Aggarwal, S. D. Kandpal, K. S. Negi, and P. Gupta, "Health seeking behaviour for RTIs/STIs: study of a rural community in Dehradun," *Health and Population: Perspectives and Issues*, vol. 32, no. 2, pp. 66–72, 2009.

[17] R. P. Ravi and R. A. Kulasekaran, "Care seeking behaviour and barriers to accessing services for sexual health problems among women in rural areas of Tamilnadu state in India," *Journal of Sexually Transmitted Diseases*, vol. 2014, Article ID 292157, 8 pages, 2014.

[18] S. Sabarwal and K. G. Santhya, "Treatment-seeking for symptoms of reproductive tract infections among young women in India," *International Perspectives on Sexual and Reproductive Health*, vol. 38, no. 2, pp. 90–98, 2012.

[19] A. Joshi, M. Dhapola, and P. J. Pelto, "Gynecological problems: perceptions and treatment-seeking behaviors of rural Gujarati-women," in *Reproductive Health in India: New Evidence*, M. A. Koenig, S. Jejeebhoy, J. C. Cleland, and B. Ganatra, Eds., pp. 133–158, Rawat Publications, New Delhi, India, 2008.

[20] J. C. Bhatia and J. C. Cleland, "Perceived gynecological morbidity, health-seeking behavior and expenditure in Karnataka," in *Reproductive Health in India: New Evidence*, M. A. Koenig, A. Michael, J. Shireen et al., Eds., pp. 266–282, Rawat Publications, New Delhi, India, 2008.

7

The Chromosomal Constitution of Embryos Arising from Monopronuclear Oocytes in Programmes of Assisted Reproduction

Bernd Rosenbusch

Department of Gynaecology and Obstetrics, University of Ulm, Prittwitzstraße 43, 89075 Ulm, Germany

Correspondence should be addressed to Bernd Rosenbusch; bernd.rosenbusch@uniklinik-ulm.de

Academic Editor: Anne Van Langendonckt

The assessment of oocytes showing only one pronucleus during assisted reproduction is associated with uncertainty. A compilation of data on the genetic constitution of different developmental stages shows that affected oocytes are able to develop into haploid, diploid, and mosaic embryos with more or less complex chromosomal compositions. In the majority of cases (~80%), haploidy appears to be caused by gynogenesis, whereas parthenogenesis or androgenesis is less common. Most of the diploid embryos result from a fertilization event involving asynchronous formation of the two pronuclei or pronuclear fusion at a very early stage. Uniparental diploidy may sometimes occur if one pronucleus fails to develop and the other pronucleus already contains a diploid genome or alternatively a haploid genome undergoes endoreduplication. In general, the chance of obtaining a biparental diploid embryo appears higher after conventional in vitro fertilization than after intracytoplasmic sperm injection. If a transfer of embryos obtained from monopronuclear oocytes is envisaged, it should be tried to culture them up to the blastocyst since most haploid embryos are not able to reach this stage. Comprehensive counselling of patients on potential risks is advisable before transfer and a preimplantation genetic diagnosis could be offered if available.

1. Introduction

The technology of assisted reproduction aims at achieving oocyte fertilization by incubation of cumulus-intact oocytes in the presence of a defined number of motile spermatozoa (conventional in vitro fertilization, IVF) or by injection of single spermatozoa into denuded, cumulus-free oocytes (intracytoplasmic sperm injection, ICSI). Both procedures are followed about 16 to 20 hours later by the so-called pronucleus check. Here, successful and normal fertilization is identified by the appearance of two pronuclei (PN) in the ooplasm and detection of two polar bodies in the perivitelline space, whereas the presence of more than two PN is considered to be associated with genetic disorders, mostly triploidy [1]. Consequently, these multipronuclear oocytes are excluded from further cell culture and embryo transfer. In contrast, recommendations on the treatment of oocytes displaying only one pronucleus are accompanied by

greater uncertainty. In case of parthenogenetic activation, one should expect the formation of a haploid embryo with exclusively maternal chromosomes and therefore transfer should be cancelled. If, however, the PN had appeared asynchronously or underwent an undetected fusion, diploid biparental and transferable embryos may be available. In fact, a few pregnancies have been reported after transfer of embryos developing from monopronuclear oocytes [2–6].

The frequency of monopronuclear oocytes among all pronuclear stages has reached 7.7% after IVF and 5.0% after ICSI in a large study evaluating more than 6,000 cells for each technique [7]. Information on the chromosomal constitution of the resulting embryos appears to be of clinical interest particularly in rare cases without regular formation of two PN. The present report therefore summarizes pertinent data, reviews possible mechanisms of origin of a single pronucleus, and tries to deduce recommendations for handling affected oocytes during assisted reproduction.

2. Material and Methods

The literature search for this review is based on PubMed and Scopus and includes results found until the end of January 2014. The key words used were "single pronucleus," "monopronuclear," "monopronucleus," "single pronucleated," "unipronucleate," "unipronuclear," "one-pronuclear," and "single-nucleated", each in combination with "oocyte(s)," "zygote(s)," and "embryo(s)." Each identified article was checked for the relevant secondary literature. If specific data were excluded from the compilation of results, the reasons have been explained in the corresponding section.

The cited studies have examined different developmental stages, including monopronuclear oocytes, zygotes, and embryos up to the blastocyst. It should be noted that a monopronuclear female gamete (Figure 1) will undergo breakdown of the pronuclear membrane after DNA replication and hence the pronucleus will disappear comparable to the situation in normally fertilized bipronuclear oocytes. The next stage is the zygote though, strictly speaking, this description does not apply to parthenogenetically activated cells because a zygote is defined to result from the union of two haploid gametes and should therefore always contain a diploid chromosome set. However, the common nomenclature has been maintained in the present review because some zygotes indeed turned out biparental diploid (see Section 3).

For cytogenetic analysis, the above-mentioned developmental stages were frequently incubated in the presence of chemicals that block mitosis, for example, colcemid. The cells were then fixed on glass slides and the chromosomes were stained in order to establish karyotypes or allow at least chromosome counting. Some zygotes that developed from monopronuclear oocytes have been fixed during our cytogenetic investigations of unfertilized and abnormally fertilized female gametes. This project had been approved by the ethical committee of the University of Ulm and details of our technique have been described elsewhere [8]. Briefly, we used a mixture of podophyllotoxin and vinblastine instead of colcemid, a gradual fixation air-drying method and homogeneous Giemsa staining of the chromosomes. The corresponding cytogenetic results included in the present review have not been published before.

Fluorescence in situ hybridization (FISH) is another approach to examine cells that had been fixed on a glass slide. The method can be applied to interphase nuclei and therefore preceding exposure to colcemid is not necessary. The most frequently used DNA probes are those for chromosomes X, Y, 18, and 13/21. FISH has been applied to intact developmental stages but also to single biopsied cells from embryos [3, 9, 10]. Levron et al. [11] isolated the karyoplast, that is, the nucleus with a small amount of cytoplasm from the remaining cytoplast in monopronuclear oocytes to analyze them separately. In one instance, polymerase chain reaction (PCR) was used in combination with FISH [9].

van der Heijden et al. [12] presented a technique based on the asymmetrical distribution of histone modifications in male and female PN. Histones are DNA-associated proteins and determination of the presence of methylated lysine residues at a certain position of the N-terminal tail of histone

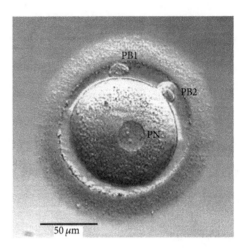

FIGURE 1: Following ICSI in our programme of assisted reproduction, this oocyte displayed a single pronucleus (PN) and two polar bodies (PB1 and PB2) on the following morning. Because another pronucleus could not be detected after a second inspection several hours later, the cell was subjected to cytogenetic analysis and revealed a haploid karyotype (23,X).

H3 by a specific antibody allows distinguishing paternal and maternal chromatin because only the latter will be stained. The method yielded information on the haploid or diploid state of monopronuclear zygotes and the parental origin of the PN but aneuploidy could not be assessed.

3. Results

Relevant information on the genetic constitution of monopronuclear oocytes and resulting developmental stages has been outlined in Table 1 according to their origin (conventional IVF or ICSI). The data provided by Balakier et al. [13] for cleavage stages have been excluded because of the low number of analyzable cells in each category (four embryos, one morula, and two blastocysts). The investigation of Munné et al. [9] was not considered because the authors themselves admitted that the applied technique would not allow clear distinction of monosomy and haploidy or trisomy and triploidy. Moreover, these authors [9] stated that "an X result by PCR could be either a haploid cell, a female diploid cell, or a trisomic or triploid female cell." From the study of Lim et al. [14], only the conventionally karyotyped embryos were included. The number of cells analyzed by FISH ($n = 14$) was low and subdividing them further (IVF or ICSI, zygotes or embryos) would have yielded very small groups without providing additional information. The study of Campos et al. [10] was excluded because diploid-aneuploid and haploid-aneuploid cases could not be distinguished.

Further difficulties encountered when trying to classify the results particularly concern cleavage stages with a larger number of analyzable blastomeres. These often show a coexistence of diploidy, haploidy, polyploidy, and superimposed numerical chromosome abnormalities. Presenting details would have been too confusing and therefore the cytogenetic terms chosen for Table 1 ("haploid," "diploid," and "other")

TABLE 1: The genetic constitution of monopronuclear oocytes and resultant developmental stages.

Material	Origin	Number of cases	Method	Cytogenetic constitution			Reference
				Haploid	Diploid	Other	
Karyoplasts	IVF	16	FISH	10 (62.5%)	6 (37.5%)	0	Levron et al. [11]
Zygotes	IVF	20	Cytogenetics/FISH	9 (45.0%)	11 (55.0%)	0	Balakier et al. [13]
Zygotes	IVF	45	Histone methylation	6 (13.3%)	39 (86.7%)	0	van der Heijden et al. [12]
Embryos	IVF	54	Cytogenetics	? (69.0%)	? (13.0%)	? (17.0%)	Plachot et al. [19]
Embryos	IVF	9	Cytogenetics	3 (33.3%)	5 (55.6%)	1 (11.1%)	Jamieson et al. [20]
Embryos	IVF	41	Cytogenetics	5 (12.2%)	33 (80.5%)	3 (7.3%)	Staessen et al. [2]
Embryos	IVF	21	FISH	3 (14.3%)	15 (71.4%)	3 (14.3%)	Sultan et al. [3]
Embryos	IVF	115	FISH	15 (13.0%)	56 (48.7%)	44 (38.3%)	Staessen and van Steirteghem [7]
Embryos	IVF	26	Cytogenetics	6 (23.1%)	19 (73.1%)	1 (3.8%)	Lim et al. [14]
Embryos	IVF	46	FISH	11 (23.9%)	25 (54.3%)	10 (21.7%)	Yan et al. [21]
Blastocysts	IVF	6	FISH	0	6 (100%)	0	Otsu et al. [22]
Zygotes	ICSI	18	Cytogenetics	18 (100%)	0	0	Rosenbusch (unpublished data)
Zygotes	ICSI	28	Cytogenetics	28 (100%)	0	0	Macas et al. [17]
Zygotes	ICSI	33	Histone methylation	23 (69.7%)	10 (30.3%)	0	van der Heijden et al. [12]
Embryos	ICSI	21	FISH	14 (66.7%)	6 (28.6%)	1 (4.8%)	Sultan et al. [3]
Embryos	ICSI	61	FISH	19 (31.2%)	17 (27.9%)	25 (41.0%)	Staessen and van Steirteghem [7]
Embryos	ICSI	24	Cytogenetics	14 (58.3%)	9 (37.5%)	1 (4.2%)	Lim et al. [14]
Embryos	ICSI	73	FISH	23 (31.5%)	23 (31.5%)	27 (37.0%)	Yan et al. [21]
Embryos	ICSI	46	FISH	8 (17.4%)	1 (2.2%)	37 (80.4%)	Mateo et al. [16]
Blastocysts	ICSI	8	FISH	1 (12.5%)	3 (37.5%)	4 (50.0%)	Mateo et al. [16]
Embryos	IVF/ICSI	95	FISH	29 (30.5%)	37 (38.9%)	29 (30.5%)	Liao et al. [15]
Blastocysts	IVF/ICSI	59	FISH	0	46 (78.0%)	13 (22.0%)	Liao et al. [15]

Embryos comprise developing or arrested cleavage stages including the morula. The category "Haploid" may contain deviations from the exact chromosome count of 23 and haploid-mosaic cells. Also, the category "Diploid" may contain deviations from the exact chromosome count of 46 and diploid-mosaic cells (see Results). "Other" cytogenetic constitutions include polyploid, mosaic, complex, and chaotic cases. ?: absolute numbers not indicated.

are simplifications. In other words, the categories "diploid" and "haploid" also contain cells with deviations from the respective exact chromosome count of 46 or 23. For instance, the diploid-aneuploid embryos and blastocysts listed by Liao et al. [15] have been counted as diploid. Concerning the study of Mateo et al. [16], it was decided to classify diploid-mosaic cells as diploid, haploid-mosaic cells as haploid, and the remainder as carrying "other" aberrations. Since the main intention of the present review was to differentiate fertilized from unfertilized cells, this subjective approach appeared justifiable. The possible biparental origin of diploid cells was not considered in Table 1 but will be addressed below.

3.1. Oocytes and Uncleaved Zygotes. The genetic constitution of monopronuclear oocytes and zygotes obtained after IVF has been examined in three studies [11–13] and it was shown that 37.5% to 86.7% of the cells were diploid (Table 1). This incidence is conspicuously different from the range of 0% to 30.3% detected in monopronuclear cells produced by ICSI ([12, 17], own unpublished results). Particularly the study of Macas et al. [17] and our own unpublished investigation, both applying conventional cytogenetics to uncleaved zygotes, failed to reveal a case of diploidy. In our material, 4 out of 18 haploid cells (22.2%) carried a chromosomal aberration (hypo- or hyperhaploidy, see Table 2), whereas Macas et al. [17] reported an incidence of 32.1%. Here, it should be

noted that cytogenetic investigations of monopronuclear zygotes are surprisingly scarce in view of the fact that these cells can inform about the total incidence of aneuploidy arising from female meioses I and II. Finally, 15 out of the 18 zygotes (83.3%) examined by us showed prematurely condensed sperm chromosomes comparable to the patterns found in unfertilized oocytes [18], indicative of correct sperm insertion into the ooplasm during ICSI.

3.2. Embryos and Blastocysts. As shown in Table 1, eight studies investigated the chromosomal constitution of embryos or blastocysts after IVF [2, 3, 7, 14, 19–22]. ICSI-derived embryos or blastocysts were included in five reports [3, 7, 14, 16, 21]. According to these data, the incidence of diploid IVF embryos varies between 13.0% [19] and 80.5% [2] and is again considerably lower after ICSI with rates between 2.2% [16] and 37.5% [14]. Whereas all six IVF blastocysts examined by Otsu et al. [22] were diploid or diploid mosaics, only three of eight (37.5%) ICSI-derived blastocysts analyzed by Mateo et al. [16] revealed diploidy. However, it is evident that both observations are based on a low number of cases. The results of Liao et al. [15] had to be considered separately because the origin of the embryos (IVF or ICSI) was not specified. Nevertheless, an important point in their study is that the rate of diploidy increases from 38.9% in early cleavage stages to 78.0% in blastocysts.

TABLE 2: A brief summary of our cytogenetic analysis of monopronuclear oocytes obtained after ICSI[a].

Number of patients	16	
Number of oocytes fixed	20	
Number of analyzable oocytes	18	
Number of diploid oocytes	0	
Number of haploid oocytes	18 (100%)	
Haploid abnormal:		
Hypohaploidy	2 (11.1%)	22,X,−B
		22,X,−D
Hyperhaploidy	2 (11.1%)	24,X,+C
		24,X,+E

[a]Previously unpublished data.

3.3. A Closer Look at Diploid Stages. As soon as a monopronuclear oocyte undergoes further development into a
diploid zygote or even an embryo, it should be ascertained
whether the diploid condition was actually caused by fertilization (= biparental or heteroparental diploidy) or by specific
mechanisms giving rise to uniparental diploidy, for instance,
endoreduplication of the haploid female chromosome set.
Pertinent information on this topic has been summarized
in Table 3. Investigating histone modifications in monopronuclear zygotes, van der Heijden et al. [12] regarded
the presence of two chromatin domains with a nonuniform
staining pattern as proof of a biparental origin. According to
this approach, all 39 diploid IVF zygotes and all 10 diploid
ICSI zygotes were classified as biparental because male and
female chromatin were detected. More common, however, is
to determine the presence of a Y-chromosome as evidence
for sperm penetration. After conventional IVF, a minimum
of 40% of diploid embryos had a Y-chromosome [20] but this
incidence even reached 66.7% both in isolated karyoplasts
[11] and in blastocysts [22]. After ICSI, the frequency of
diploid embryos with a Y-chromosome ranged from 16.7%
[3] to 52.2% [21]. Mateo et al. [16] found a Y-chromosome
in 19/54 (35.2%) ICSI embryos but these data could not
be included in Table 3 because it was not clear whether
mosaic haploid embryos were involved. Finally, it should be
added that 15/31 (48.4%) complex mosaic IVF embryos and
12/16 (75.0%) complex mosaic ICSI embryos revealed a Y-
chromosome [7]. The latter authors [7] also reported one
diploid ICSI embryo with a YY-chromosome constitution.
Taken together, these figures support the former statement
by Munné et al. [9] who, having found a Y-chromosome in
41% (9/22) of the embryos, suggested that approximately 80%
may have originated from fertilized eggs. The authors [9]
arrived at this value by doubling the percentage of Y-bearing
embryos because it is assumed that X- and Y-spermatozoa
participate equally in fertilization. With this formula in mind,
some of the data shown in Table 3 suggest an even higher
incidence of biparental diploidy that may reach nearly 100%
independent of IVF or ICSI, whereas uniparental diploidy in
cleavage stages arising from monopronuclear oocytes appears
to be an exception.

4. Discussion

Up to now, the transfer of embryos that developed from
monopronuclear IVF oocytes resulted in one pregnancy with
unknown outcome [3], the birth of two healthy children
and one biochemical pregnancy [2], and the birth of a
normal healthy boy [5]. Moreover, even the birth of normal
twin boys following transfer of a single embryo has been
reported [6]. In contrast, only Barak et al. [4] achieved
the birth of a normal healthy boy after round spermatid
injection accompanied by formation of one pronucleus. It
should also be mentioned that a diploid (46,XX) human
embryonic stem cell (hESC) line could be derived from a
monopronuclear ICSI zygote [23], whereas another group
[15] established 33 hESC lines. The latter authors [15] who did
not indicate the origin of the monopronuclear oocytes (IVF
or ICSI) obtained a diploidy rate of 97% (32/33) and only one
abnormal (47,XY,+16) cell line. In contrast to these successes,
Petignat et al. [24] described a twin pregnancy combining
a complete hydatidiform mole and normal pregnancy that
had to be terminated. This pregnancy occurred after transfer
of two embryos, one obtained from a normally fertilized
oocyte with two PN and the other from a monopronuclear
oocyte. The authors [24] hypothesized that the oocyte with
one pronucleus gave rise to the hydatidiform mole and
emphasized the danger of transferring the corresponding
embryos. The underlying mechanism in this peculiar case
would involve fertilization by a haploid spermatozoon with
subsequent chromosome duplication or fertilization by a
diploid spermatozoon, always accompanied by failed formation of the female pronucleus. This annotation shows that
it must be clarified which mechanisms are responsible for
the different genetic compositions, particularly haploidy and
diploidy.

4.1. Haploid Embryos. Haploidy is generally attributed to
parthenogenesis, gynogenesis, or androgenesis and these
terms have been explained in detail elsewhere [25, 26]. Briefly,
parthenogenesis means the development of an embryo from
an oocyte without any intervention of a male gamete. Oocytes
can, for instance, be activated by heat or mechanical means.
It is evident that these embryos contain only the female
genome. The same is true in the case of gynogenesis but
here the oocyte has been stimulated by a spermatozoon to
undergo the second meiotic division. Cleavage then proceeds
without participation of the male genome. On the other
hand, androgenesis also starts with oocyte activation by a
spermatozoon but the female genome will be genetically
inactivated or completely extruded and only the male genome
is involved during subsequent development.

About 45% of monopronuclear IVF zygotes showed signs
of sperm penetration [13] and the authors surmised that, in
oocytes without visible sperm heads or nucleus-like structures, the sperm chromatin might have undergone complete
disintegration or extrusion to form observed but undefined
"extra bodies." Thus, the incidence of sperm penetration
could even be higher. More data are available for monopronuclear ICSI zygotes. Here, intact sperm heads or decondensed
sperm chromatin was found in 76 to 86.5% of examined cases

TABLE 3: The origin of diploidy in monopronuclear oocytes and ensuing developmental stages.

Material	Origin	Method	Diploid cells	Heteroparental cells	Reference
Karyoplasts	IVF	Y-detection by FISH	6	4 (66.7%)	Levron et al. [11]
Zygotes	IVF	Histone methylation patterns[a]	39	39 (100%)	van der Heijden et al. [12]
Embryos	IVF	Cytogenetics/karyotyping	5	2 (40.0%)	Jamieson et al. [20]
Embryos	IVF	Y-detection by FISH	15	9 (60.0%)	Sultan et al. [3]
Embryos	IVF	Y-detection by FISH	56	25 (44.6%)	Staessen and van Steirteghem [7]
Embryos	IVF	Y-detection by FISH	25	15 (60.0%)	Yan et al. [21]
Blastocysts	IVF	Y-detection by FISH	6	4 (66.7%)	Otsu et al. [22]
Zygotes	ICSI	Histone methylation patterns[a]	10	10 (100%)	van der Heijden et al. [12]
Embryos	ICSI	Y-detection by FISH	6	1 (16.7%)	Sultan et al. [3]
Embryos	ICSI	Y-detection by FISH	17	6 (35.3%)	Staessen and van Steirteghem [7]
Embryos	ICSI	Y-detection by FISH	23	12 (52.2%)	Yan et al. [21]

[a]Note that this is a nongenetic method that distinguishes maternal and paternal chromatin independent of the occurrence of specific chromosomes. Under the assumption that X- and Y-spermatozoa participate equally in fertilization, the figures obtained by detection of a Y-chromosome should be doubled [9] and then yield percentages of heteroparental cells that are comparable to the findings of van der Heijden et al. [12].

[27–29]. Our own unpublished results of 83.3% are in good agreement with these figures. In one study [29], a male origin of the single pronucleus was determined in only 4% of the examined oocytes due to the presence of a sperm tail and it was assumed that the entire maternal chromatin had been extruded into a polar body (PB) or did not succeed in forming a pronucleus. Oocytes in which the meiotic spindle cannot be detected at the time of ICSI appear to be more susceptible to formation of a single male pronucleus [30]. Assessing histone methylation patterns in uncleaved zygotes, van der Heijden et al. [12] arrive at different figures. In their study, only paternal chromatin was found in 24.2% of ICSI zygotes and in 4.4% of IVF zygotes. These authors concluded that complete extrusion of the maternal chromatin during formation of the second PB might be a quite frequent event. It remains to be determined whether the applied detection methods are responsible for the varying rates of male PN reported by Kovacic and Vlaisavljevic [29] and van der Heijden et al. [12] for ICSI zygotes.

In the discussion on causative mechanisms, ICSI could indeed be regarded as a separate phenomenon because it involves both a mechanical stimulus and participation of a spermatozoon that is inserted into the ooplasm. Most probably, however, a sperm factor activates the oocyte and then sperm chromatin decondensation stops [29], whereas female pronucleus formation proceeds normally. This would again comply with the definition of gynogenesis. Taken together, most of the available data support the opinion that the majority (~80%) of haploid monopronuclear oocytes and resulting embryos are produced by gynogenesis and that parthenogenesis or androgenesis is less common.

4.2. Biparental Diploid Embryos. An asynchronous appearance of PN is the first possibility to explain the existence of biparental diploidy in embryos that develop from monopronuclear oocytes. For instance, Staessen et al. [2] performed a second observation of 312 single-pronucleated oocytes 4 to 6 hours after the initial assessment and detected a second pronucleus in 25% of these cases. The authors concluded that a single observation of an oocyte with one pronucleus does not allow differentiating between asynchrony of pronuclear development and parthenogenetic activation. Since delayed formation of the second pronucleus may not be a rare event, monopronuclear oocytes should therefore be rechecked after some hours. Consequently, a proportion of diploid embryos could have arisen from fertilized oocytes in which the asynchronous pronuclear formation had been overlooked. These embryos would be characterized by a diploid, 46,XX or 46,XY chromosome constitution.

However, how does diploidy arise if definitely only one pronucleus persists during the whole observation period? A solution is offered by the concept of pronuclear fusion that has been put forward by Levron et al. [11]. These authors suggested that monospermic diploid monopronuclear zygotes may be formed by a fusion of the paternal and maternal genomes during syngamy, most probably by very early enclosure in a common pronuclear envelope rather than by fusion of pronuclear membranes at a later stage. It was further assumed that sperm penetration close to the metaphase plate of the oocyte might predispose to this modified fertilization process. Pronuclear fusion was not observed in an investigation using time-lapse video cinematography [31] but the number of examined oocytes (43 with formation of PN) appears too low for definite conclusions. Whereas Levron et al. [11] did not address the question whether fused PN possibly show an increase in size, Otsu et al. [22] differentiated between large (29–34 μm) and small (23–26 μm) PN. Only some oocytes (6/34) from the group with larger PN were able to reach the blastocyst stage and these blastocysts were diploid or diploid mosaic. Otsu et al. [22] suggested that larger PN might be a product of pronuclear fusion before nuclear membrane breakdown. In contrast, others [16] could not demonstrate a correlation between pronuclear size and chromosomal constitution and also denied the existence of pronuclear fusion at a later stage.

The only possibility for formation of a diploid heteroparental pronucleus would consist in an irregular membrane formation enclosing maternal and paternal genomes [16].

Prior to these investigations, however, Tesarik and Mendoza [32] had reported that oocytes injected with spermatids may develop two PN that later fuse to form a "syngamy nucleus." This nucleus was described to be only slightly larger than a pronucleus. It is currently not clear whether the described phenomenon is restricted to the use of sperm precursor cells for injection. Further confirmatory observations are rare and spermatid injections have apparently been abandoned during the past years. Obviously, there is a need for more basic research concerning the dynamics of pronuclear development, fusion events, and pronuclear size. Comparable to cases of asynchronous pronuclear formation, embryos resulting from fertilization and early fusion of the genomes or later pronuclear fusion should reveal a diploid, 46,XX or 46,XY chromosome constitution.

4.3. Uniparental Diploid Embryos.

4.3. Uniparental Diploid Embryos. An embryo within this category can carry a diploid 46,XX genome which is exclusively composed of female chromosomes as soon as a diploid oocyte starts to cleave without participation of a male genome. If on the other hand the genome is exclusively derived from the male gamete, the following chromosome complements can occur in embryos: 46,XY (first meiotic nondisjunction during spermatogenesis) and 46,XX or 46,YY (second meiotic nondisjunction). In each case, a diploid spermatozoon would fertilize an oocyte and cleavage would commence without participation of the female genome. As already mentioned above, Staessen and van Steirteghem [7] detected one diploid ICSI embryo with two Y-chromosomes. This observation can be explained by a failed formation of the female pronucleus and development of a diploid male pronucleus due to injection of a diploid spermatozoon. Alternatively, however, injection of a haploid spermatozoon might have been accompanied by suppression of the female and endoreduplication in the male pronucleus. Endoreduplication has been reported to affect not only single chromosomes but also complete chromosome sets and may in the latter case contribute to the development of triploidy if it occurs in one of the two PN of a regularly fertilized oocyte [33]. It is therefore conceivable that endoreduplication in a monopronuclear oocyte produces uniparental diploid embryos but clear evidence for this assumption is lacking.

Nonextrusion of the second PB has been discussed as another mechanism that may cause uniparental diploidy in embryos arising from monopronuclear oocytes [19]. In such cases, the 23 oocyte chromosomes should separate into single chromatids but all 46 chromatids will remain within the ooplasm, become enclosed by a pronuclear membrane, and undergo DNA replication, thus restoring a diploid female chromosome set. A male pronucleus will not be formed. This concept has been described as one of the mechanisms for diploid parthenogenesis [26] but it appears questionable in view of the findings for tripronuclear ICSI oocytes. Here, it is generally accepted that nonextrusion of the second PB leads to two individual haploid female PN and not to a single diploid female pronucleus [33]. More data are therefore needed to verify a participation of the second PB in producing monopronuclear diploid oocytes and embryos.

From these considerations, it becomes evident that a variety of mechanisms can influence the genetic composition of zygotes and embryos obtained from monopronuclear oocytes. In addition, mitotic nondisjunction of single chromosomes or whole chromosome sets may occur in cleavage stages and thus explain the observation of polyploid, mosaic, complex, and chaotic cases.

4.4. Additional Remarks. From the preceding compilation of published results, two important points can be condensed: (a) monopronuclear oocytes are able to develop into embryos with variable chromosomal constitutions and (b) the majority of diploid embryos obviously result from a fertilization event. How should clinicians proceed with monopronuclear oocytes in view of this conflicting information? First, monopronuclear oocytes should be rechecked after the first assessment of pronuclear formation to detect delayed appearance of a second pronucleus. If this is not the case, one may follow Sultan et al. [3] who recommended that embryos developing from monopronuclear IVF oocytes may be replaced, whereas those obtained after ICSI would not be suitable. Nowadays, however, the frequently used transfer of blastocysts may provide an additional option. As discussed by Feenan and Herbert [1], human parthenotes are capable of cleaving to the 8-cell stage but they rarely seem to develop up to the blastocyst (Table 1). Liao et al. [15] added that, besides haploidy, autosomal aneuploidy and polyploidy were eliminated in blastocysts and they concluded that blastocyst formation would be a useful indicator for normal fertilization and chromosomal constitution. Thus, monopronuclear IVF and ICSI oocytes in which the single pronucleus persists after a second assessment might be used for transfer when they are able to reach the blastocyst stage and when no other embryo is available. Of course, each institution will have to clarify whether this approach should be accompanied by adequate counselling on potential genetic risks and written consent of the patients and whether a preimplantation genetic diagnosis could be offered. Finally, though Mateo et al. [16] discourage from the use of diploid-mosaic blastocysts, it should be considered that a high rate of aneuploidy and mosaicism even occurs in high quality embryos derived from normally fertilized ICSI oocytes [34]. Therefore, the implantation potential of such embryos and possible mechanisms of self-correction of abnormal chromosome complements are topics of future research. Another important question may concern the epigenetic status of fertilized monopronuclear oocytes, particularly whether the interaction between paternal and maternal chromatin is disturbed when they are prematurely enclosed within one pronuclear envelope [12].

5. Conclusions

Oocytes in which a single pronucleus persists might be considered for transfer if they reach a good-quality blastocyst stage but this remains an individual decision of the IVF laboratory. More data on the morphologic quality, developmental ability, and genetic constitution of affected embryos are undoubtedly needed before a general consent can be achieved that should include recommendations on counselling of the patients and the role of preimplantation genetic diagnosis. The incidence and significance of early pronuclear fusion events or an immediate enclosure of paternal and maternal chromatin within a single pronuclear envelope might be an interesting topic of future research, particularly in view of genetic and epigenetic implications.

Conflict of Interests

The author declares that there is no conflict of interests regarding the publication of this paper.

References

[1] K. Feenan and M. Herbert, "Can "abnormally" fertilized zygotes give rise to viable embryos?" *Human Fertility*, vol. 9, no. 3, pp. 157–169, 2006.

[2] C. Staessen, C. Janssenswillen, P. Devroey, and A. C. van Steirteghem, "Cytogenetic and morphological observations of single pronucleated human oocytes after in-vitro fertilization," *Human Reproduction*, vol. 8, no. 2, pp. 221–223, 1993.

[3] K. M. Sultan, S. Munné, G. D. Palermo, M. Alikani, and J. Cohen, "Chromosomsal status of uni-pronuclear human zygotes following in-vitro fertilization and intracytoplasmic sperm injection," *Human Reproduction*, vol. 10, no. 1, pp. 132–136, 1995.

[4] Y. Barak, A. Kogosowski, S. Goldman, Y. Soffer, Y. Gonen, and J. Tesarik, "Pregnancy and birth after transfer of embryos that developed from single-nucleated zygotes obtained by injection of round spermatids into oocytes," *Fertility and Sterility*, vol. 70, no. 1, pp. 67–70, 1998.

[5] L. Gras and A. O. Trounson, "Pregnancy and birth resulting from transfer of a blastocyst observed to have one pronucleus at the time of examination for fertilization," *Human Reproduction*, vol. 14, no. 7, pp. 1869–1871, 1999.

[6] D. Dasig, J. Lyon, B. Behr, and A. A. Milki, "Monozygotic twin birth after the transfer of a cleavage stage embryo resulting from a single pronucleated oocyte," *Journal of Assisted Reproduction and Genetics*, vol. 21, no. 12, pp. 427–429, 2004.

[7] C. Staessen and A. C. van Steirteghem, "The chromosomal constitution of embryos developing from abnormally fertilized oocytes after intracytoplasmic sperm injection and conventional in-vitro fertilization," *Human Reproduction*, vol. 12, no. 2, pp. 321–327, 1997.

[8] B. Rosenbusch, M. Schneider, B. Gläser, and C. Brucker, "Cytogenetic analysis of giant oocytes and zygotes to assess their relevance for the development of digynic triploidy," *Human Reproduction*, vol. 17, no. 9, pp. 2388–2393, 2002.

[9] S. Munné, Y.-X. Tang, J. Grifo, and J. Cohen, "Origin of single pronucleated human zygotes," *Journal of Assisted Reproduction and Genetics*, vol. 10, no. 4, pp. 276–279, 1993.

[10] G. Campos, M. Parriego, F. Vidal, B. Coroleu, and A. Veiga, "Cytogenetic constitution and developmental potential of embryos derived from apronuclear and monopronuclear zygotes," *Revista Iberoamericana de Fertilidad y Reproduccion Humana*, vol. 24, no. 1, pp. 29–34, 2007.

[11] J. Levron, S. Munné, S. Willadsen, Z. Rosenwaks, and J. Cohen, "Male and female genomes associated in a single pronucleus in human zygotes," *Biology of Reproduction*, vol. 52, no. 3, pp. 653–657, 1995.

[12] G. W. van der Heijden, I. M. van den Berg, E. B. Baart, A. A. H. A. Derijck, E. Martini, and P. de Boer, "Parental origin of chromatin in human monopronuclear zygotes revealed by asymmetric histone methylation patterns, differs between IVF and ICSI," *Molecular Reproduction and Development*, vol. 76, no. 1, pp. 101–108, 2009.

[13] H. Balakier, J. Squire, and R. F. Casper, "Characterization of abnormal one pronuclear human oocytes by morphology, cytogenetics and in-situ hybridization," *Human Reproduction*, vol. 8, no. 3, pp. 402–408, 1993.

[14] A. S. T. Lim, V. H. H. Goh, C. L. Su, and S. L. Yu, "Microscopic assessment of pronuclear embryos is not definitive," *Human Genetics*, vol. 107, no. 1, pp. 62–68, 2000.

[15] H. Liao, S. Zhang, D. Cheng et al., "Cytogenetic analysis of human embryos and embryonic stem cells derived from monopronuclear zygotes," *Journal of Assisted Reproduction and Genetics*, vol. 26, no. 11-12, pp. 583–589, 2009.

[16] S. Mateo, M. Parriego, M. Boada, F. Vidal, B. Coroleu, and A. Veiga, "In vitro development and chromosome constitution of embryos derived from monopronucleated zygotes after intracytoplasmic sperm injection," *Fertility and Sterility*, vol. 99, no. 3, pp. 897–902.e1, 2013.

[17] E. Macas, B. Imthurn, M. Roselli, and P. J. Keller, "Chromosome analysis of single- and multipronucleated human zygotes proceeded after the intracytoplasmic sperm injection procedure," *Journal of Assisted Reproduction and Genetics*, vol. 13, no. 4, pp. 345–350, 1996.

[18] B. E. Rosenbusch, "Frequency and patterns of premature sperm chromosome condensation in oocytes failing to fertilize after intracytoplasmic sperm injection," *Journal of Assisted Reproduction and Genetics*, vol. 17, no. 5, pp. 253–259, 2000.

[19] M. Plachot, J. Mandelbaum, A. M. Junca, J. de Grouchy, J. Salat-Baroux, and J. Cohen, "Cytogenetic analysis and developmental capacity of normal and abnormal embryos after IVF," *Human Reproduction*, vol. 4, supplement, pp. 99–103, 1989.

[20] M. E. Jamieson, J. R. T. Coutts, and J. M. Connor, "The chromosome constitution of human preimplantation embryos fertilized in vitro," *Human Reproduction*, vol. 9, no. 4, pp. 709–715, 1994.

[21] J. Yan, Y. Li, Y. Shi, H. L. Feng, S. Gao, and Z.-J. Chen, "Assessment of sex chromosomes of human embryos arising from monopronucleus zygotes in in vitro fertilization and intracytoplasmic sperm injection cycles of chinese women," *Gynecologic and Obstetric Investigation*, vol. 69, no. 1, pp. 20–23, 2010.

[22] E. Otsu, A. Sato, M. Nagaki, Y. Araki, and T. Utsunomiya, "Developmental potential and chromosomal constitution of embryos derived from larger single pronuclei of human zygotes used in in vitro fertilization," *Fertility and Sterility*, vol. 81, no. 3, pp. 723–724, 2004.

[23] E. Suss-Toby, S. Gerecht-Nir, M. Amit, D. Manor, and J. Itskovitz-Eldor, "Derivation of a diploid human embryonic stem cell line from a mononuclear zygote," *Human Reproduction*, vol. 19, no. 3, pp. 670–675, 2004.

[24] P. Petignat, A. Senn, P. Hohlfeld, S. A. Blant, R. Laurini, and M. Germond, "Molar pregnancy with a coexistent fetus after intracytoplasmic sperm injection: a case report," *The Journal of Reproductive Medicine*, vol. 46, no. 3, pp. 270–274, 2001.

[25] U. Mittwoch, "Parthenogenesis," *Journal of Medical Genetics*, vol. 15, no. 3, pp. 165–181, 1978.

[26] N. Rougier and Z. Werb, "Minireview: parthenogenesis in mammals," *Molecular Reproduction and Development*, vol. 59, no. 4, pp. 468–474, 2001.

[27] D. Dozortsev, P. de Sutter, and M. Dhont, "Behaviour of spermatozoa in human oocytes displaying no or one pronucleus after intracytoplasmic sperm injection," *Human Reproduction*, vol. 9, no. 11, pp. 2139–2144, 1994.

[28] S. P. Flaherty, D. Payne, and C. D. Matthews, "Fertilization failures and abnormal fertilization after intracytoplasmic sperm injection," *Human Reproduction*, vol. 13, supplement 1, pp. 155–164, 1998.

[29] B. Kovacic and V. Vlaisavljevic, "Configuration of maternal and paternal chromatin and pertaining microtubules in human oocytes failing to fertilize after intracytoplasmic sperm injection," *Molecular Reproduction and Development*, vol. 55, no. 2, pp. 197–204, 2000.

[30] L. Rienzi, F. Ubaldi, F. Martinez et al., "Relationship between meiotic spindle location with regard to the polar body position and oocyte developmental potential after ICSI," *Human Reproduction*, vol. 18, no. 6, pp. 1289–1293, 2003.

[31] D. Payne, S. P. Flaherty, M. F. Barry, and C. D. Matthews, "Preliminary observations on polar body extrusion and pronuclear formation in human oocytes using time-lapse video cinematography," *Human Reproduction*, vol. 12, no. 3, pp. 532–541, 1997.

[32] J. Tesarik and C. Mendoza, "Spermatid injection into human oocytes. I. Laboratory techniques and special features of zygote development," *Human Reproduction*, vol. 11, no. 4, pp. 772–779, 1996.

[33] B. E. Rosenbusch, "Mechanisms giving rise to triploid zygotes during assisted reproduction," *Fertility and Sterility*, vol. 90, no. 1, pp. 49–55, 2008.

[34] A. Mertzanidou, L. Wilton, J. Cheng et al., "Microarray analysis reveals abnormal chromosomal complements in over 70% of 14 normally developing human embryos," *Human Reproduction*, vol. 28, no. 1, pp. 256–264, 2013.

8

The Effects of Interpregnancy Intervals and Previous Pregnancy Outcome on Fetal Loss in Rwanda (1996–2010)

Ignace Habimana-Kabano,[1,2] **Annelet Broekhuis,**[2] **and Pieter Hooimeijer**[2]

[1]*Demography and Statistics, University of Rwanda, P.O. Box 117, Huye, Rwanda*
[2]*Utrecht University, P.O. Box 80115, 3508 TC Utrecht, Netherlands*

Correspondence should be addressed to Ignace Habimana-Kabano; kabanoignace@gmail.com

Academic Editor: Hind A. Beydoun

In 2005, a WHO consultation meeting on pregnancy intervals recommended a minimum interval of 6 months after a pregnancy disruption and an interval of two years after a live birth before attempting another pregnancy. Since then, studies have found contradictory evidence on the effect of shorter intervals after a pregnancy disruption. A binary regression analysis on 21532 last pregnancy outcomes from the 2000, 2005, and 2010 Rwanda Demographic and Health Surveys was done to assess the combined effects of the preceding pregnancy outcome and the interpregnancy intervals (IPIs) on fetal mortality in Rwanda. Risks of pregnancy loss are higher for primigravida and for mothers who lost the previous pregnancy and conceived again within 24 months. After a live birth, interpregnancy intervals less than two years do not increase the risk of a pregnancy loss. This study also confirms higher risks of fetal death when IPIs are beyond 5 years. An IPI of longer than 12 months after a fetal death is recommended in Rwanda. Particular attention needs to be directed to postpregnancy abortion care and family planning programs geared to spacing pregnancies should also include spacing after a fetal death.

1. Introduction

An expert consultation organized by the World Health Organization in 2005 made an inventory of available research on births spacing. The experts recommended an interpregnancy interval (IPI) of at least 6 months after a miscarriage before attempting a next pregnancy, in order to reduce morbidity and mortality risks for mother, fetus, and newborn. An IPI of at least 24 months was recommended after a live birth, corresponding to a birth interval of at least 33 months. The consultation team also concluded that future research is needed on the mechanisms underlying the relation between interval length and pregnancy outcomes. More studies using datasets from both rich and poor countries could contribute to more in-depth knowledge [1]. Contradicting results of research on the effect of short intervals on the risk of adverse pregnancy outcomes [1–6] conducted after 2005 confirmed the relevance of these statements. The few studies on the effect of intervals after a previous pregnancy disruption show a large

variation by country. DaVanzo and colleagues [4] emphasized that studies on the effects of interpregnancy intervals should take into account the outcome of the previous pregnancy.

Our study contributes to the debate on pregnancy loss and interpregnancy intervals (IPIs) in line with these recommendations. We focus on the effect of the duration of the IPI on pregnancy losses by combining the effect of the interval duration and the type of previous pregnancy outcome (pregnancy loss, live births that survived infancy or died in the first year), and controlling for important confounders. In this study, the term pregnancy loss includes all pregnancy outcomes (spontaneous and induced abortion, fetal death, and stillbirth) opposite to a live birth.

Fetal loss has got limited attention [7] compared to other issues, neither in the field of reproductive health nor in development debates among policy makers, nor in debates among scholars in population studies. This lack of attention is regrettable, because for many women the loss of a pregnancy is an emotional experience which affects their subsequent reproductive health and behavior. Fetal loss and stillbirths constitute the majority of the world's perinatal deaths and, yet, the absence of easy accessible and reliable secondary data on pregnancy loss is mentioned as a reason for neglecting the topic of fetal deaths by scientists [7, 8].

Reducing adverse pregnancy outcomes contributes to the health of the mother. Contrary to the reduction of maternal morbidity and of infant mortality, reducing pregnancy loss is not a policy objective but should become so in the future.

The outcome of our analysis will be discussed in the framework of results of a few [1, 4, 7, 9–11] available studies that followed the same approach by including the IPI duration and the previous pregnancy outcome to estimate the risk of a pregnancy loss. The majority of these studies focus on the effect of IPI duration on adverse pregnancy outcomes after a previous spontaneous or induced abortion while only a few have a broader perspective and include also other prior pregnancy outcomes (see Table 4). The studies differ on essential points, such as various types of mothers in the sample, nulliparous or multiparous women; various types of adverse pregnancy outcomes, pregnancy loss, preterm births, and low birth weight; reference group; categories of IPI; data collection method; and geographical region, which could contribute to explain the variety in the findings.

Only two studies, one from the USA and the other from Latin America, did not find significant associations between IPI duration and a fetal or neonatal death after a spontaneous or induced abortion [7, 9]. The other studies do find an association between IPI duration and adverse maternal and pregnancy outcomes after a previous fetal loss, but the associations between IPI duration and recurrent pregnancy losses are weak or nonexistent for late fetal deaths (stillbirths) [9–11]. Some results from USA and Scotland are even the opposite of what is expected on the WHO recommendations after early fetal deaths (miscarriages) [5, 6]. They find that, after a previous early fetal loss, short IPI intervals are associated with a higher likelihood on a live birth compared to longer IPIs. For Bangladesh [4], no differences between these likelihoods were found after a fetal loss according to IPI length except after very long IPI (>74 months).

However, the studies [10, 11] that focus on the association between IPI duration and the risk of a fetal death (and other adverse pregnancy outcomes) show higher risks of an adverse outcome after a fetal loss and a short IPI relative to a previous live birth combined with a healthy IPI. The meta-analyses [10] included many countries from all over the world and consequently examples with good and poor health care systems. A study on Sweden [12], a country with an advanced medical health care system, however, stated that risks are only found for long intervals and that the impact of short intervals may have been overestimated in other studies. From all those studies, we learn that it is important to include the outcome of the previous pregnancy in the analysis and to focus on several previous pregnancy outcomes when analyzing the effect of short IPIs on fetal losses. Therefore, we will follow this approach in our analysis about pregnancy loss in Rwanda.

Since 2000, Rwanda is experiencing a steady economic growth and after 2005 a rapid demographic and health transition [13, 14] thanks to the extension of access to reproductive health facilities [15]. The health service infrastructure, which was badly damaged during the civil war of the ninety-nineties, has been rebuilt to a large extent. At local level, community health centers are established and more than 45,000 community health care workers, male and female, have been trained to provide basic medical care and drugs and to give information on health matters. A third of those health care workers were trained in midwifery. The number of qualified medical staffs increased yet is still insufficient according to international standards: one medical doctor and one professional midwife per 16,500 and 23,400 inhabitants, respectively [16].

The government improved access to community health care also by introducing a community based insurance system. Today, more than 90% of the population participates in these *Mutuelles de Santé* "Health Mutualities" which give access to community level health services and, with additional payment, to a package of extra health care at district hospitals. This percentage of more than 90% explains an impressive increase in access to health care, given the fact that this percentage was only 7% in 2003. The prenatal checks and the costs of a normal delivery assisted by a nurse or midwife are covered by the basic health insurance schemes but exclude the 200 RwF per visit to a health center.

Yet, the health-seeking behavior among pregnant women still needs improvement although, according to the 2010 Demographic and Health Survey (DHS), less than two percent of the women did not have any antenatal medical test before the delivery. However, only 35 percent of them went for four antenatal checks, as recommended by the WHO. Most pregnant women got their first medical examination in the second trimester of their pregnancy and some even later [16–19].

2. Material and Method

The Demographic and Health Survey (DHS) is an internationally recognized data collection method that provides current and reliable data based on a national representative sample. Data from three successive Rwanda Demographic and Health Surveys (RDHS 2000, RDHS 2005, and RDHS 2010) were merged in this study to analyze the last pregnancy outcome of women within the DHS calendar periods of five years preceding the moment of interview.

Pregnancies and pregnancy outcomes that occurred in the eight months before the month of the interview were not included in our analysis to be sure that all pregnancies in the analysis had the same probability of ending in a pregnancy termination or a live birth after nine months. To identify the moment of the start of the last pregnancy, we used the detailed recording in the "calendar" of the DHS, which gives the pregnancy status for each month over a period of 59 months before the month of the interview. The nature and timing of the previous event are then defined. The exact months of all births, deaths, and pregnancy terminations are recorded in the DHS. The duration of the IPI is measured by subtracting the date of the previous pregnancy outcome from the date of the start of the last pregnancy.

The month of the previous outcome is registered at any time before the start of the last pregnancy. In total, 21532 women had at least one pregnancy outcome in the three reduced calendar periods before 2000, 2005, and 2010; for 3631 women, it was their first pregnancy (primigravida); for the other 17901 women, we calculated the date and type of the previous pregnancy outcome. In case of a long interpregnancy interval, this previous pregnancy outcome could have occurred before the five-year calendar period.

The DHS datasets enable the calculation of the exact date (in terms of month and year) of the events in the reproductive history of women in the sample if one combines answers to various questions in the questionnaire. We constructed Century Month Codes (CMC), the number of months elapsed since January 1900, of the pregnancy outcomes (pregnancy loss, infant death, and live birth) reported by the mothers to calculate the IPIs. In case of a live birth as last pregnancy outcome, the pregnancy was supposed to start 9 months before the CMC of the birth. In case of a fetal loss as last pregnancy outcome, the mother did report the duration of the pregnancy in months. Data from retrospective studies, like the Demographic and Health Surveys, are biased by errors due to memory lapses as the respondents have to report the number and date of the events in the past [20]. This is in particular the case when one asks for matters as pregnancy losses and induced abortions. Early pregnancy losses may not be noted or easily forgotten and induced abortions may not be reported as these are illegal in many societies. By focusing on the two last pregnancies of which the last one (and in many cases the previous as well) occurred during the calendar period, we reduced the risk of memory errors.

For our analysis, we calibrated a binary logistic regression model using the statistical package STATA 12. The dependent variable is the outcome of the last pregnancy (fetal loss coded as 1, live birth coded as 0). We checked whether a distinction between early and late losses gave different results, but this turned out not to be the case. To construct a more powerful model, we decided to take all fetal deaths together.

We defined the two main independent variables: length of the interpregnancy interval and previous pregnancy outcome as follows. Interpregnancy intervals (IPI) were calculated as the time between the outcome of the previous pregnancy that ended either in a pregnancy loss or live birth and the last conception. Short intervals are defined as shorter than 4 months or 4 up to 12 months after a previous pregnancy loss and shorter than 1 year or between 1 and 2 years after a live birth. A healthy interval after a live birth is an interval of at least two years and less than 5 years.

We categorized the live births of the previous pregnancy in two groups: infants that survived the first year of their life or infants that did not survive. The reason behind this categorization relates to the maternal depletion hypothesis and the quick return of the ovulation combined with the replacement strategy. In regard to the maternal depletion, the idea is to test whether a surviving breastfed infant will increase the depletion of maternal resources and therefore affect the survival of the next pregnancy that is conceived after a short IPI. Secondly, the death of the previous infant might be related to an unhealthy physiological status of the mother and the wish to quickly replace the infant, thus shortening the IPI.

We did not exclude multiple gestations, but we considered them as one birth. Subsequently, we constructed variables to represent the interaction between those two main independent variables in which we used different classifications for the IPI duration after the previous pregnancy outcomes. We tested for several confounding factors but, in the final model, included only four control variables that turned out to be of significance. The first is the inevitable biodemographic control variable age of the mother at conception which is an indicator for her physiological condition at the start of and during her pregnancy. We specified mother's age as a categorical variable to allow for nonlinear effects as we will focus on broad age categories and compare young (below the age of 21) and especially older mothers (over the age of 35) with women of a more optimal reproductive age. Age refers to the reproductive condition that contributes to a healthy pregnancy and the birth of a healthy infant. In particular, we want to test if older mothers have higher pregnancy loss risks compared to younger ones. The second control variable is the pregnancy wish. Question V228 of the DHS women's questionnaire asks the responding woman whether, at the time she became pregnant for the last pregnancy, she wished to become pregnant, she wished to wait until later, or she did not want to have any more children at all. Response categories included the following: wanting pregnancy then, wanting pregnancy later, wanting no more children, or unknown/vague answer. The latter category is used as a proxy for intended pregnancy losses together with the third included variable: place of residence that distinguishes between urban and rural residence.

The available dataset does not make a distinction between induced and spontaneous pregnancy losses, which is an omission seen in the different relations between the two types of abortions at the beginning of the IPI, length of the IPI, and pregnancy outcome found in other researches. However, we expect that Rwandan women will not easily indicate that they had an induced abortion as it is illegal, except when the physical health of the mother is in great danger. The study of Basinga and colleagues [21] estimated the rate of induced abortion in Rwanda in 2009 between 18 and 31 per 1,000 women in the 15–44-year-old group. Their study also revealed that the induced abortion rate was remarkably higher in the capital city Kigali compared to the situation in the provinces. In most African rural settings, induced abortion remains a taboo and social control in communities that watch over virginity as a core value, the reason why in particular rural women support legalization of abortion less compared to urban women [22]. As far as Rwanda is concerned, May et al. [23] stated that in the early nineties induced abortion did not occur traditionally in this country. For that reason, we expected that in case this situation changed during the last two decades abortions will be chiefly an urban phenomenon. We tried to control for it by including place of residence (urban versus rural) in the analysis. The percentages of unknown/vague answers in our dataset were, respectively, 27.9 and 23.6 for urban and rural women.

TABLE 1: Descriptive statistics: last pregnancy outcomes in percentages and in total numbers (pooled data from DHS 2000, DHS 2005, and DHS 2010).

Variable names	Latest pregnancy outcome (N = 21532)	
	Pregnancy loss (%)	Total number
First pregnancy (primigravida)	3.3	3631
Previous pregnancy outcome and IPI		
Pregnancy loss		
IPI ≤3 months	10.6	161
IPI ≥4 months and ≤12 months	7.9	381
IPI ≥13 months and ≤24 months	8.0	217
IPI ≥25 months	4.7	149
Live birth (child died in infancy)		
IPI ≤12 months	3.3	662
IPI ≥13 months and ≤24 months	2.6	582
IPI ≥25 months	5.5	513
Surviving live birth		
IPI ≤12 months	2.3	1594
IPI ≥13 months and ≤24 months	2.7	5580
IPI ≥60 months	7.6	1314
IPI ≥24 and ≤59 months	3.5	6740
Age of mother at the latest conception		
20 years and younger	2.7	2075
36 years and older	6.8	4780
21 to 35 years	2.7	14677
Pregnancy timing		
Mistimed (later)	1.7	4116
Unwanted (no more)	1.4	2786
Unknown/vague answer	8.7	5246
Wanted (then)	2.2	9368
Type of place of residence		
Urban	4.2	4125
Rural	3.5	17407
Year of interview		
2000	4.1	6383
2005	3.6	6816
2010	3.3	8333
Total	3.6	21532

Sources: RDHS 2000, RDHS 2005, and RDHS 2010.

Finally, we included the year of the interview to check for changes over time in reproductive health: notably, the extent of the possible reduction of fetal mortality. Table 1 gives the descriptive statistics of the research population.

3. Results and Discussion

The results presented in Table 1 illustrate that many Rwandan women still have to deal with pregnancy losses, the death of an infant, and unwanted pregnancies: 36 out of 1000 last pregnancies in our sample population ended in a pregnancy loss. Among the women with at least two pregnancies, 15 percent mourned a fatal outcome of the previous pregnancy: five percent had a pregnancy loss and nearly ten percent got a child that died in infancy. The results indicate also that the percentages of pregnancies ending in a pregnancy loss are the highest after an IPI shorter than 24 months that started after a pregnancy loss. Higher percentages of pregnancy loss than the mean of 3.6 per cent were found after a live-born infant that died in its infancy and an IPI of more than two years and after a surviving live birth and a very long IPI (>60 months).

The descriptive statistics in Table 1 show a modest decline of the rate of fetal losses during the period under study. For the three consecutive research periods, the rate of pregnancy loss diminished from 41 out of 1000 pregnancies (1996–2000) to 36 (2001–2005) and finally to 33 in the most recent period 2006–2010. It is difficult to assess if the total number of reported pregnancy losses in the three DHSs used in this study, 36 per 1000 pregnancies, is in line with expectations or not. It is a result of measurements over a rather diffuse period of time. The frequency fits within an indication given in medical literature that states that the number of fetal losses in the month after conception is high but that after a gestation of 8 weeks the loss is about 3 percent [21]. This could mean that women in Rwanda did not mention losses that occurred in the first one or two months of a pregnancy, when they were not fully aware of being pregnant. The early pregnancy losses reported in the DHS are probably underestimated as in poor countries the number of stillbirths (after a gestation of 28 weeks) is higher compared to that of rich countries and the stillbirth rate in countries in the central part of Sub-Saharan Africa varies between 25 and 40 or more per 1000 births [24]. With the number of early miscarriages added, the final rate must be even higher.

Women who were pregnant for the first time reported the highest percentage of wanted pregnancies (nearly 60%, see Table 2). Of all last pregnancies by the other women, only 40 percent were wanted at that time, while more than a third were unwanted or the mother gave an unclear answer (or answer not known). The cross tabulation presented in Table 2 shows that after a pregnancy loss or the loss of an infant a large portion of the women want to replace this loss. The percentages of wanted pregnancies extend the average of 40 percent. Very low numbers of wanted pregnancies are found among women who became pregnant within two years after the birth of the previous child that survived the first year of its life. Those two groups of women had liked to become pregnant later in time (indicated by 40 and 31%, resp.).

A large portion of the women became pregnant again before the recommended time (by WHO) for recovery was over. From the women whose previous pregnancy ended with a fetal loss, 43 percent were expecting a child again within half a year. For women who had a live-born child that died afterwards in infancy, 71 percent were pregnant again within two years after the last delivery, which could point at a replacement effect or at a lack of protection against pregnancy. For women whose child survived the first year of its life, this percentage was much lower (47%). This group

TABLE 2: Wanted the last pregnancy (in %) according to previous pregnancy outcome and IPI duration.

Prev. outc.	IPI	Vague	Unwanted	Mistimed	Wanted		Tot. no.
Primigr.	—	19.6	8.3	13.4	58.8	100.0	3631
Fetal loss	<3	24.8	14.3	14.9	46.0	100.0	161
	4 ≤ 12	20.2	12.9	12.9	54.9	100.0	381
	13–24	37.3	14.2	5.3	43.1	100.0	225
	25+	28.9	14.1	4.0	53.0	100.0	149
Live born died	≤12	23.9	9.8	13.7	52.6	100.0	662
	13–24	27.0	10.5	9.6	52.9	100.0	582
	≥25	31.6	11.8	6.3	49.7	100.0	513
Surviving live born	<12	28.4	11.2	39.7	20.7	100.0	1594
	13–24	21.1	13.5	31.5	34.0	100.0	5580
	25–59	25.1	15.2	14.0	45.7	100.0	6740
	60+	38.8	16.5	2.2	42.5	100.0	1314
Total		24.4	12.9	19.0	43.5	99.9	21532

Sources: RDHS 2000, RDHS 2005, and RDHS 2010.

of women is probably temporarily subfecund due to a longer amenorrhea period caused by lactation.

The constant (Table 3) reflects the risk of a pregnancy loss for the reference category: rural women in 2000, in age category of 21–35 years at the time of the last conception, whose last pregnancy was wanted and started after a healthy IPI (25–59 months), and whose previous pregnancy resulted in a child that survived its infancy. The estimate of the risk of experiencing a pregnancy termination for these women is very low (2%). The other variables Exp(β) give the odds ratios for women in the categories that deviate from the reference category.

Linking the risk of a pregnancy termination with both the outcome of the previous pregnancy and the length of the IPI (interaction variables) shows significant deviations from the risk estimated for the reference group: all except one point at a higher risk. The highest odds are found for women who became pregnant shortly after a previous pregnancy loss. Women who conceived again within 3 months after the previous pregnancy loss are 3.68 times more likely to lose the next pregnancy than the reference group with a healthy interval. The odds ratio is 2.648 for those that waited 4–12 months and even women who waited 12–14 months were almost twice as likely to lose the next pregnancy. Women with an IPI of more than two years after a previous fetal loss had a lower risk compared to the reference group, but the association is not significant. The higher odds of pregnancy loss for all groups with a previous pregnancy loss suggest that some women are prone to repeated losses, regardless of IPI duration. Repeated or recurrent pregnancy loss is phenomenon that puzzles medical experts like gynecologist already for decades and that is probably associated with more than genetic factors of the woman alone [25, 26].

After a live birth, regardless of whether the newborn survived its infancy or not, the likelihood of a pregnancy loss after an IPI considered as unhealthy (<2 years) is not higher compared to the reference group with a recommended

IPI duration. For the mother that became pregnant within, respectively, one to two years after the previous birth, the signs of the coefficients are negative but only significant for women whose infant stayed alive and conceived within one year. Any pregnancy after a live birth seems to prepare for a successful next pregnancy, regardless of the interpregnancy interval.

This mechanism vanishes after some years, as an IPI of more than 5 years results in a substantial higher likelihood of a pregnancy loss (1.6 times more likely). This result is found in other studies as well. The risk of a pregnancy loss for mothers who are pregnant for the first time is of the same magnitude (1.5 times more likely). The physiological regression hypothesis states that after a very long IPI the body of a women has lost the beneficial physiological adaptations in her reproductive system that occur after a pregnancy [10, 12]. Her condition then resembles that of a primigravida.

According to the literature, a higher age at conception relates to lower fecundity and consequently longer IPI. Higher age is associated as well with physiological problems of the mother. This is reflected in the higher likelihood of a pregnancy loss (2.3 times more likely) for women who were older than 35 years when they became pregnant. The positive coefficients found for urban women and for women who gave a vague answer or did not answer the question on whether they wanted the last pregnancy could point at the occurrence of induced pregnancy terminations. As induced abortions are prohibited and a taboo, women who had an illegal abortion will probably answer evasively when asked for their pregnancy timing. The higher risk of pregnancy losses among urban women in our sample fits in with research findings by Basinga and colleagues [21] who calculated that induced abortions occur more frequently in the capital city of Kigali compared to other regions of Rwanda.

The finding that women who explicitly declared that the last pregnancy was not wanted have a significant lower

TABLE 3: Binary logistic coefficients on the risk of pregnancy loss in Rwanda (pooled data 2000, 2005, and 2010).

Log likelihood = −3038.95	LR χ^2 (19)			642.2
	Prob. > χ^2			0.000
	Pseudo $R2$			0.096
Variable names	N = 21532	B	P > z	Exp(B)
Previous pregnancy outcome and IPI				
Previous live birth and IPI ≥25 and ≤59 months (Ref.)	6,740			
Pregnancy termination				
IPI ≥3 months	161	**1.303**	* * *	**3.680**
IPI ≥4 months and ≤12 months	381	**0.974**	**	**2.648**
IPI ≥13 months and ≤24 months	225	**0.663**	*	**1.940**
IPI ≥25 months	149	0.102		1.107
Previous infant death				
IPI ≤12 months	662	−0.014		0.986
IPI ≥13 months and ≤24 months	582	−0.401		0.670
IPI ≥25 months	513	0.257		1.292
Previous surviving live birth				
IPI ≤12 months	1,594	**−0.410**	*	**0.664**
IPI ≥13 months and ≤24 months	5,580	−0.083		0.920
IPI ≥60 months	1,314	**0.494**	**	**1.639**
Primigravida	3,631	**0.400**	*	**1.492**
Age of mother at the latest conception				
21 to 35 years (ref.)	14,677			
20 years and younger	2,075	−0.199		0.819
36 years and older	4,780	**0.843**	* * *	**2.323**
Pregnancy timing				
Wanted (ref.)	9,368			
Untimed (later)	4,116	−0.108		0.898
Unwanted (no more)	2,786	**−0.751**	* * *	**0.472**
Unknown/vague answer	5,262	**1.308**	* * *	**3.698**
Place of residence				
Rural (ref.)	17,407			
Urban	4,125	**0.217**	*	**1.243**
Year of interview				
2000 (ref.)	6,383			
2005	6,816	−0.117		0.889
2010	8,333	**−0.259**	**	**0.772**
Constant		**−4.004**	* * *	**0.018**

Significance: * <0.05, ** <0.01, and *** 0.001.
Sources: RDHS 2000, RDHS 2005, and RDHS 2010.

risk of losing the next pregnancy gives food for thought. Maybe these are highly fecund women who become pregnant easily and therefore more often unwanted, and who do not encounter pregnancy problems.

We remark that the likelihood of a pregnancy termination decreased significantly between 2000 and 2010. For 2005, the sign of the coefficient (β) is negative, but the decrease is not significant. In 2010, however, the decrease is significant. Further analyses, not shown here, showed that this decrease pertained to late pregnancy loss only. This may be seen as an indication that improved health-seeking behaviour among pregnant women in particular during the second half of their pregnancy contributed to less pregnancy losses.

4. Conclusion and Policy Recommendations

The first important result of our analyses is that one needs to take the previous pregnancy outcome into account when estimating the effects of IPIs on the risk of a pregnancy loss. The second main finding is that negative outcomes (in terms of a higher risk of recurrent pregnancy loss) were found for IPIs up to 24 months after a prior pregnancy loss, a period four times as long as the recommended healthy IPI of only 6 months. In contrast, an IPI shorter than 2 years after a live birth does not seem to increase significantly the risk of a pregnancy loss. We are aware that a pregnancy loss is not the only possible adverse pregnancy outcome. Shorter IPIs

TABLE 4: (a) Results from other studies concerning the effect of IPI duration on pregnancy loss after a previous spontaneous or induced termination. (b) Results from studies concerning the effect of IPI duration on pregnancy outcomes.

(a)

Study period/country	Sample	Effect of IPI	Reference category for statistical analysis	Controlled for
Wong et al. 2015 [6] USA (EAGeR trial) period 2006–2012	724 pregnant women with 1-2 prior pregnancy losses	No association between adverse pregnancy outcomes including pregnancy loss and IPI (<3 months or > 3 months)	Unknown	Demographic and reproductive history characteristics
Makhlouf et al. 2014 [7] USA, period 2003–2008	Nulliparous women 7681 primigravida 1240 with 1-2 previous spontaneous pregnancy losses (SAB) 817 with a previous induced abortion (IAB)	On fetal/neonatal death and other adverse outcomes after SAB and IAB No statistically significant difference for various IPI (<6, 6–12, >12 months) on risk of fetal loss and neonatal death	Primigravida Women with one previous SAB and IPI < 6 months	Maternal age, race, education, smoking, marital status, BMI, and use of vitamins C and E
DaVanzo et al. 2012 [4] Bangladesh (Matlab), period 1977–2008	9214 women with a miscarriage (spontaneous abortion prior to gestation of 28 weeks)	The shorter the IPI following a miscarriage is, the more likely the next pregnancy results in a live birth No significant effects of IPI duration on risks of a stillbirth Relative risk of a subsequent miscarriage increases with IPI duration	Women with a previous miscarriage and IPI of 6–12 months	Maternal age, education, gravidity, and calendar year
Love et al. 2010 [5] Scottish hospital data, period 1981–2000	30,937 women with a miscarriage in first recorded pregnancy	On miscarriage, ectopic pregnancy, IAB, and stillbirth Women with IPI < 6 months had less likely a miscarriage, highest sign Risk for women with IPI > 24 months No significant effect of IPI duration on risk of stillbirth	Women with a miscarriage and IPI of 6–12 months	Maternal age, socioeconomic status, year of first conception, and smoking
Conde-Agudelo et al. 2005 [9] Latin America period 1985–2002	258,108 women with a previous abortion	On fetal death and other adverse outcomes No significant difference of effect of IPI on fetal death or on neonatal death	Women with an IPI of 18–23 months	Maternal age, parity, education, smoking, marital status, BMI, year of delivery, hypertension, nbr antenatal checks, hospital type, and geographical area

(b)

IPI = interpregnancy interval, SAB = spontaneous abortion, IAB = induced abortion, and BMI = Body Mass Index.

Study	Sample	Effect of IPI	Reference category	Controlled for
Conde-Agudelo et al. 2006 [3] Rich and poor countries from all over the world	Meta-analysis	On various adverse perinatal outcomes Less clear is the association between pregnancy spacing and the risk of fetal (and neonatal) death Curves suggest that IPI < 6 months and IPI > 50 months are associated with increased risks	Differs per included study	Various factors Not standard for previous pregnancy outcome

(b) Continued.

Study	Sample	Effect of IPI	Reference category	Controlled for
DaVanzo et al. 2007 [11] Bangladesh (Matlab) period 1982–2002	66759 pregnancies including multiple births of 28540 women	On various pregnancy outcomes. An IPI < 6 months after a live birth lead to a 7.5 fold increase for miscarriages, and 1.6 fold increase for stillbirths. An IPI >75 months showed a less increased risk on fetal losses. After a fetal loss a subsequent same fetal loss regardless of the IPI duration. Highest OR on a miscarriage after IPI < 6 months after a life birth	Women with live birth after IPI of 27–50 months	Socioeconomic status, maternal age, education both spouses, religion, and calendar year
Stephansson et al. 2003 [12] Sweden, period 1983–1997	410,021 women with two deliveries	Stillbirths and early neonatal death. Previous reproductive history and maternal characteristics substantially confounded the association between IPI and risks of stillbirth. Risks are only found for long intervals. Role of short intervals may have been overestimated in previous studies	IPI of 12–35 months	Outcome of first pregnancy (*stillbirth/early neonatal death, preterm delivery,* etc.) Maternal age, education, presence of partner, country of origin, diabetes, hypertension, period of delivery, and smoking

than two years after a live birth do not give higher risks of a pregnancy loss, but they will affect other pregnancy outcomes such as preterm birth, low birth weight, low Apgar scores, and a higher neonatal death.

We found clear indications for negative effects of the replacement mechanism after the loss of a pregnancy. The replacement wish after a fetal death leads to shorter IPIs and therefore to a higher risk of another pregnancy loss [12]. Finally, the results of our study confirm the physiological regression hypothesis: a higher risk of a fetal death when IPIs are longer than 5 years. Also older women have a higher likelihood of a pregnancy loss compared to younger ones.

Our results are partially in line with the ones from DaVanzo and colleagues in Bangladesh [1, 11] based also on a general sample of women with all types of prior pregnancy outcomes. To avoid a higher risk of a next miscarriage or stillbirth also in Bangladesh, women should wait longer than the recommended 6 months (up to 15 months) to become pregnant again after a former pregnancy loss. The researchers found a significant increased risk of a pregnancy loss after a live birth and an IPI < 6 months. For longer IPI durations up to 74 months after a live birth, no significant higher risks of a pregnancy loss were found. After a duration of 74 months, the risk was again significantly higher.

Based on the results of this study on Bangladesh and ours on Rwanda, one could conclude that, in societies without an advanced health care system, the WHO recommendations concerning spacing after a fetal loss still count. Workers in the health care system should advise women, even if they are eager to become pregnant again, to take actions to prevent a quick new pregnancy and wait even longer than a year to become pregnant again.

The improvements in the Rwandan health care system between 2000 and 2010 and in particular the increased access to this system contributed to a lower pregnancy loss frequency. Probably, the increased antenatal checks during the last pregnancy period had an impact, as the significant decrease in pregnancy losses between 2000 and 2010 resulted in particular in fewer late fetal losses (after a pregnancy duration of 20 weeks). With a policy that recommends to women an IPI of at least a year to two years after a fetal death and more early pregnancy visits to the community health facility, a decrease in an early fetal death could be achieved as well.

Conflict of Interests

The authors declare that there is no conflict of interests regarding the publication of this paper.

Acknowledgment

The authors thank the William and Flora Hewlett Foundation and The Netherlands Organization for Scientific Research for their financial support (Grant no. W07 40 202 00).

References

[1] J. DaVanzo, L. Hale, A. Razzaque, and M. Rahman, "The effects of pregnancy spacing on infant and child mortality in Matlab, Bangladesh: how they vary by the type of pregnancy outcome that began the interval," *Population Studies*, vol. 62, no. 2, pp. 131–154, 2008.

[2] E. M. McClure, M. Nalubamba-Phiri, and R. L. Goldenberg, "Stillbirth in developing countries," *International Journal of Gynecology and Obstetrics*, vol. 94, no. 2, pp. 82–90, 2006.

[3] A. Conde-Agudelo, A. Rosas-Bermúdez, and A. C. Kafury-Goeta, "Birth spacing and risk of adverse perinatal outcomes: a meta-analysis," *The Journal of the American Medical Association*, vol. 295, no. 15, pp. 1809–1823, 2006.

[4] J. DaVanzo, L. Hale, and M. Rahman, "How long after a miscarriage should women wait before becoming pregnant again? Multivariate analysis of cohort data from Matlab, Bangladesh," *BMJ Open*, vol. 2, no. 4, Article ID e001591, 2012.

[5] E. R. Love, S. Bhattacharya, N. C. Smith, and S. Bhattacharya, "Effect of interpregnancy interval on outcomes of pregnancy after miscarriage: retrospective analysis of hospital episode statistics in Scotland," *British Medical Journal*, vol. 341, Article ID c3967, 2010.

[6] L. F. Wong, K. C. Schliep, R. M. Silver et al., "The effect of a very short interpregnancy interval and pregnancy outcomes following a previous pregnancy loss," *American Journal of Obstetrics & Gynecology*, vol. 212, no. 3, pp. 375.e1–375.e11, 2015.

[7] M. A. Makhlouf, R. G. Clifton, J. M. Roberts et al., "Adverse pregnancy outcomes among women with prior spontaneous or induced abortions," *American Journal of Perinatology*, vol. 31, no. 9, pp. 765–772, 2014.

[8] J. Frederik Frøen, S. J. Gordijn, H. Abdel-Aleem et al., "Making stillbirths count, making numbers talk—issues in data collection for stillbirths," *BMC Pregnancy and Childbirth*, vol. 9, article 58, 2009.

[9] A. Conde-Agudelo, J. M. Belizán, R. Breman, S. C. Brockman, and A. Rosas-Bermudez, "Effect of the interpregnancy interval after an abortion on maternal and perinatal health in Latin America," *International Journal of Gynecology and Obstetrics*, vol. 89, no. 1, pp. S34–S40, 2005.

[10] A. Conde-Agudelo, A. Rosas-Bermúdez, F. Castaño, and M. H. Norton, "Effects of birth spacing on maternal, perinatal, infant, and child health: a systematic review of causal mechanisms," *Studies in Family Planning*, vol. 43, no. 2, pp. 93–114, 2012.

[11] J. DaVanzo, L. Hale, A. Razzaque, and M. Rahman, "Effects of interpregnancy interval and outcome of the preceding pregnancy on pregnancy outcomes in Matlab, Bangladesh," *BJOG: An International Journal of Obstetrics and Gynaecology*, vol. 114, no. 9, pp. 1079–1087, 2007.

[12] O. Stephansson, P. W. Dickman, and S. Cnattingius, "The influence of interpregnancy interval on the subsequent risk of stillbirth and early neonatal death," *Obstetrics & Gynecology*, vol. 102, no. 1, pp. 101–108, 2003.

[13] D. Malunda and S. S. Musana, "Rwanda case study on economic transformation," Report for the African Centre for Economic Transformation, Institute of Policy Analysis and Research, Kigali, Rwanda, 2012.

[14] UNDP, *Human Development Report*, United Nations Development Program, New York, NY, USA, 2013.

[15] E. M. Leahy, "Rwanda: Dramatic Uptake in Contraceptive Use Spurs Unprecedented Fertility Decline," 2011, http://www.newsecuritybeat.org/2011/11/building-commitment-to-family-planning-rwanda/.

[16] A. Binagwaho, R. Hartwig, D. Ingeri, and A. Makaka, *Mutual Health Insurance and Its Contribution to Improving Child Health In Rwanda*, Passauer Diskussionspapiere: Volkswirtschaftliche Reihe no. V-66-12, Ministry of Health, Family Planning Strategic Plan, Kigali, Rwanda, 2012.

[17] Office National de la Population (ONAPO) and Macro International, *Enquete Demographique et de Sante (Demographic and Health Survey) (DHS 2000), Rwanda 2000*, Ministère de la Sante, Office National de la Population and ORC Macro, Calverton, Md, USA, 2001.

[18] National Institute of Statistics of Rwanda (INSR) and ORC Macro, *(DHS 2005). Rwanda Demographic and Health Survey 2005*, National Institute of Statistics of Rwanda, ORC Macro, Calverton, Md, USA, 2006.

[19] National Institute of Statistics of Rwanda (INSR) and ORC Macro, *(DHS 2010). Rwanda Demographic and Health Survey 2010*, National Institute of Statistics of Rwanda, ORC Macro, Calverton, Md, USA, 2010.

[20] N. Auriat, "Who forgets? An analysis of memory effects in a retrospective survey on migration history," *European Journal of Population*, vol. 7, no. 4, pp. 311–342, 1991.

[21] P. Basinga, A. M. Moore, S. D. Singh, E. E. Carlin, F. Birungi, and F. Ngabo, "Abortion incidence and post-abortion care in Rwanda," *Studies in Family Planning*, vol. 43, no. 1, pp. 11–20, 2012.

[22] F. E. Okonofua, C. Odimegwu, B. Aina, P. H. Daru, and A. Johnson, *Women's Experiences of Unwanted Pregnancy and Induced Abortion in Nigeria*, The Population Council, The Robert H. Ebert Program, 1996.

[23] J. F. May, M. Mukamanzi, and M. Vekemans, "Family planning in Rwanda, status and prospects," *Studies in Family Planning*, vol. 21, no. 1, pp. 20–32, 1990.

[24] J. L. Simpson and S. A. Carson, *Genetic and Nongenetic Causes of Pregnancy Loss*, The Global Library of Women's Medicine, 2013.

[25] J. Schneider, "Repeated pregnancy loss," *Clinical Obstetrics and Gynecology*, vol. 16, no. 1, pp. 120–133, 1973.

[26] K. A. Rao and J. R. Pillai, "Recurrent pregnancy loss," *Journal of the Indian Medical Association*, vol. 104, no. 8, pp. 458–461, 2006.

9

Predictive Value of Middle Cerebral Artery to Uterine Artery Pulsatility Index Ratio in Hypertensive Disorders of Pregnancy

Prashanth Adiga, Indumathi Kantharaja, Shripad Hebbar, Lavanya Rai, Shyamala Guruvare, and Anjali Mundkur

Department of Obstetrics and Gynaecology, Kasturba Medical College, Manipal University, Manipal 576104, India

Correspondence should be addressed to Shripad Hebbar; drshripadhebbar@yahoo.co.in

Academic Editor: Padma Murthi

Aims and Objectives. (i) To determine the predictive value of cerebrouterine (CU) ratio (middle cerebral artery to uterine artery pulsatility index, MCA/UT PI) in assessing perinatal outcome among hypertensive disorders of pregnancy. (ii) To compare between CU ratio and CP ratio (MCA/Umbilical artery PI) as a predictor of adverse perinatal outcome. *Methods.* A prospective observational study was done in a tertiary medical college hospital, from September 2012 to August 2013. One hundred singleton pregnancies complicated by hypertension peculiar to pregnancy were enrolled. Both CU and CP ratios were estimated. The perinatal outcomes were studied. *Results.* Both cerebrouterine and cerebroplacental ratios had a better negative predictive value in predicting adverse perinatal outcome. However, both CU and CP ratios when applied together were able to predict adverse outcomes better than individual ratios. The sensitivity, specificity, positive predictive value, and the negative predictive values for an adverse neonatal outcome with CU ratio were 61.3%, 70.3%, 56%, and 78.9%, respectively, compared to 42%, 57.5%, 62%, and 76% as with CP ratio. *Conclusion.* Cerebrouterine ratio and cerebroplacental ratio were complementary to each other in predicting the adverse perinatal outcomes. Individually, both ratios were reassuring for favorable perinatal outcome with high negative predictive value.

1. Introduction

Hypertension peculiar to pregnancy (preeclampsia and gestational hypertension) is a pregnancy specific syndrome characterized by reduced organ perfusion secondary to vasospasm and endothelial pathology. There are several hall mark studies which have already established the two arms of the fetal circulation (middle cerebral artery pulsatility index and umbilical artery pulsatility index) both in normal and compromised fetuses. We felt that the actual problem starts from uterine vessels and finally the changes are reflected in the cerebral circulation. We wanted to compare whether alterations in uterocerebral ratio reflect the flow dynamics better than umbilical-cerebral ratio. The vascular changes in these conditions can be reflected in Doppler studies well in advance compared to the conventional antenatal tests of fetal well-being. The brain sparing effect is maximum 2 or 3 weeks before the occurrence of late decelerations on cardiotocogram, suggesting that patient with a high risk for unfavorable pregnancy outcome may have alteration in the blood flow in the middle cerebral artery 2-3 weeks prior to the delivery [1, 2]. As placental insufficiency occurs, several changes occur in fetal circulation, culminating with the brain sparing, characterized by blood flow redistribution with priority to important organs like brain and heart adrenals at the expense of spleen, kidney, and peripheral circulation.

Cerebroplacental (CP) ratio is a well-established predictor of unfavorable pregnancy outcomes, while cerebrouterine (CU) ratio is fairly new ratio of vascular impedance between MCA and uterine arteries, which has not been commonly evaluated [3]. The intent of this study was to know which of the two parameters would help us to predict the perinatal outcome better. Our hypothesis was, therefore, that MCA/uterine artery PI ratio could have a better predictive value for unfavorable outcome than the CP ratio.

TABLE 1: Modified Tchirikov Composite score for perinatal outcome.

Outcome	0	1	2
Birth weight	>90th centile	10th–90th centile	<10th centile
Perinatal death	Absent	—	Present
APGAR	>7	5–7	<5
Respiratory problems	Grunting	Ventilator support	Hyaline membrane disease
Acidemia	>7.2	7.1-7.2	<7.2
Seizure	Absent	—	Present

>/=2: unfavourable score, <2: favourable score.

2. Methodology

This was a prospective observational study, which was carried out over a period from September 2012 to September 2013, in the Department of Obstetrics and Gynecology, in tertiary care center. Eligible participants were those women with singleton pregnancy diagnosed with "hypertension peculiar to pregnancy" (preeclampsia and gestational hypertension), after 26 weeks of gestation. Women with history of chronic hypertension, chronic renal disease, diabetes mellitus, and secondary hypertension due to immunological disease such as SLE and APLA syndrome and women in active labor or those with premature rupture of membranes were excluded. Serial scans by transabdominal route were performed for interval growth and Doppler parameters (umbilical, middle cerebral artery, and uterine artery Doppler). The last Doppler values before the delivery were considered for the study. The biometric parameters were plotted on a customized growth chart to look for any evidence of intrauterine growth restriction. All the ultrasound scans were performed by the first author. Doppler ultrasound was performed as soon as the diagnosis of preeclampsia/gestational hypertension was made. The procedures followed were in accord with the ethical standards of the committee on human experimentation of our institution. Written informed consent was taken from all patients after hospital ethical committee approval.

Preeclampsia was defined as a pregnancy specific syndrome characterized by blood pressure > 140/90 mm of Hg after 20 weeks of gestation with proteinuria > 300 mg/24 hrs or persistent 1+ random dipstick proteinuria and was considered to be severe when associated with blood pressure > 160/110 mm, thrombocytopenia (platelets less than 100,000/μL), renal insufficiency (creatinine greater than 1.1 mg/dL or doubling of baseline), liver involvement (serum transaminases levels twice the normal), cerebral involvement (headache, visual disturbances, persistent nausea or vomiting), or pulmonary edema. Gestational hypertension was defined as blood pressure > 140/90 mm of Hg after 20-week period of gestation with no proteinuria, and blood pressure returns to normal in less than 12 weeks postpartum [4].

Fetal hypoxia was said to exist antenatally, whenever there was absent end diastolic flow or reversal of flow in the umbilical artery, suboptimal NST, and intranatally, when there was thick meconium staining of the amniotic fluid and ominous cardiotocographic changes (persistent and prolonged bradycardia, loss of beat to beat variability, etc.).

Scan was done in recruited patients using Philips HD 11XE machine using 3–5 MHz transabdominal probe.

Doppler velocity of uterine artery was recorded at the point at which they crossed over the external iliac artery cranial to crossing of iliac artery. Mean of the PI of both uterine arteries was taken for ratio estimation. The middle cerebral artery was located by color Doppler in a transverse view of fetal brain. The pulsed Doppler sample gate was placed on the vessel about 1 cm of the origin of MCA from the circle of Willis towards lateral edge of orbit. The Umbilical artery PI was obtained from free loop of umbilical cord during fetal apnea. Cerebrouterine ratio (middle cerebral artery to uterine artery PI ratio) and cerebroplacental ratio (middle cerebral artery to umbilical artery PI ratio) were estimated. Cerebrouterine (CU) ratio was plotted on the chart; < 5_{th} percentile was considered as decreased or abnormal [3]. Cerebroplacental (CP) ratio was considered as abnormal or to have brain sparing effect, when ratio was <1.08. Patients were followed up till delivery and perinatal outcome was analyzed [3]. The abnormal outcomes studied were small for gestational age, low APGAR, preterm delivery, hyaline membrane disease, assisted ventilation, academia, and overall perinatal outcome.

Table 1 shows the composite score used to calculate the overall perinatal outcome, as more than one adverse outcome was present in many cases. Basic score values of 0, 1, or 2 were assigned to the five outcome variables (birth weight, perinatal death, APGAR at 5 min, respiratory problems, acidemia, and seizure), and the basic score values were summed to obtain an "outcome score" which was called as Modified Tchirikov Composite score for perinatal outcome [5]. This score was constructed after the data had been collected for each new born before further statistical evaluation of overall perinatal outcome. Neonates with scores of more than 2 made up the group of compromised neonates. The data collected was analyzed using Statistical Package for Social Sciences (SPSS, version 16). The validity of the predictive values was analyzed using sensitivity, specificity, and positive and negative predictive values and Chi-square test was used for testing statistical significance. P value < 0.05 was considered significant.

Patange and Goel [6] have reported that the cerebroumbilical ratio in normal pregnancy is 1.77 ± 0.43. They noticed that this ratio is reduced to 1.47 (difference of 0.3) when there was placental insufficiency. Based on this information, we calculated sample size with the formula

$$n = \frac{2\left(z_{1-\alpha/2} + z_{1-\beta}\right)^2}{\left(\left(\mu_0 - \mu_1\right)/\sigma\right)^2}, \qquad (1)$$

TABLE 2: Patient profile ($n = 95$).

Maternal age in years	28.45 ± 4.665 (20–41)
Gestation in weeks at examination	33.82 ± 3.473 (26–39)
Gestation in weeks at delivery	35.47 ± 2.752 (27–40)
Uterine artery pulsatility index	1.02 ± 0.496 (0.35–2.7)
Middle cerebral artery pulsatility index	1.52 ± 0.661 (0.6–6)
Umbilical artery pulsatility index	1.09 ± 0.582 (0.30–3.7)

Values are given as mean ± standard deviation (range).

where $z_{1-\alpha/2}$ is equal to 1.96 (for $\alpha = 0.05$, i.e., type I error), $z_{1-\beta}$ is equal to 0.84 (for $\beta = 0.20$, i.e., type II error), $\mu_0 - \mu_1$ is equal to the difference of means (0.3 as in quoted study), and σ is the standard deviation. This equation will give expected power of 0.80. Accordingly, the sample size required is 32 and our sample size of 100 is far more than adequate.

3. Results

The patient profile has been described in Table 2. There were a total of 100 cases at initial recruitment (72 primigravidae and 28 multigravidae), gestational hypertension was seen in 64 patients, and 36 had preeclampsia. Out of these 100 cases, 5 cases were lost for followup; thus, perinatal outcome was analysed in 95 patients. Each outcome measure and its relation to cerebrouterine ratio and cerebroplacental ratio were analysed. As prematurity and intrauterine growth restriction can be confounding factors for NICU admission and hyperbilirubinemia; these outcomes were neither correlated with Doppler findings nor were they considered for composite scoring. Out of 95 babies, 48 (50.5%) babies required NICU admission for more than 24 hours. There were 53/95 (55.7%) premature babies of which 34/95 (68%) were below 34 weeks of gestation. Small for gestational age (SGA) neonates were 33/95 (34.7%). Low APGAR (less than 7 at 5 minutes of birth) was seen in 16/95 babies (16.8%), 23/95 babies (24.2%) required assisted respiration, acidemia was present in 10/95 babies (10.5%), hyperbilirubinemia was present in 33/95 (34.7%), and neonatal seizures were seen in only 1/95 (1.05%). Perinatal mortality was present in 5/95 (5.2%) cases of which one was intrauterine fetal death.

When CU and CP ratios were compared, in abnormal CU ratio group, SGA (47.4% versus 26.3%), acidemia (18.4% versus 5.3%), fetal hypoxia (50% versus 22.8%), low APGAR (26.3% versus 10.5%), and adverse perinatal outcome (50% versus 21.1%) were present, which was statistically significant (Table 3). In abnormal CP ratio group, SGA (52.4% versus 29.3%), acidemia (23.8% versus 6.8%), low APGAR (42.7% versus 9.5%), and perinatal outcome (61.9% versus 24.3%) were present, which was also statistically significant. This shows that both of these ratios are fairly accurate in predicting adverse neonatal outcomes. However, CU ratio was better in predicting fetal hypoxia than CP ratio.

Table 4 shows overall performance of CU and CP ratio in predicting perinatal outcome. In the prediction of SGA by CU ratio, the specificity was 67.7%, but negative predictive value

(NPV) was higher (73.7%). In prediction of poor APGAR, the NPV of the test was good with 89.5%, whereas the sensitivity and specificity was comparatively lower (i.e., 62.5% and 64.6% resp.). Even for the prediction of the need for assisted ventilation, the NPV of the test was higher (80.7%). In 94.7%, if the cerebrouterine ratio was normal, less likelihood of acidemia was seen. In predicting overall adverse perinatal outcome, specificity was 70.3% and NPV was 78.9%, with low sensitivity and positive predictive value.

In the prediction of SGA with CP ratio, the specificity was higher (83.9%) and NPV was 70.3%. The test had a good specificity of 84.8% and NPV of 90.5%, in ruling out poor APGARs. In prediction of need for assisted respiration, specificity and NPV were higher. In overall prediction of adverse perinatal outcomes, specificity was 87.5% and negative predictive value was 75.7%, indicating that if CP ratio is normal, the likelihood of adverse perinatal outcome is less.

Table 5 shows perinatal outcome for four possible combinations of normal and abnormal CU and CP ratios. It is interesting to note that when both ratios were normal, 76.9% had favorable outcome and when both were abnormal, 81.2% had adverse outcome. Thus it can be inferred that both ratios are complementary to each other in predicting perinatal outcome.

4. Discussion

The prevalence of preeclampsia was more in primigravida in our study as is also seen in general. Nulliparous women are at increased risk, which is related to maternal first exposure to chorionic villi [7]. In the present study, abnormal CU ratio was present in 38/95 (40%) cases and abnormal CP ratio (brain sparing) was seen in 21/95 (22%) cases. The mean gestational age of delivery was comparable with that of a study done by as Eser et al. which indicates that gestational age at delivery was significantly lower in group with abnormal CU ratio [8]. When CU ratio was abnormal, SGA was present in 47.4% (18/38) babies and AGA in 52.6% (20/38) babies. However, when CU ratio was normal, 73.7% of the babies were AGA. Thus, with the ratio being normal, the chance of SGA was less likely. Simanaviciute and Gudmundsson found significant correlation with SGA newborn independently with abnormal CP ratio and bilateral uterine artery notching [3]. However, the abnormal CU ratio was not found to be associated with an SGA in the newborn in their study.

The need of an assisted respiration such as continuous positive airway pressure (CPAP) and ventilatory support was studied in relation to CU ratio. Those admitted to NICU with respiratory morbidity were seen in 31.6% (12/38) of babies. When CU ratio was normal, 80.7% (46/57) did not require respiratory assistance. There are no studies available in the current literature which have evaluated the correlation between CU and need for assisted respiration.

Those with normal CU ratio 89.5% (51/57) had good APGARs, indicating that normal CU ratio is reassuring. Simanaviciute and Gudmundsson found no significant correlation between abnormal CU ratio and poor Apgar score [3]. Similar finding was noted in a study by Eser et al. [8].

TABLE 3: Comparison between CP and CU ratios in predicting perinatal outcomes.

Outcome	CU ratio			CP ratio		
	Abnormal n (%)	Normal n (%)	P value	Abnormal n (%)	Normal n (%)	P value
SGA	18 (47.4)	15 (26.3)	**0.035**	11 (52.4)	22 (29.3)	**0.054**
Acidemia	7 (18.4)	3 (5.3)	**0.041**	5 (23.8)	5 (6.80)	**0.025**
Fetal hypoxia	19 (50)	13 (22.8)	**0.006**	9 (42.9)	23 (31.1)	0.314
Low Apgar	10 (26.3)	6 (10.5)	**0.044**	9 (42.7)	7 (9.5)	**0.000**
HMD	6 (15.8)	5 (8.8)	0.295	5 (23.8)	6 (8.1)	**0.025**
Assisted respiration	12 (31.6)	11 (19.3)	0.171	7 (33.3)	16 (21.6)	0.269
Perinatal outcome	19 (50)	12 (21.1)	**0.003**	13 (61.9)	18 (24.3)	**0.001**

$P < 0.05$ significant.

TABLE 4: Overall performance of CU and CP ratios in predicting perinatal outcome (based on Modified Tchirikov Composite score).

Outcome	CU ratio					CP ratio				
	Sensitivity (%)	Specificity (%)	PPV (%)	NPV (%)	Accuracy (%)	Sensitivity (%)	Specificity (%)	PPV (%)	NPV (%)	Accuracy (%)
SGA	54.5	67.7	47.4	73.7	63.2	33.3	83.9	52.4	70.3	66.3
Poor Apgar	62.5	64.6	26.2	89.5	64.2	56.3	84.8	42.9	90.5	80.0
Assisted respiration	52.2	63.9	31.6	80.7	61.1	30.4	80.6	33.3	78.4	68.9
Acidemia	70	63.5	18.4	94.7	64.2	50	81.2	23.8	93.2	77.9
Adverse perinatal outcome	61.3	70.3	50.0	78.9	67.4	41.9	87.5	61.9	75.7	72.6

TABLE 5: Perinatal outcome in relation to both CU and CP ratios (based on Modified Tchirikov Composite score).

Perinatal outcome	CU and CP ratio			
	Both ratios normal n (%)	Only CU ratio abnormal n (%)	Only CP ratio abnormal n (%)	Both ratios abnormal n (%)
Adverse outcome n = 31	12 (23.1)	6 (27.3)	0	13 (81.2)
Favourable outcome n = 64	40 (76.9)	16 (72.7)	5 (100)	3 (18.8)

To study the overall outcome, Modified Tchirikov Composite score for perinatal outcome was used. CU ratio was helpful in ruling out compromised fetus. Preterm delivery was high in those patients with abnormal CU ratio. In cases of severe preeclampsia or imminent eclampsia, the threshold for caesarean delivery was also low. In 11 cases, absent end diastolic flow was noted, of which 2 cases also had severe olighydramnios. Pregnancy was terminated for both maternal and fetal causes, which led to premature delivery in preeclampsia cases. Thus, abnormal CU ratio could not be directly attributed to preterm delivery. In Eser et al. study, CU ratio was independently associated with delivery before 37 weeks, whereas CP ratio was not [8].

Even with severe preeclampsia, some cases had normal CU ratio which can be due to the maternal intake of antihypertensive drug. In a study done by Günenç et al., treatment with methyldopa lowered the uterine artery resistance in preeclamptic patients but did not affect the resistance of umbilical and fetal middle cerebral artery [9]. In two separate studies done by Khalil et al. and Muračević et al., they did not find change in flow resistance of umbilical artery after administration of methyldopa [10, 11].

In our study, 28 patients were on methyldopa and 16 patients were on combination of antihypertensives. CU ratio was abnormal in 17/44 (38.6%) and normal in 27/44 (61.3%). We found that SGA, poor Apgar scores, and preterm delivery rates were higher in the group with abnormal CU ratio than those with normal CU ratio, but poor outcomes were also seen in those with normal ratio, which indicates that there was not much change in fetal hemodynamic changes before and after treatment in cases of severe preeclampsia. Normalization of the Doppler velocimetric indices of the fetal MCA has also been reported in terminal cases [12, 13]. This could have also resulted in normal CU ratio in patients with severe preeclampsia, although the pathological changes would have already occurred.

5. Conclusion

The current study found that in the diagnosis of the complications of hypertension peculiar to pregnancy (preeclampsia and gestational hypertension), CU ratio and CP ratio were complimentary to each other in predicting adverse perinatal outcomes than the independent ratios alone.

Strength and Limitations of the Study

The strength of the study is the adequacy of the sample size. There are few studies in the past which have studied the comparison of these parameters. However, the limitation of this study is the confounding factors like the use of antihypertensive agents and gestational age for more than 37 weeks. We know that the addition of antihypertensives may to some extent bring about resistance changes in the uterine vessel. We are also aware that beyond 37 weeks, the placenta tries to compensate for the placental insufficiency by remodeling itself.

Conflict of Interests

The authors declare that there is no conflict of interests regarding the publication of this paper.

References

[1] D. Arduini and G. Rizzo, "Prediction of fetal outcome in small for gestational age fetuses: comparison of Doppler measurements obtained from different fetal vessels," *Journal of Perinatal Medicine*, vol. 20, no. 1, pp. 29–38, 1992.

[2] K. Harrington, M. O. Thompson, R. G. Carpenter, M. Nguyen, and S. Campbell, "Doppler fetal circulation in pregnancies complicated by pre-eclampsia or delivery of a small for gestational age baby: 2. Longitudinal analysis," *BJOG: An International Journal of Obstetrics & Gynaecology*, vol. 106, no. 5, pp. 453–466, 1999.

[3] D. Simanaviciute and S. Gudmundsson, "Fetal middle cerebral to uterine artery pulsatility index ratios in normal and preeclamptic pregnancies," *Ultrasound in Obstetrics and Gynecology*, vol. 28, no. 6, pp. 794–801, 2006.

[4] "Report of the National High Blood Pressure Education Program Working Group on High Blood Pressure in Pregnancy," *American Journal of Obstetrics and Gynecology*, vol. 183, no. 1, pp. S1–S22, 2000.

[5] M. Tchirikov, C. Rybakowski, B. Hüneke, V. Schoder, and H. J. Schröder, "Umbilical vein blood volume flow rate and umbilical artery pulsatility as 'venous-arterial index' in the prediction of neonatal compromise," *Ultrasound in Obstetrics and Gynecology*, vol. 20, no. 6, pp. 580–585, 2002.

[6] R. P. Patange and N. Goel, "Role of colour Doppler: cerebral and umbilical arterial blood flow velocity in normal and growth restricted pregnancy," *Journal of Evolution of Medical and Dental Sciences*, vol. 3, no. 13, pp. 3310–3320, 2014.

[7] C.-J. Lee, T.-T. Hsieh, T.-H. Chiu, K.-C. Chen, L.-M. Lo, and T.-H. Hung, "Risk factors for pre-eclampsia in an Asian population," *International Journal of Gynecology and Obstetrics*, vol. 70, no. 3, pp. 327–333, 2000.

[8] A. Eser, E. Zulfikaroglu, S. Eserdag, S. Kilic, and N. Danisman, "Predictive value of middle cerebral artery to uterine artery pulsatility index ratio in preeclampsia," *Archives of Gynecology and Obstetrics*, vol. 284, no. 2, pp. 307–311, 2011.

[9] O. Günenç, N. Çiçek, H. Görkemli, Ç. Çelik, A. Acar, and C. Akyürek, "The effect of methyldopa treatment on uterine, umblical and fetal middle cerebral artery blood flows in preeclamptic patients," *Archives of Gynecology and Obstetrics*, vol. 266, no. 3, pp. 141–144, 2002.

[10] A. Khalil, K. Harrington, S. Muttukrishna, and E. Jauniaux, "Effect of antihypertensive therapy with alpha-methyldopa on uterine artery Doppler in pregnancies with hypertensive disorders," *Ultrasound in Obstetrics and Gynecology*, vol. 35, no. 6, pp. 688–694, 2010.

[11] B. Muračević, J. Hodžić, J. Badir, and L. Muhamedagić, "Effect of antihypertensive therapy with alpha-methyldopa on umbilical artery Doppler in pregnancies with hypertensive disorders," *Medicinski Glasnik*, vol. 10, no. 2, pp. 278–282, 2013.

[12] S. Vyas, K. H. Nicolaides, S. Bower, and S. Campbell, "Middle cerebral artery flow velocity waveforms in fetal hypoxaemia," *British Journal of Obstetrics and Gynaecology*, vol. 97, no. 9, pp. 797–803, 1990.

[13] P. Johnson, T. Stojilkovic, and P. Sarkar, "Middle cerebral artery Doppler in severe intrauterine growth restriction," *Ultrasound in Obstetrics and Gynecology*, vol. 17, no. 5, pp. 416–420, 2001.

10

Feasibility, Acceptability, and Programme Effectiveness of Misoprostol for Prevention of Postpartum Haemorrhage in Rural Bangladesh: A Quasiexperimental Study

Abdul Quaiyum,[1] Rukhsana Gazi,[2] Shahed Hossain,[2] Andrea Wirtz,[3] and Nirod Chandra Saha[4]

[1] Centre for Reproductive Health, icddr,b, Bangladesh
[2] Centre for Equity and Health Systems, icddr,b, Mohakhali C/A, Dhaka 1212, Bangladesh
[3] Department of Epidemiology, The Centre for Public Health and Human Rights, Johns Hopkins Bloomberg School of Public Health, 615 North Wolfe Street/E7144, Baltimore, MD 21205, USA
[4] Health Systems and Infectious Diseases Division, icddr,b, Bangladesh

Correspondence should be addressed to Rukhsana Gazi; rukhsana@icddrb.org

Academic Editor: Stefan P. Renner

We explored the feasibility of distributing misoprostol tablets using two strategies in prevention of postpartum haemorrhage (PPH) among women residing in the Abhoynagar subdistrict of Bangladesh. We conducted a quasiexperimental study with a posttest design and nonequivalent comparison and intervention groups. Paramedics distributed three misoprostol tablets, one delivery mat (Quaiyum's delivery mat), a packet of five standardized sanitary pads, and one lidded plastic container with detailed counseling on their use. All materials except misoprostol were also provided with counseling sessions to the control group participants. Postpartum blood loss was measured by paramedics using standardized method. This study has demonstrated community acceptability to misoprostol tablets for the prevention of PPH that reduced overall volume of blood loss after childbirth. Likewise, the delivery mat and pad were found to be useful to mothers as tools for assessing the amount of blood loss after delivery and informing care-seeking decisions. Further studies should be undertaken to explore whether government outreach health workers can be trained to effectively distribute misoprostol tablets among rural women of Bangladesh. Such a study should explore and identify the programmatic requirements to integrate this within the existing reproductive health program of the Government of Bangladesh.

1. Introduction

Globally, postpartum haemorrhage (PPH) has been identified as one of the leading causes of maternal mortality and morbidity and approximately one-third of total maternal deaths occur in Asia [1]. We learned from both national DHS surveys [2, 3] and individual studies [4, 5] that haemorrhage has been one of the major causes of maternal deaths in Bangladesh during this last decade. PPH is unpredictable, catastrophic, and may occur even among women who are considered to be at low risk [6]. As a result, experts have concluded that the millennium development goals will not successfully be achieved without reducing deaths attributable to PPH, particularly those that occur in resource poor settings [7].

Several causes are attributable to the development of PPH, most commonly reported is uterine atony, as well as surgical incisions or lacerations and coagulation disorders [8]. Investigators of a study conducted in Pakistan identified two major causes of primary PPH: uterine atony (70.5%) and traumatic lesions of genital tract (29.4%) [9]. The investigators of this study further suggested that uterine atony was associated with augmented labor, prolonged labor, retention of placenta, and multiple pregnancies [9]. The consequences of primary PPH are serious in nature and may include hypovolemic shock, cerebral anoxia, renal failure, anemia, puerperal sepsis, and Sheehan's syndrome [10].

Although effective clinical treatments for PPH are available, these are not practical for use in developing countries where the majority of births occur at home and are overseen by the untrained attendants. Following literature reviews, we have learned that active management of third stage of labour, especially the administration of uterotonic drugs, may reduce the risk of PPH due to uterine atony without increasing the incidence of retained placenta or other serious complications [11]. Although active management of third stage of labour has proven efficacious in the management of PPH, the challenge is translating active management into general use in rural settings. For example, oxytocin and syntometrine are preferred uterotonic drugs but are not useful in the situation of home deliveries where parenteral administration is unsuitable and drug storage is a problem as it requires refrigeration [12].

An alternative drug, misoprostol, a prostaglandin, has been proven to be practical and effective in developing countries to reduce PPH [12–15]. Misoprostol is low cost, stable at room temperature, and easy to administer [16]. Misoprostol can be effectively administrated sublingually [17], orally [14, 18], or rectally [19, 20]. Researchers in prior studies have demonstrated some side effects of misoprostol, which include postpartum maternal shivering and fever while no side effects have been reported for the newborn [21]. The benefits of misoprostol, however, should be weighed against reported side effects, particularly in the resources poor settings where there is no other alternative.

In Bangladesh, wide geographical variation exists in the availability of emergency obstetric care facilities in the public sectors [22]. From a national survey done in both rural and urban areas of Bangladesh we learned that there are challenges related to health access and uptake and barriers related to economic cost; more than 75% of women experiencing delivery related complications such as convulsion or haemorrhage either failed to seek treatment or were treated by an unqualified provider [23]. Further exploration by researchers suggested that the principal reasons for not seeking care were related to concerns over medical costs and severe socioeconomic disparities [23]. Gross misunderstandings and misconceptions regarding PPH at the community level in Bangladesh also contribute to low access and uptake of care [24–26]. Among service providers, current methods to assess PPH are also suboptimal. In Bangladesh, visual assessments are used to estimate postpartum blood loss even in the clinical settings. By conducting a review of published studies, researchers have confirmed that visual assessments of postpartum blood loss significantly underestimate blood loss, compared to direct estimation and other methods [27]. Investigators in a randomized control trial done in India assessed that visual assessment was 33% less accurate than blood loss estimated by a blood collection drape [28]. In Bangladesh, the absence of any suitable tool available to identify a case of suspected PPH at the community level may result in delays to accessing health care facilities during obstetric emergencies.

Distribution of misoprostol for prevention of PPH has been identified as one of the most cost effective interventions for safe motherhood in resource poor settings [29]. A cost-effectiveness analysis has led experts to emphasize that training of traditional birth attendants (TBAs) to administer

misoprostol for the treatment of PPH has the potential to both save money and improve the health of mothers in resource poor settings [30].

The objective of this study to test the feasibility, acceptability, and program effectiveness of misoprostol distributed by different cadres of health providers in the prevention of PPH after delivery of the baby. This was a collaborative effort by the International Centre for Diarrhoeal Disease Research, Bangladesh (icddr,b), the Obstetric and Gynaecological Society of Bangladesh (OGSB), and the government's Reproductive Health Program (RHP). In the same study researchers found that the use of a delivery mat (Quaiyum's mat) can guide women and community people about the amount of blood loss after delivery [31].

2. Materials and Methods

We conducted a quasiexperimental study with a posttest design and nonequivalent comparison and intervention groups. Research activities were conducted between July 2006 and December 2007 in Abhoynagar subdistrict of Jessore district of Bangladesh, which has a population of 240,000.

The study assessed two strategies for distribution of tablets (Table 1). In Strategy 1, trained study paramedics distributed misoprostol and provided counseling on use and potential side effects. In Strategy 2, distribution and counseling on misoprostol use were done by the participant's intended TBA. Three randomly selected subdistricts were assigned to two-distribution strategies or control area. Pregnancies in each union were identified and enumerated based on the expected date of delivery (EDD) falling between July 16, 2006 and May 2007. Other eligibility criteria included local residents, married women of reproductive age group, and no prior reported complications like heart diseases. Women with expected delivery dates between these dates and who met the other inclusion criteria were informed of the study activities and asked for their consent to participate. Those who gave an informed consent to participate were enrolled and followed for to 24 hours postdelivery. All participating women in the intervention areas (both distribution strategies) were provided with 600 μg (3 tablets of 200 μg) misoprostol oral doses. This dosage was recommended and found to be effective in previous research [29, 32, 33]. All enrolled women, their intended delivery attendant, and at least one nearest kin of the pregnant women were counseled on misoprostol use: how and when to take tablets, potential side effects, methods to remedy side effects, and danger of swallowing the tablets prior to delivery. Women were also counseled on the danger signs of pregnancy and delivery and were informed of where to go if danger signs appear. Counseling occurred at least three times during the course of follow-up: at enrollment, during follow-up visits, and 4 weeks before the expected date of delivery.

In Table 1, research activities are described for the three study areas. During the visit, 4 weeks before the expected delivery date, paramedics distributed three misoprostol tablets, one delivery mat (Quaiyum's delivery mat), a packet of five standardized sanitary pads, and one lidded plastic

TABLE 1: Project activities by study areas.

Activity	Strategy 1	Strategy 2	Control
Distribution of mat and pad with counseling on methods of use and preservation	Conducted by project staff (paramedics). Provided to women, family members, and intended birth attendant	Conducted by the intended TBAs. Provided to women and family members	Conducted by project staff (paramedics). Provided to women, family members, and intended birth attendant
Distribution of misoprostol tablets and detailed counseling on misoprostol use, side effects, and remedies	Conducted by paramedics	Conducted by intended TBAs	No misoprostol tablets distributed
Measurements of blood loss within 24 hours of delivery	Conducted by paramedics		
Interview of participants	Conducted by project staff members		
Establishment of referral mechanism for complications	Standard for all sites		

container with detailed counseling on their use. All materials except misoprostol were also provided in the control group participants. All women were provided with a study identification card that included the cell phone numbers of the study medical officer and field supervisors. The family member or attendant was reminded to save the used mat and pads after delivery in the lidded container until a study personnel came for collection. During the postdelivery visit (24 hours after delivery), the study paramedics weighed the used mat and pads by a calibrated digital scale. The study paramedics also conducted visual assessment of blood loss and completed the structured questionnaire to collect information on the delivery and misoprostol use. All complicated medical cases were referred to appropriate facilities.

The standard dry weight of a Quaiyum's delivery mat is 40 ± 2 grams and sanitary pads weigh 16 ± 1 gram. A fully soaked mat can retain 448.0 ± 58.2 mL of blood and a fully soaked pad may retain 60.2 ± 2.1 mL of blood. To estimate blood loss and identify possible cases of PPH, the soaked mat and all soaked pads were weighed after 24 hours of delivery using a calibrated, electronic postal scale prior to disposal. PPH was defined as blood loss >500 mL after birth, as per international protocol [32]. Blood loss was calculated by subtracting the dry weight of the mat and pads from total weight of the soaked mat and pads.

An additional qualitative assessment included subgroups of female participants (22), their husbands (22), and mothers-in-law (15) who were selected to take part in in-depth interviews. The female participants included women who experienced PPH (15) and women who did not experience PPH (7). Qualitative data was collected using an open-ended interview guide. In-depth interviews were audio recorded and later transcribed for content analysis. The study was approved by the Research Review Committee (RRC) and Ethical Review Committee (ERC) of icddr,b. All severe adverse effects were reported to the Data Safety Monitoring Board under the Ethical Review Committee of icddr,b. Two professors of obstetrics and gynaecology of Bangladesh served as technical advisers during study.

3. Results

3.1. Sociodemographic Characteristics of Participants.
Sociodemographic characteristics of female participants are shown in Table 2. There were no major differences in characteristics of women in intervention A, intervention B, and control area. Overall, 17.1 to 22.4% women had no formal education. A higher proportion of husbands in control areas reported having no formal education compared to intervention areas A and B. The majority of the women in both intervention and the control areas were from low income families. Overall, two percent of the women in both areas were nulliparous.

3.2. History of Current Pregnancy and Delivery by Intervention and Control Areas.
Table 3 displays pregnancy and delivery outcomes of participants during the study. In intervention areas, 22.7 to 38% women received ANC visits compared to 27.2% women in control area who received ANC. Few women experienced vaginal bleeding during the current pregnancy (0.6 to 1.8%). Significantly higher proportions of women in control area (49.5%) than intervention areas (41% in intervention A and 45.9% in intervention B) mentioned reported medication use to mitigate labor pains. Medication included intramuscular injections, intravenous infusion, and oral tablets. Irrespective of study area, most deliveries were assisted by traditional, untrained TBAs. In all study areas, approximately two percent of deliveries were still-births.

3.3. Feasibility of Distribution of Misoprostol Tablets and Its Acceptability to Women.
Figure 1 shows enrollment and distribution of misoprostol tablets in intervention and control areas. For instance, in intervention area A, 1307 pregnant women were identified, of which 1121 women were enrolled into the study, and 795 mothers delivered at home. A total of 709 (89%) mothers consumed misoprostol tablets in intervention area A. In intervention area B, 758 (92%) mothers took misoprostol tablets. There was no statistical significant difference between intervention area A and intervention area B

TABLE 2: Profile of the mothers by areas.

	Intervention area-A n = 795 %	Intervention area-B n = 824 %	Control area n = 648 %
Age in years			
<20	22.1	26.5	20.5
20–24	33.5	33.1	32.4
25–34	40.0	35.7	40.7
35+	4.4	4.7	6.3
Women's education			
No education	22.4	17.1	20.1
1–5	30.9	32.2	33.5
6–10	44.4	47.7	45.7
11+	2.3	3.0	0.8
Husbands education			
No education	26.7	28.4	35.6
1–5	30.8	33.1	29.5
6–10	35.8	31.6	29.5
11+	6.7	6.9	5.4
Monthly family income in Taka (1 USD = 51 Taka)			
<4000 Taka	74.0*	74.5*	82.2
4000 and above	23.6*	24.9*	8.1
Do not know	2.4	0.6	9.7
Parity of the mothers			
0	1.8	1.7	1.8
1	48.4	47.9	45.0
2	26.2	27.8	31.1
3	13.2	14.9	11.4
4	7.0	4.0	6.6
5+	3.4	3.7	4.2

Note: *shows statistical significant difference between intervention and control; $P < 0.001$ at 95% level.

TABLE 3: Current pregnancy and delivery related characteristics.

	Intervention area-A n = 795 %	Intervention area-B n = 824 %	Control area n = 648 %
Duration of pregnancy in weeks			
35 to 39	39.7	35.0	40.9
40	40.8	43.4*	33.8
41 to 44	19.5	21.6	25.1
Women received ANC	38.0*	22.7	27.2
Women experienced vaginal bleeding during pregnancy	1.8	1.8	0.6
Labour pain was augmented by medication	41.0	45.9	49.5*
Types of birth attendants			
Relatives	3.9*	1.2*	10.0
Untrained birth attendant	54.6	50.6	49.5
Trained birth attendant	38.6	47.2*	38.0
Nurse/midwife	1.9	0.7	0.8
No birth attendant	1.0	0.2*	1.7
Outcome of pregnancy			
Live birth	97.9	98.2	97.7
Still birth	2.1	1.8	2.3

Note: *shows statistically significant difference between intervention and control; $P < 0.001$ at 95% level.

B ($P = .09$) regarding tablet consumption. Participants who did not take misoprostol tablets cited the following reasons: the placenta was out simultaneously with delivery of baby (13%), the person who had been informed about misoprostol tablets was absent at the time of delivery (33%), and somebody from the family was opposed to taking the tablets (41%).

3.4. Consumption of Misoprostol Tablets and Perceived Benefits. Irrespective of distribution of tablets by TBAs or paramedics (Strategy 1 or 2), there was no reported mistiming of tablet consumption by participants; all participants reported taking misoprostol tables postdelivery. Over 70% of the women consumed the misoprostol within 1 to 3 minutes after delivery. Another 15% women took it instantly after delivery. Among those who consumed the tablets, 80% believed that misoprostol tablets were beneficial to them. The benefits cited include placenta was expelled quickly (61.8%), bleeding was reduced (74.8%), pain was minimized (6.2%), and physical weakness was reduced (6.1%). Almost all (98.0%) of these participants indicated they would advise other pregnant women to use misoprostol tablets following delivery. The majority of the participants (85.8%) indicated willingness to buy tablets during future pregnancies.

During in-depth interviews with female participants, mothers-in-law, and husbands, participants discussed their perspectives on the use of misoprostol tablets. Almost all of the interviewed women including mother in-laws believed that misoprostol tablets were beneficial for a newly delivered mother. The commonly cited expressions were "as mother took the tablets," "there was less bleeding," "placenta came out quickly," "mother recovered soon," and "mothers felt well quickly after childbirth." Most husbands viewed treatment by misoprostol as "one type of *prathomic* (primary) treatment at home." Perceived benefits among husbands included that misoprostol was "free of cost," and "saves life and money."

3.5. Reported Side Effects of Misoprostol Tablets. Of 1459 intervention participants who took misoprostol tablets, 558 (38.2%) reported at least one side effect. Among those reporting any side effects, 75.4% women had shivering and 37.8% experienced low grade fever (Table 4). Few reported nausea (4.8%) and/or vomiting (8.6%). Of 10 participants who experienced shivering and needed any measures, seven

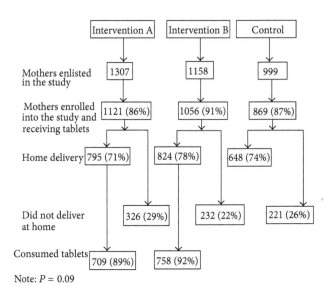

Note: $P = 0.09$

FIGURE 1: Distribution and consumption of misoprostol tablets for prevention of postpartum haemorrhage in intervention and control areas.

TABLE 4: Side effect experienced by mothers who took misoprostol.

	Intervention area-A $n = 281$	Intervention area-B $n = 277$	Total $n = 558$
Nausea	5.3	4.3	4.8
Shivering	77.9	72.9	75.4
Vomiting	8.9	8.3	8.6
Low grade fever	50.5	24.9	37.8

Note: multiple responses considered.

women had this problem for 30 minutes or less and three women reported to have it for two hours or more. Among four participants who suffered from fever and needed any measures, two women had this for 30 minutes and another 2 women had this for one hour or more.

3.6. Measures Taken for Side Effects. Of total 558 women who reported having any of the side effects, only 13 required or sought any additional treatment or care; these included two participants consulted with doctors, one participant was self-referred to Thana Health Complex, one consulted neighbors, and another 9 women were self-referred to Khulna Hospital. Additional care resulted from shivering (76.9%, 10/13), fever (23.1%, 3/10), and combined shivering and fever (8%, 1/13). However, no women required hospitalization for any adverse effects. Among women, those who reported side effects but did not seek additional care ($n = 545$), mentioned that they didn't consider these as serious problems thus, didn't require any additional care.

3.7. Assessments on Amount of Blood Loss after Childbirth. Table 5 displays the postpartum blood loss across the three areas. Overall postpartum blood losses in intervention areas

were significantly lower compared to control area. In Intervention area A, mean blood loss was 437.1 ± 171.2 (95% CI 425.1–448.9) and 478.1 ± 194.5 (CI 464.7–491.3) in intervention area B, compared to 486 ± 194.8 (CI 471.0–500.9) in control area ($P < .001$). The prevalence of PPH per area was 4.7% (38/794), 10.3% (85/824), and 12.5% (81/648) in areas A, B, and control, respectively.

3.8. Reported Benefits of Delivery Mat and Pad. Over 90% of the participants reported opined that delivery mat and pads had been beneficial during delivery. Table 6 presents perceived benefits of the mat and/or pad. Frequently reported benefits included comfort (72.3%), no need of additional cloth (47.7%), and no need to wash the mat or pad (38.5%) (Table 6).

The participants of the qualitative component (women and their husbands) also provided perspectives on the benefits of the mat and pad. Most of the women indicated that the delivery mat and pads were "hygienic, clean, and soft." Women preferred the delivery mat for the following reasons: the amount of blood loss was visible to them, they did not require extra clothes for collecting postpartum blood, and no washing was required. Husbands appreciated using delivery mat and pads because they thought "it kept the environment clean," "it helped the village doctor to give proper treatment to the mother," "quick decisions were made for hospitalization," and "supply was free of cost."

4. Discussion

In the present study, we explored the feasibility of distributing misoprostol tablets to prevent PPH among women residing in rural settings of Bangladesh. We further explored alternative methods of distribution, comparing distribution and counseling through paramedics with distribution and counseling through TBAs. Study findings suggest that community-based distribution of misoprostol tablets through minimally trained TBAs and paramedics can be a feasible strategy for reducing PPH in the resource poor settings and settings where there are limited health care facilities or absence of other alternatives.

Irrespective of the distribution strategy, the overwhelming majority (90%) of participants consumed the misoprostol, reflecting acceptability of the treatment. Based on the fact that misoprostol was consumed at the time directed by TBAs or paramedics, immediately following delivery (meaning no mistiming of consumption of tablets), we believe this study demonstrates the viability of employing TBAs and paramedics for such distribution efforts. Similar results have been demonstrated in settings comparable to Bangladesh; for example, investigators from a study in India reported that paramedical workers from rural primary health centers were able to administer oral misoprostol for active management of third stage of labor for prevention of PPH [18]. Another randomized double-blind placebo-controlled trial conducted in India has also confirmed that oral misoprostol can safely and effectively be distributed by skilled TBAs for home deliveries [33]. Community-based distribution such as this may also be cost effective as misoprostol is a lower-cost alternative to

TABLE 5: Assessments on amount of blood loss after childbirth.

	Intervention area-A (mean ± SD)	Intervention area-B (mean ± SD)	Control area (mean ± SD)
Mean blood loss in three areas	437.1 ± 171.2*	478.1 ± 194.5*	486 ± 194.8
95% CI	425.1–448.9	464.7–491.3	471.0–500.9
Mean blood loss among mothers who developed PPH in three areas	678.4 ± 213.7	684.7 ± 193.9	689.8 ± 186.1
95% CI	628.6–727.3	649.3–720.6	654.5–725.5

Note: *shows statistical significant difference between intervention and control; $P < 0.001$ at 95% level.

TABLE 6: Perceived benefits of delivery mat and pads supplied among women.

	Intervention area-A $n = 739$	Intervention area-B $n = 795$	Control area $n = 625$	Total $n = 2159$
No need to wash	33.0	43.6	38.9	38.6
Comfortable	79.5	65.5	82.2	75.2
No need for extra clothes	38.7	56.1	47.0	47.5
Easy to move/walk	21.8	18.4	16.6	19.0
Hygienic/safe	20.7	18.5	5.9	15.6
All blood remains in one place	8.4	2.0	3.5	4.6
Amount of blood is assessable	19.1	15.1	27.5	20.1
Keep body warm	1.2	0.9	2.7	1.5

Note: multiple responses considered.

other PPH treatments, community-level distribution requires minimal training, distribution can be implemented outside of the clinical infrastructure, and community-level activities are already core components of TBA and paramedic responsibilities. Further research that would examine cost-effectiveness of misoprostol through alternative delivery methods might be beneficial.

This study adds to the body of knowledge on the benefits of the use of misoprostol to reduce PPH. When compared to either intervention area, participants of the control area experienced greater blood loss following childbirth. Derman and colleagues (2006) also found that misoprostol was associated with a decrease in mean postpartum blood loss and reported that one case of PPH was prevented for every 18 women treated [33]. Among female participants who consumed the misoprostol tablets, reported side effects were minimal but did include shivering and fever for which some sought additional care. Shivering and fever are known side effects of misoprostol and have been reported by other researchers [14, 34, 35]. In general, those who experienced the side effects considered these to be minor and the majority did not seek additional care. In fact, only 13 women sought medical attention for shivering and fever but no hospitalization was indicated for any of these side effects. Overall, among participants of the intervention areas and including those who developed PPH, about 80% of the participants perceived the treatment as beneficial for them. Qualitative findings supported this evidence: many women in intervention areas suggested that with consumption of the tablets, the placenta expelled quickly and bleeding was less. The majority of the women expressed willingness to misoprostol during future pregnancies and they would recommend it to others

for use, reflecting positive perceptions and acceptability on the use and benefits of misoprostol tablets. Husbands and mothers-in-law, who are key individuals in decisions related to reproductive health, also supported these perceptions. Provision of misoprostol to all women who participated in the intervention areas of the study was not superfluous as it reduced overall volume of blood loss in these areas and may also confer secondary benefits. For example, reduction of volume of blood loss is also particularly important in the context of Bangladesh, where 49 to 50% of pregnant women were found to be anemic in rural areas [36, 37] and iron and folate status is found to be particularly low among women during the periconception period [38].

We also assessed the acceptability of misoprostol tablets and delivery mat and pads among women and their husbands. This study is a pioneer one that estimated blood loss after childbirth among women at the rural communities of Bangladesh using an easy blood collection method. Participants of the study felt that delivery mat and pads were very useful and convenient to them. With the ability to visually assess the amount of blood loss, collected by the delivery mat and pads, participants and family members believed they could make timely decisions of whether to seek care at formal health facilities. This increased capacity is extremely important in the context of rural Bangladesh where more than 80% of deliveries take place at home situations [3]. In a randomized control trial, the use of a medical drape to assess blood loss after delivery [18, 39] was demonstrably more efficient for measuring blood loss and identifying PPH, as compared to visual assessments [28]. However, the method requires trained personal for implementation and blood volume measurement. In Africa, one study reported that "Kanga", rectangular cotton made fabric that is normally used as a skirt or head wrap or to carry a baby on a mother's back, was effectively used as a postpartum blood collection towel [29]. However, there must be standardized means to assess blood loss at the community level. In rural Bangladesh, a delivery mat will be very suitable because local women use similar materials, such as folds of old cloths, for the purpose of postpartum blood collection. Women found the delivery mat and pads useful and convenient for such use, as did the family decision makers (mother-in-law and husbands), who are important as these individuals must be motivated to support women's use of the delivery mat and pad.

One of the limitations of the study was our inability to track those female participants who delivered outside the study areas. There is a common tradition in Bangladesh that women usually deliver at their parental home, particularly with respect to the first child. Many women in our study were pregnant for the first time, so we were unable to follow those women through delivery. A second limitation was the use of a nonequivalent control group; this was due to scarcity of resources, though we do not believe nonequivalency changes the findings of the feasibility of misoprostol distribution.

5. Conclusions

This study highlighted the programmatic feasibility of distributing misoprostol tablets for prevention of PPH, through paramedics as well as TBAs in rural communities of Bangladesh. This study has demonstrated acceptability to misoprostol tablets for the prevention of PPH, and participants perceived these as generally beneficial to their health. Likewise, the delivery mat and pad were found to be useful to mothers as tools for assessing the amount of blood loss after delivery and informing care-seeking decisions. For scale-up of such programs, we recommend that TBAs should be properly educated on the correct administration and common side effects of this drug. Future research should explore the possibility of misoprostol distribution via TBA delivery kits during future PPH intervention studies. As we found, some family members were not convinced of the benefits of misoprostol tablets and prevented women from taking the tablets; it is suggestive that behavioral change and communication (BCC) activities should complement misoprostol distribution to build awareness among community members, particularly among husbands and in-laws. Further studies should be undertaken to explore whether government outreach health workers can be trained to effectively distribute misoprostol tablets among rural women of Bangladesh. Such a study should explore and identify the programmatic requirements to integrate this within the existing reproductive health program of the Government of Bangladesh.

Conflict of Interests

The authors declare that there is no conflict of interests regarding the publication of this paper.

Acknowledgments

This research study was funded by icddr,b's core donors and the United States Agency for International Development (USAID) under the Cooperative Agreement no. 388-A-00-97-00032-00. icddr,b acknowledges with gratitude the commitment of USAID to its research efforts. icddr,b also gratefully acknowledges the following donors who provided unrestricted support: Australian Agency for International Development (AusAID), Government of the People's Republic of Bangladesh, Canadian International Development Agency (CIDA), Swedish International Development Cooperation Agency (Sida), and the Department for International Development, UK (DFID).

References

[1] World Health Organization, *Cause of Maternal Death: Epidemiology of Major Maternal Perinatal Conditions*, WHO, Geneva, Switzerland, 2009.

[2] National Institute of Population and Training (NIPORT), ORC Macro, John Hopkins University, and ICDDRB, *Bangladesh Maternal Health Services and Maternal Mortality Survey 2001*, NIPORT, ORC Macro, Jhon Hopkins University, ICDDRB, Dhaka, Calverton, 2003.

[3] National Institute of Population and Training (NIPORT), Mitra and Associates, and Macro International, *Bangladesh Demographic and Health Survey 2007*, NIPORT, Mitra and Associates, Macro International, Dhaka, Calverton, 2009.

[4] A. R. Khan, F. A. Jahan, and S. F. Begum, "Maternal mortality in rural Bangladesh: the Jamalpur district," *Studies in Family Planning*, vol. 17, no. 1, pp. 7–12, 1986.

[5] M. H. Rahman, H. H. Akhter, M. E. K. Chowdhury, H. R. Yusuf, and R. W. Rochat, "Obstetric deaths in Bangladesh, 1996-1997," *International Journal of Gynecology and Obstetrics*, vol. 77, no. 2, pp. 161–169, 2002.

[6] S. E. Geller, S. S. Goudar, M. G. Adams, V. A. Naik, A. Patel, and M. B. Bellad, "Factors associated with acute postpartum hemorrhage in low-risk women delivering in rural India," *International Journal of Gynecology and Obstetrics*, vol. 101, no. 1, pp. 94–99, 2008.

[7] M. Potts and M. Campbell, "Three meetings and fewer funerals—misoprostol in postpartum haemorrhage," *The Lancet*, vol. 364, no. 9440, pp. 1110–1111, 2004.

[8] N. M. de Lange, M. D. Lance, R. de Groot, E. A. Beckers, Y. M. Henskens, and H. C. Scheepers, "Obstetric hemorrhage and coagulation: an update. Thromboelastography, thromboelastometry, and conventional coagulation tests in the diagnosis and prediction of postpartum hemorrhage," *Obstetrical & Gynecological Survey*, vol. 67, no. 7, pp. 426–435, 2012.

[9] S. Bibi, N. Danish, A. Fawad, and M. Jamil, "An audit of primary post partum hemorrhage," *Journal of Ayub Medical College, Abbottabad*, vol. 19, no. 4, pp. 102–106, 2007.

[10] C. A. Klufio, A. B. Amoa, and G. Kariwiga, "Primary postpartum haemorrhage: causes, aetiological risk factors, prevention and management," *Papua and New Guinea Medical Journal*, vol. 38, no. 2, pp. 133–149, 1995.

[11] M. L. McCormick, H. C. G. Sanghvi, B. Kinzie, and N. McIntosh, "Preventing postpartum hemorrhage in low-resource settings," *International Journal of Gynecology and Obstetrics*, vol. 77, no. 3, pp. 267–275, 2002.

[12] Z. Alfirevic, J. Blum, G. Walraven, A. Weeks, and B. Winikoff, "Prevention of postpartum hemorrhage with misoprostol," *International Journal of Gynecology and Obstetrics*, vol. 99, supplement 2, pp. S198–S201, 2007.

[13] C. Langenbach, "Misoprostol in preventing postpartum hemorrhage: a meta-analysis," *International Journal of Gynecology and Obstetrics*, vol. 92, no. 1, pp. 10–18, 2006.

[14] G. Walraven, J. Blum, Y. Dampha et al., "Misoprostol in the management of the third stage of labour in the home delivery setting in rural Gambia: a randomised controlled trial," *International Journal of Obstetrics and Gynaecology*, vol. 112, no. 9, pp. 1277–1283, 2005.

[15] J. Walder, "Misoprostol: preventing postpartum haemorrhage," *Modern Midwife*, vol. 7, no. 9, pp. 23–27, 1997.

[16] J. V. Lazarus and A. Lalonde, "Reducing postpartum hemorrhage in Africa," *International Journal of Gynecology and Obstetrics*, vol. 88, no. 1, pp. 89–90, 2005.

[17] A. H. Al-Harazi and K. A. Frass, "Sublingual misoprostol for the prevention of postpartum hemorrhage," *Saudi Medical Journal*, vol. 30, no. 7, pp. 912–916, 2009.

[18] N. Chandhiok, B. S. Dhillon, S. Datey, A. Mathur, and N. C. Saxena, "Oral misoprostol for prevention of postpartum hemorrhage by paramedical workers in India," *International Journal of Gynecology and Obstetrics*, vol. 92, no. 2, pp. 170–175, 2006.

[19] N. Haque, L. Bilkis, N. Haque, M. S. Bari, and S. Haque, "Comparative study between rectally administered misoprostol as a prophylaxis versus conventional intramuscular oxytocin in post partum hemorrhage," *Mymensingh Medical Journal*, vol. 18, supplement 1, pp. S40–S44, 2009.

[20] N. Prata, G. Mbaruku, M. Campbell, M. Potts, and F. Vahidnia, "Controlling postpartum hemorrhage after home births in Tanzania," *International Journal of Gynecology and Obstetrics*, vol. 90, no. 1, pp. 51–55, 2005.

[21] G. J. Hofmeyr and A. M. Gulmezoglu, "Misoprostol for the prevention and treatment of postpartum haemorrhage," *Best Practice & Research Clinical Obstetrics & Gynaecology*, vol. 22, no. 6, pp. 1025–1041, 2008.

[22] M. K. Mridha, I. Anwar, and M. Koblinsky, "Public-sector maternal health programmes and services for rural Bangladesh," *Journal of Health, Population and Nutrition*, vol. 27, no. 2, pp. 124–138, 2009.

[23] M. A. Koenig, K. Jamil, P. K. Streatfield et al., "Maternal health and care-seeking behavior in Bangladesh: findings from a national survey," *International Family Planning Perspectives*, vol. 33, no. 2, pp. 75–82, 2007.

[24] E. A. Goodburn, R. Gazi, and M. Chowdhury, "Beliefs and practices regarding delivery and postpartum maternal morbidity in rural Bangladesh," *Studies in Family Planning*, vol. 26, no. 1, pp. 22–32, 1995.

[25] N. Kalim, I. Anwar, J. Khan et al., "Postpartum haemorrhage and eclampsia: differences in knowledge and care-seeking behaviour in two districts of Bangladesh," *Journal of Health, Population and Nutrition*, vol. 27, no. 2, pp. 156–169, 2009.

[26] L. M. Sibley, D. Hruschka, N. Kalim et al., "Cultural theories of postpartum bleeding in Matlab, Bangladesh: implications for community health intervention," *Journal of Health, Population and Nutrition*, vol. 27, no. 3, pp. 379–390, 2009.

[27] M. N. Schorn, "Measurement of blood loss: review of the literature," *Journal of Midwifery and Women's Health*, vol. 55, no. 1, pp. 20–27, 2010.

[28] A. Patel, S. S. Goudar, S. E. Geller et al., "Drape estimation versus visual assessment for estimating postpartum hemorrhage," *International Journal of Gynecology and Obstetrics*, vol. 93, no. 3, pp. 220–224, 2006.

[29] N. Prata, S. Hamza, R. Gypson, K. Nada, F. Vahidnia, and M. Potts, "Misoprostol and active management of the third stage of labor," *International Journal of Gynecology and Obstetrics*, vol. 94, no. 2, pp. 149–155, 2006.

[30] S. E. K. Bradley, N. Prata, N. Young-Lin, and D. M. Bishai, "Cost-effectiveness of misoprostol to control postpartum hemorrhage in low-resource settings," *International Journal of Gynecology and Obstetrics*, vol. 97, no. 1, pp. 52–56, 2007.

[31] R. Gazi, A. Quaiyum, M. Islam, S. Hossain, A. Wirtz, and C. Nirod, "Post-partum excessive bleeding among Bangladeshi women: determinants, perceptions, recognition, responses," *Reproductive System & Sexual Disorders*, vol. 1, no. 4, p. 115, 2012.

[32] World Health Organization, *Guidelines for the Management of Postpartum Haemorrhage and Retained Placenta*, WHO, Geneva, Switzerland, 2009.

[33] R. J. Derman, B. S. Kodkany, S. S. Goudar et al., "Oral misoprostol in preventing postpartum haemorrhage in resource-poor communities: a randomised controlled trial," *The Lancet*, vol. 368, no. 9543, pp. 1248–1253, 2006.

[34] S. D. Joy, L. Sanchez-Ramos, and A. M. Kaunitz, "Misoprostol use during the third stage of labor," *International Journal of Gynecology and Obstetrics*, vol. 82, no. 2, pp. 143–152, 2003.

[35] P. Danielian, B. Porter, N. Ferri, J. Summers, and A. Templeton, "Misoprostol for induction of labour at term: a more effective agent than dinoprostone vaginal gel," *British Journal of Obstetrics and Gynaecology*, vol. 106, no. 8, pp. 793–797, 1999.

[36] F. Ahmed, "Anaemia in Bangladesh: a review of prevalence and aetiology," *Public Health Nutrition*, vol. 3, no. 4, pp. 385–393, 2000.

[37] S. M. Hyder, L. A. Persson, M. Chowdhury, B. O. Lonnerdal, and E. C. Ekstrom, "Anaemia and iron deficiency during pregnancy in rural Bangladesh," *Public Health Nutrition*, vol. 7, no. 8, pp. 1065–1070, 2004.

[38] A. Khambalia, D. L. O'Connor, and S. Zlotkin, "Periconceptional iron and folate status is inadequate among married, nulliparous women in rural Bangladesh," *Journal of Nutrition*, vol. 139, no. 6, pp. 1179–1184, 2009.

[39] H. Tixier, C. Boucard, C. Ferdynus, S. Douvier, and P. Sagot, "Interest of using an underbuttocks drape with collection pouch for early diagnosis of postpartum hemorrhage," *Archives of Gynecology and Obstetrics*, vol. 283, no. 1, pp. 25–29, 2011.

11

Knowledge, Attitude, and Preventive Practices among Prison Inmates in Ogbomoso Prison at Oyo State, South West Nigeria

Abdulsalam Saliu and Babatunde Akintunde

Department of Community Medicine, Ladoke Akintola University of Technology Teaching Hospital, Ogbomoso 201, Oyo State, Nigeria

Correspondence should be addressed to Abdulsalam Saliu; saliu_abdulsalam@yahoo.co.uk

Academic Editor: Yves Jacquemyn

Prisoners are at special risk for infection with human immunodeficiency virus (HIV) because of overcrowded prisons, unprotected sex and sexual assault, occurrence of sexual practices that are risky to health, unsafe injecting practices, and inadequate HIV prevention, care, and support services. This study aimed to describe the knowledge, attitude, and preventive practices towards HIV/AIDS by male inmates in Ogbomoso Prison at Oyo State, South West Nigeria. This was a cross-sectional study. A simple random sampling method was employed to select 167 male participants and data were collected using pretested structured interviewer-administered questionnaire. The data were collated and analyzed using the Statistical Package for Social Sciences version 17. Fifty (29.9%) were in the age group 20–24 years with mean age of 30.99 ± 11.41. About half (50.3%) had been married before incarceration. Family and friends (30%), health care workers (25%), prison staff (20%), and mass media (25%) were the commonest sources of information on HIV/AIDS. Knowledge about HIV was found to be high (94.6%). About 68.9% believed that people with the disease should be avoided. The knowledge about HIV/AIDS among inmates was high, but misconceptions about HIV/AIDS are still rife among the prisoners and educational programs would be required to correct this.

1. Introduction

Globally, many studies on human immunodeficiency virus/ acquired immunodeficiency disease syndrome (HIV/AIDS) have been undertaken by various government and non-governmental organizations among the general public. There are certain high risk groups in well-defined but restricted settings who are usually left out from the interventions they deserve especially in developing countries. Inmates of prisons are example of this left out population [1]. Prisoners worldwide have a significantly higher prevalence of HIV than in the community [2, 3]. Prisoners are at a special risk for HIV infection because of overcrowded prisons, unprotected sex and sexual assault, occurrence of sexual practices that are risky to health, unsafe injecting practices, and inadequate HIV prevention, care, and support services [4].

Generally in Africa, existing data on HIV/AIDS in prison are not recent or accurate enough to provide a real picture of the current situation [5]. Of particular importance is that documentation of research studies on HIV/AIDS among prison inmates in Nigeria is very scanty and limited [5]. However, there is growing concern over the HIV status of inmates in Nigeria prisons as a report showed that there is an increase in the number of prisoners who are affected with the disease [6]. One of the previous studies found out that HIV is not a silent issue to Nigeria prison inmates which may be a reflection of the generally high level of knowledge of HIV/AIDS among the general population [7]. Other studies equally showed a very high awareness of HIV/AIDS among prison inmates in Nigeria [1–3]. However, despite the high knowledge, misconceptions of various degrees concerning HIV/AIDS were documented in Nigeria and also elsewhere in Africa [7–9].

The common high risk behaviors in the prison environment include rampart use of drugs, practice of tattooing and toothbrush sharing, prison marriages, unprotected violence, rape, sex bartering, sexual assault, and sex among inmates (mostly anal and between males) [10]. Homosexual activity which is culturally, religiously, and politically unacceptable by most societies is widely spread behind the wall and Nigerian prisoners are not an exception [2]. This is because prisons, being unisexual institutions, create an ideal environment for various sexual activities between men [11]. Some inmates are lured by other inmates to have conceptual anal intercourse in exchange for food and toiletries probably due to lack of basic sanitary materials and adequate nutrition in prison [2]. The majority of inmates who engaged in homosexual activities in the prisons are actually circumstantial homosexuals who would not have become involved in the practice if they were not confined [12–14]. A previous study reported that very few of the inmates knew that HIV/AIDS could be contacted through homosexual intercourse [9].

These sexual encounters are fraught with the risk of contracting HIV because of the frequent tearing of sensitive anal membranes. Prisoners are most at risk population not only for HIV and other sexually transmitted infections (STIs) but also for tuberculosis (TB) due to overcrowding, lack of ventilation, and poor prevention practices. TB is the most opportunistic infection among people living with HIV in Africa resulting in high mortality rates among prisoners with HIV/AIDS. Despite the necessity of providing targeted HIV-prevention interventions for prison inmates, institutional and access barriers have impeded the development and evaluation of such programmes [15].

HIV prevalence in the prisons is usually higher than that in the population at large. It could be 5, 6, or even as much as 10 times higher than the values obtained in the general population [15–17]. A rapid assessment on HIV/AIDS in Nigeria prisons revealed a prevalence rate of 8.7% compared to the national figure of 4.6%. Some other countries in Africa even have higher prevalence with Cote d'Ivoire (27.5%), Zambia (26.7%), and South Africa (15%) [17].

Even though inmates may know that HIV/AIDS could be prevented with the use of condoms, it may not be readily available or affordable [18]. There are considerable proportions of receptive naïve inmates who stand the risk of being infected due to their level of ignorance about HIV/AIDS. Another study stated that there were gaps, misconceptions, and high risk behaviors among prisoners [12]. In a study in Lagos, Nigeria, it was found out that despite the fact that many of these prison inmates knew the correct modes of transmission, many still indulged in high risk behaviors for AIDS transmission [19]. Some studies reported that there are unsafe injecting practices among injecting drug users and the use of nonsterile needles and other cutting instruments is high [20]. Some prison inmates who are professional barbers used unsterilized barbing instruments to barb prisoners because they were unaware of the need for sterilizing these instruments [21].

This study aimed to describe the knowledge, attitude, and preventive practices of male inmates with a view to identify the gaps, misconceptions, and the high risk behaviors towards HIV/AIDS among Ogbomoso Prison inmates in South West Nigeria.

2. Materials and Methods

The Ogbomoso Prison is one of the 86 satellite prisons in Nigeria. The satellite prisons are set up mainly in areas with courts that are far from the main prisons. They serve the purpose of providing remand centers especially for whose cases are going on in courts within the area. When convicted, long-term prisoners could be moved to appropriate convict prisons to serve their terms [22].

The study was a descriptive cross-sectional survey conducted in December 2013. The total number of inmates in the prison during the study period was 256 comprising 250 males and 6 females. A total of 167 inmates were recruited for the study after calculating the sample size assuming that 50% of inmates had correct knowledge about HIV in prison using the formula $4pq/L^2$ and 10% degree precision at 95% confidence interval [23]. Respondents were chosen using simple random sampling method until desired sample size was obtained. None of the females consented to participate in the study. The Survey Select Procedure was used to randomly sample 167 respondents of the 250 males using the full listing of inmates available with prison authority at the time of survey. None of the selected male respondents declined to participate in the study.

Approval for the study was sought from the ethical review committee of Ladoke Akintola University of Technology (LAUTECH) Teaching Hospital (LTH), Ogbomoso, Nigeria. Written permission to interview the inmates was obtained from the prison authorities before the interview. Written informed consent was also obtained from the inmates by signing of the consent forms after the contents of the form had been clearly explained to them. They were also told that the study was voluntary and that individuals who agreed to participate will be allowed to withdraw from the study at any stage of the research.

The instrument for data collection was a pretested structured interviewer-administered questionnaire. A pretest of the instruments was carried out with 17 inmates (10% of the calculated sample size) in Ilorin Prison (about 50 Km from Ogbomoso) with similar sociodemographic characteristics as those of respondents. The questionnaire was adopted from knowledge, attitudes, beliefs, and practices survey of the WHO HIV/AIDS programme and previous literatures [2, 19, 23]. The questionnaire consisted of 39 questions in 4 broad four sections. The first section collected information on sociodemographic profile of the respondents (6 items); the second section obtained information about HIV/AIDS related knowledge (10 items); statements about individual's attitude covering sociocultural issues (7 items); and 16 items about the individual's practices concerning HIV/AIDS. In order to militate against social desirability bias, the indirect questioning was employed where socially desirable response was of special concern especially on sexual behaviors. The questionnaire was written in English but was translated into the three major languages in Nigeria, that is, Yoruba, Hausa, and Igbo languages, to enable the respondents to understand the questions clearly.

The questionnaires were administered by trained research assistants in private rooms made available by the prison authority. The research assistant received one-day training on how to use the questionnaire. The field workers included a resident doctor and undergraduate medical students of the

Department of Community Medicine of LTH, Ogbomoso, Nigeria. The researcher spent about two hours with the prison inmates to explain to them the nature of the study. The research assistants helped to fill in the responses of the inmates. Strict confidentiality was maintained.

Evaluation of knowledge of respondents about HIV/AIDS was assessed based on scoring of ten [10] questions that were asked in the questionnaire; a score of one is administered for every right answer while zero is allocated to every wrong answer. The overall mean score obtained was 10 and respondents who scored 10 and above were adjudged to have good knowledge while respondents that scored below ten were said to have poor knowledge.

Data collected were checked for completeness before they were entered into the computer. The data were analyzed using Statistical Package for Social Sciences (SPSS) version 17. Descriptive statistics were applied to determine frequency of relevant variables in the study while Fisher's exact test using a Monte Carlo approach was used to test associations between sociodemographic characteristics and knowledge of the respondents.

The study was limited by being done in only one prison due to logistics and financial constraints; however the findings in this work are expected to give an insight into what prevails in other prisons in Nigeria. Equally, lack of consent by the females' prisoners prevented gender comparison.

3. Results

The age range of the respondents was 20–59 years (mean = 30.99 ± 11.41). Fifty (29.9%) were in the age group 20–24 years. All the respondents were males. Only 53 (31.7%) had secondary education, 83 (50.3%) were married, and about 67 (40.1%) were drivers before incarceration (Table 1). The highest age groups were found among the age group 20–24 (29.9%) and 35–39 (24.6%) respectively (Figure 1).

All the inmates did not know the meaning of HIV. About 158 (94.6%) of the inmates were aware of HIV/AIDS. Among these, 118 (70.7%) knew that HIV is a virus and 68 (40.7%) knew it is mainly transmitted through unprotected sexual intercourse. About 133 (80%) knew that HIV is transmissible through other modes citing at least one mode of transmission: 139 (83.2%) through infected surgical needles and 75% by using unsterilized sharps such as clippers and blades and infected mother to a child during pregnancy 34 (20.4%). On the risk of HIV infection only 53 (31.7%) believed that the risk of HIV could be reduced by having one faithful partner. About 119 (71.3%) of the respondents believed that a condom protect from both pregnancy and HIV infection (Table 2).

Only 66 (39.5%) of the respondents will offer support and feel sorry for an HIV infected friend, but 115 (68.9%) will avoid an HIV infected friend. About 40 (24%) believed a condom spoil sexual pleasure (Table 3).

Ninety-two (51.1%) believed that HIV infection exists in the prisons. Only 72 (43.1%) believed they are at risk of HIV infection, but most 141 (84.4%) of the respondents are willing to have HIV testing. About 105 (62.9%) of the respondents have had sexual relations; 58 (34.7%) had sexual relation with

TABLE 1: Sociodemographic characteristics of respondents.

Variables	Frequency	%
Age group (years)		
20–24	50	29.9
25–29	25	15.0
30–34	17	10.2
35–39	41	24.6
40–44	17	10.2
>45	17	10.2
Marital status		
Single	83	49.7
Married	84	50.3
Educational status		
None	8	4.8
Primary school	50	29.9
Completed secondary school	53	31.7
Secondary school dropout	48	28.7
Other	8	4.8
Religion		
Islam	25	15.0
Christianity	134	80.2
Traditional	8	4.8
Ethnicity		
Yoruba	107	64.1
Hausa/Fulani	26	15.6
Igbo	16	9.6
Others	18	10.8

one regular partner while 44 (26.3%) had sexual relations with more than one partner in the past. As shown in Table 4, about 53 (34.1%) confirmed that the risk of HIV infection can be reduced by having one regular partner. Homosexuality, 124 (74.3%), was recognized as the commonest sexual practice in the prison by respondents. Others include masturbation 34 (20.4%) and intravenous drug injection 9 (5.4%).

Table 5 shows a cross tabulation of the socio-demographic characteristics of respondents with their knowledge about HIV/AIDS and its preventive practices.

4. Discussion

The 20–24 years age group represents the largest age group similar to previous studies conducted in South West Nigeria [11, 12] (Figure 1). The religion of the prison inmates does not mirror the general South West population with 80% of the inmates being Christians. Religious beliefs of individuals do have significant bearings on the knowledge and attitudes and beliefs that affect the transmission of HIV/AIDS in both positive and negative ways; for example, the Catholic Christians frown at the use of condoms [13].

Most of the respondents, 158 (94.6%), are aware of HIV/AIDS, with family and friends, 50 (30%), being their main source of information followed by mass media, 42 (25%). The print media, healthcare workers, and the prison

TABLE 2: Knowledge of HIV/AIDS by respondents.

Questions	Frequency of "Yes answers"	%
Have you ever received information on HIV/AIDS?	158	94.6
What do you think causes HIV/AIDS?		
Virus	118	70.7
Punishment from God	41	25.0
Is HIV transmissible?	133	80
Can HIV/AIDS be cured?	60	35.9
Can healthy-looking person have HIV?	159	90.2
Will a condom protect from pregnancy and HIV?	119	71.3
Will a condom protect from pregnancy but not HIV?	53	31.7
*Mode of transmission of HIV mode		
Hugging or shaking of hands	74	44.3
Having sexual intercourse without a condom	68	40.7
Sharing a meal with an infected person	118	70.7
Mosquito bites	98	58.7
A mother infected with HIV to unborn baby	34	20.4
Kissing someone infected with HIV	120	71.9
Do you know that you can be infected with HIV/AIDS during injection?	165	90.8
Spiritual/witchcraft	35	21.0
Using surgical needles containing infected blood	139	83.2
Using of unsterilized sharps (clippers and blades)	36	21.6
Risk of HIV infection can be reduced by having one faithful partner	53	31.7

*Multiple answers.

TABLE 3: Attitudes towards HIV prevention by respondents.

Questions	Frequency of "Yes answers"	%
Do you know anyone infected with HIV?	143	85.6
Would you offer support to an HIV infected friend?	66	39.5
Would you avoid an HIV infected friend?	115	68.9
Would you use the same WC with HIV infected person?	61	70
Will a condom spoil sexual pleasure?	40	24.0

TABLE 4: HIV prevention practices by respondents.

Questions	Frequency of "Yes answers"	%
Have you ever used a condom?	83	49.7
In the past year have you had sexual relations?	105	62.9
Did you use a condom last time you had sex?	47	28.1
In the past year have you had sexual relation with one regular partner?	58	34.7
In the past year have you had sexual relations with more than one partner?	44	26.3
Do you feel you are at risk of an HIV/AIDS infection?	72	43.1
Have you ever had an HIV test?	26	15.5
Would you like to have an HIV test?	141	84.4
Do you know where to have HIV test?	115	68.9
Do you believe HIV/AIDS exist in prison?	92	55.1
Which of these risky behaviors exist in this prison?		
Homosexuality	124	74.3
Masturbation	34	20.4
Intravenous drug injection	9	5.4
Do you know inmate who has used hard drugs?	113	67.3
Do you know of the inmates who practice anal sex in the prison?	25	15.0
Do you partake in any of the risky behaviors mentioned above?	9	5.4

TABLE 5: Sociodemographic characteristics of respondents and knowledge about HIV/AIDS.

Variables	Good knowledge	Poor knowledge
Age groups (years)		
20–24	50	0
25–29	16	9
30–34	17	0
35–39	41	0
40–44	17	0
>45	17	0
Marital status		
Single	83	0
Married	75	9
Educational status		
None	8	0
Primary	50	0
Completed secondary school	44	9
Secondary school dropout	48	0
Others	8	0
Occupation before incarceration		
Driving	67	0
Schooling	25	0
Mechanic	8	0
Farming	8	0
Carpentry	8	0
Others	42	9

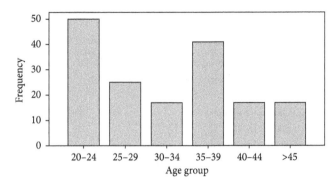

FIGURE 1: Age groups of inmates in the Ogbomoso Prison, 2013.

officials still have a major role to play in the dissemination of information regarding HIV/AIDS. More programmes concerning HIV/AIDS should be discussed on radio and television frequently since they are major sources of information about health issues in Nigeria.

One hundred and thirty-three (80%) had knowledge that HIV is transmissible. Many of them also know the possible routes of transmission of the virus and identify the sexual route as the commonest route of transmission. Their knowledge is however shallow in some aspects as some believe that hugging (15%), sharing a meal with infected person (25%), mosquito bites (25%), kissing (30%) and witchcraft (20%) were routes of transmission.

About 70% also believed that AIDS can be cured. The more people believe that HIV/AIDS could be cured, the less likely they are to practice safe sex or abstain from risky behavior that increases transmission of the infection [13]. The nonavailability of cure for HIV/AIDS creates fear in the minds of people and motivates them to protect themselves against the disease. Some of the information available to some of the inmates about HIV/AIDS has been incorrect. The primary goal of HIV/AIDS education within the prison systems is to prevent the transmission of HIV as prisoners are potential vector for increased transmission within prison and eventually in the society after their release.

About 65% of the respondents believed that people living with HIV/AIDS (PLWHA) should be avoided. This sort of attitude will enhance stigmatization and discrimination against PLWHA. This will further reduce the rate of voluntary testing for the HIV and militate against self-reporting of status, thereby promoting the spread of HIV infection. About 85% of the respondents would like to be tested for HIV. Voluntary testing and counseling is crucial to the prevention of HIV/AIDS and it is crucial among high risk groups.

Homosexuality is a common sexual practice among the respondents as 75% claimed that it is one of the risky behaviors being practiced in this particular prison although only 5.4% of respondents admitted partaking in any of the risky behaviors including homosexuality. The 5.4% of the respondents that admitted partaking in any of the risky behaviors (including homosexuality) are likely to be severe underestimates considering percentage that claimed that homosexuality is one of the common sexual behaviors practiced in this prison. The practice of homosexuality is a criminal offence in Nigeria unlike many Western countries where it is legal; it carries an additional 14-year jail term in Nigeria when an inmate is convicted. In Nigeria prisons, same sex practices are made possible because inmates of the same sex sleep together in the same cell due to overcrowding which militate against the HIV/AIDS and tuberculosis prevention campaign. Previous studies reported more of such sexual activities in prisons [20, 24, 25]. Prison's officials had acknowledged that homosexuality accounts for over 90% of HIV/AIDS transmission in Nigeria prisons [26]. Previous studies reported that very few of the inmates knew that HIV/AIDS could be contacted through homosexual intercourse [1, 10, 18]. There is the risk of higher rate of HIV transmission in homosexuals compared with heterosexuals, and prisoners engaged in homosexuality are capable of transmitting HIV infection more than those who are not.

5. Conclusion and Recommendation

The knowledge about HIV/AIDS among inmates was high, but misconceptions about HIV/AIDS are still rife among the prisoners and educational programs would be required to correct this. Most of the inmates still display negative attitudes that are likely to encourage stigmatization and discrimination against the PLWHA. This will militate against voluntary counseling and testing as fear of isolation will prevent individuals from being tested. Efforts should be made by Nigeria Prison Service to comply with United Nations Committee on crime prevention and control that recommended that each prisoner should be made to occupy by night a cell or room by himself [27]. The sharing of sharp shaving instruments like razor blades should be discouraged in the prison to prevent the spread of HIV among inmates if an instrument got contaminated with blood infected with HIV.

Conflict of Interests

The authors declare that there is no conflict of interests regarding the publication of this paper.

Acknowledgments

The authors would like to acknowledge the staff and inmates of the Ogbomoso Prison for their cooperation. Their thanks also go to the wife of the Chairman Care Taker Committee and the Medical Officer of Health of Orire Local Government Area, Oyo State, Nigeria, for their support.

References

[1] O. O. Taiwo and A. Bukar, "Knowledge and attitude of prisoners towards HIV/AIDS infection," *Research Center for Oral Health Research and Training Initiative for Africa*, vol. 1, no. 1, pp. 31–34, 2006.

[2] K. Sabitu, Z. Iliyasu, and I. A. Joshua, "An assessment of knowledge of HIV/AIDS and associated Risky Behavior among inmates of Kaduna convict prison, the implications for prevention programs in Nigerian prisons," *Nigerian Journal of Medicine*, vol. 18, no. 1, pp. 52–58, 2009.

[3] National Population Commission (NPC) and ICF Macro, *Nigeria Demographic and Health Survey 2008*, National Population Commission (NPC) and ICF Macro, Abuja, Nigeria, 2009.

[4] K. C. Goyer, "HIV/AIDS in prisons: problems, policies, and potentials," Paper presented at the Institute for Security Studies, February 2003.

[5] United Nations office on Drugs and Crime, "HIV and Prisons in Sub-Saharan Africa: Opportunities for Action," 2006, http://www-wds.worldbank.org/.

[6] L. Fadeyi, "HIV scares in local prisons," *Daily Independent Nigeria*, 2009.

[7] O. Audu, S. J. Ogboi, A. U. Abdullahi, K. Sabitu, E. R. Abah, and O. P. Enokela, "Sexual risk behaviour and knowledge of HIV/AIDS among male prison inmates in Kaduna State, North Western Nigeria," *International Journal of Tropical Disease & Health*, vol. 3, no. 1, pp. 57–67, 2013.

[8] O. Simooya and N. Sanjobo, ""In but free"—an HIV/AIDS intervention in an African prison," *Culture, Health and Sexuality*, vol. 3, no. 2, pp. 241–251, 2001.

[9] H. Gayle, "An overview of the global HIV/AIDS epidemic, with a focus on the United States," *AIDS*, vol. 14, no. 2, pp. S8–S17, 2000.

[10] H. S. Labo, "A rapid assessment of the Knowledge, Attitude and Practice on HIV/AIDS and seroprevalence amongst staff and prisoners in paramilitary services survey in the Nigerian Para-Military," 2002.

[11] O. L. Ikuteyijo and M. O. Agunbiade, "Prison reforms and HIV/AIDS in selected Nigerian prisons," *The Journal of International Social Research*, vol. 1, no. 4, pp. 279–289, 2008.

[12] N. Awofeso and R. Naoum, "Sex in prisons—a management guide," *Australian Health Review*, vol. 25, no. 4, pp. 149–158, 2002.

[13] I. A. Joshua and S. J. Ogboi, "Sero-prevalence of HIV amongst inmates of Kaduna prison, Nigeria," *Science World Journal*, vol. 3, no. 1, pp. 17–19, 2008.

[14] L. Olusegun and O. A. Melvin, "Prison reform and HIV/AIDS in selected Nigeria prisons," *Journal of International Social Research*, vol. 1–4, 2008.

[15] J. Pont, H. Strutz, W. Kahl, and G. Salzner, "HIV epidemiology and risk behavior promoting HIV transmission in Austrian prisons," *European Journal of Epidemiology*, vol. 10, no. 3, pp. 285–289, 1994.

[16] E. Kantor, "HIV transmission and prevention in prisons. HIV in site knowledge base Chapter," 2003, http://hivinsite.ucsf.edu/.

[17] E. Malignity and G. B. Alvarez, "Preventive HIV/AIDS education for prisons," in *Proceedings of the 12th International Conference on AIDS*, vol. 12, p. 1018, Geneva, Switzerland, June–July 1998, abstract 60100.

[18] Avert, "Prisoners and HIV/AIDS," 2014, http://www.avert.org/prisoners-hivaids.htm.

[19] M. T. Odujinrin and S. B. Adebajo, "Social characteristics, HIV/AIDS knowledge, preventive practices and risk factors elicitation among prisoners in Lagos, Nigeria," *West African Journal of Medicine*, vol. 20, no. 3, pp. 191–198, 2001.

[20] Y. Hutin, A. Hauri, L. Chiarello et al., "Best infection control practices for intradermal, subcutaneous, and intramuscular needle injections," *Bulletin of the World Health Organization*, vol. 81, no. 7, pp. 491–500, 2003.

[21] Population Services International & Metrics Nigeria, "HIV/AIDS TRaC study evaluating behavior among risk groups in Nigeria Prisons Service. Roud one," PSI TRaC Summary Report, 2010, http://www.psi.org/resources/publications.

[22] Ministry of Interior Abuja Nigeria, Prison Service Information, 2013, http://interior.gov.ng/.

[23] *Interview Schedule on Knowledge, Attitudes, Beliefs, and Practices on AIDS/KABP Survey*, World Health Organization, Geneva, Switzerland, 1988.

[24] V. A. Akeke, M. Mokgatle, and O. O. Oguntibeju, "Assessment of knowledge and attitudes about HIV/AIDS among inmates of Quthing Prison, Lesotho," *West Indian Medical Journal*, vol. 56, no. 1, pp. 48–54, 2007.

[25] A. I. Olugbenga-Bello, O. A. Adeoye, and K. G. Osagbemi, "Assessment of the reproductive health status of adult prison inmates in Osun State, Nigeria," *International Journal of Reproductive Medicine*, vol. 2013, Article ID 451460, 9 pages, 2013.

[26] United Nation Integrated Regional Information Network, "Prison authorities free HIV positive inmates," August 2001.

[27] "First United Nations Congress on the Prevention of Crime and the Treatment of the Offenders: standard minimum rules for the treatment of prisoners," 2014, http://www.ohchr.org/EN/Pages/WelcomePage.aspx.

12

Determinants of Method Switching among Social Franchise Clients Who Discontinued the Use of Intrauterine Contraceptive Device

Waqas Hameed,[1] Syed Khurram Azmat,[1,2] Moazzam Ali,[3] Wajahat Hussain,[1] Ghulam Mustafa,[1] Muhammad Ishaque,[1] Safdar Ali,[1] Aftab Ahmed,[1] and Marleen Temmerman[2,3]

[1]*Marie Stopes Society, Research, Monitoring & Evaluation Department-Technical Services, Karachi, Sindh 75500, Pakistan*
[2]*Department of Uro-Gynecology, University of Ghent, 9000 East Flanders, Belgium*
[3]*Department of Reproductive Health and Research, World Health Organization, 1211 Geneva, Switzerland*

Correspondence should be addressed to Waqas Hameed; waqas.hameed1@gmail.com

Academic Editor: Hind A. Beydoun

Introduction. Women who do not switch to alternate methods after contraceptive discontinuation, for reasons other than the desire to get pregnant or not needing it, are at obvious risk for unplanned pregnancies or unwanted births. This paper examines the factors that influence women to switch from Intrauterine Contraceptive Device (IUCD) to other methods instead of terminating contraceptive usage altogether. *Methods.* The data used for this study comes from a larger cross-sectional survey conducted in nine (9) randomly selected districts of Sindh and Punjab provinces of Pakistan, during January 2011. Using Stata 11.2, we analyzed data on 333 women, who reported the removal of IUCDs due to reasons other than the desire to get pregnant. *Results.* We found that 39.9% of the women do not switch to another method of contraception within one month after IUCD discontinuation. Use of contraception before IUCD insertion increases the odds for method switching by 2.26 times after removal. Similarly, postremoval follow-up by community health worker doubles (OR = 2.0) the chances of method switching. Compared with women who received free IUCD service (via voucher scheme), the method switching is 2.01 times higher among women who had paid for IUCD insertion. *Conclusion.* To increase the likelihood of method switching among IUCD discontinuers this study emphasizes the need for postremoval client counseling, follow-up by healthcare provider, improved choices to a wider range of contraceptives for poor clients, and user satisfaction.

1. Introduction

Contraceptive discontinuation is not uncommon, though the rates vary from country to country [1, 2]. On average, 38% of women discontinue using reversible method by the 12th month. The discontinuation of any modern contraceptive is 13% (IUCD) to 50% (condom) within the first 12 months of its use [3]. According to a report based on developing countries, 13.1% of IUCD users discontinue its use during the first 12 months, 26.3% within 24 months, and 36.7% by the third year of its use [2]. Research evidence shows that contraceptive users are less likely to discontinue the method for which they are required to visit a clinic or need assistance from health professionals such as IUCD and implants, compared to discontinuation of short-term or traditional methods [3–6].

Not all women who discontinue contraception become nonusers; some switch to other contraceptive methods [1]. It has been estimated that approximately half of the women that discontinue IUCDs switch to another method within a 3-month period [4] and about 35.6% switch to short-term contraceptive methods. This indicates that those who switch are likely to be highly motivated to restrict fertility whereas others may be intimidated by its side effects, which can be the main reason behind IUCD removal [7].

Women who do not switch to alternate methods after the discontinuation of IUCDs for reasons other than the desire to get pregnant are at risk of having unplanned pregnancies or unwanted births [8–10]. Also, method switching is indicative of strong family planning programs that have an adequate range of available methods coupled with a service environment flexible to women's needs [11]. Women when not satisfied with quality of care often consider method switching [12]. However, woman's age, parity, geographic location (urban versus rural), and education are the most consistent predictors of method switching [4, 13, 14].

High rates of contraceptive discontinuation (for reasons other than the desire to get pregnant) are highlighted as a public health concern due to their association with negative reproductive health outcomes [10]. It has been recommended that healthcare providers should be motivated to encourage women that had discontinued a method to opt for another method of their choice [15]. Discontinuation and low rates of switching to alternate methods have been neglected by family planning programs in many developing countries [5]. The increased contraceptive use in developing countries has cut the number of maternal deaths by 40% over the past 20 years, by merely reducing the number of unintended pregnancies. Increased contraceptive use has reduced the maternal mortality ratio by about 26% in little more than a decade; a further 30% of maternal deaths could be avoided by fulfillment of unmet need for contraception [16]. Yet, in order to understand the mechanisms through which contraceptive usage contributes to fertility decline, it is important to first understand and examine contraceptive dynamics, including contraceptive failure and method switching [17].

2. Rationale

Pakistan has a population of over 184 million [18] where 65% of the people live in rural areas [19]. Each year, over 12,000 women die due to preventable pregnancy-related complications [20] and nearly 2.2 million cases of induced abortions are reported [21, 22]. Modern contraceptive use is only 26% with a majority using either permanent or less effective methods, while the use of long-term methods is negligible (IUCD = 2.3% and implant is negligible). More specifically, the use of IUCD remains unchanged since 2006-2007 [23, 24]. The overall situation in the rural terrains of Pakistan is far worse with respect to the aforementioned health indicators. Generally, factors affecting method switching vary from country to country [6]. The latest national Demographic Health Survey (DHS 2012-13) reveals that overall 37% of contraceptive usage episodes are discontinued within 12 months for any particular reason, while side effects or health concerns are the most often cited reason for stopping use of the pill, IUCDs, and injection. Only 8% of IUCD users switch to another method [24].

Marie Stopes Society "*Suraj*" Social Franchise Network: *Suraj* Social Franchise (SF) is essentially a partnership between Marie Stopes Society (a nongovernment organization) and local health providers, aiming to increase demand, access, choices, and provision of quality family planning services in rural, underserved, and poor communities. The model uses a two-pronged approach: demand side and supply side. The demand side includes the provision of local area

female health educators (FHEs) for raising awareness in communities regarding family planning and the referral of clients to service providers. Other components include free vouchers for long-term contraceptive method (IUCD) for the poor and comprehensive training of service providers on short-term (oral pill, condom, injectable, and emergency contraceptives) and long-term (IUCD insertion and removal) contraceptive methods and infection prevention.

The service providers mainly belong to midlevel providers category including lady health visitor, nurse, or community midwife. In each district the network ranged from 4 to 7 service providers practicing in the far-flung areas, each covering a total of 20,000–25,000 population.

There is very little evidence available in Pakistan with regard to this context. Therefore, in order to fill the gap in the existing body of knowledge, this paper reports on the cross-sectional data collected from women who received IUCD services from Marie Stopes Society's (MSS) Social Franchise providers in Pakistan, branded as "*Suraj*" (meaning "sun" in English) [15, 25].

This paper attempts to examine the factors that affect women's decision to switch to other contraceptive methods after the removal of IUCDs, instead of terminating usage altogether. The findings are also expected to be used for enhancing programme efficiency.

3. Methods

3.1. Data. The data used for this study come from a larger cross-sectional survey conducted by Marie Stopes Society in nine (9) randomly selected districts of Sindh and Punjab provinces during January 2011. The districts included Bahawalnagar, Jhang, Kasur, Lodhran, Sheikhupura, and Sialkot from Punjab and Umerkot, Hala/Matiari, and Tando Muhammad Khan from Sindh. The key objective of that survey was to estimate IUCD discontinuation rates and its determinants [15].

Participants were selected employing a multistage sampling with stratification. The first stage included district selection, the second stage included *Suraj* providers, and the final stage included selection of IUCD clients. The sampling details can be found elsewhere [15].

Women who received IUCD services (through *Suraj* providers) 6, 12, and 24 months prior to the survey were selected for this study. Women aged between 15 and 49 years and willing to give informed consent were invited to participate in the survey.

Face-to-face interviews were conducted with study participants using an adapted structured questionnaire that had previously been used in Philippines [26]. On an average, each interview took 20–25 minutes. The questionnaire covered sociodemographic characteristics (women's age, education, and number of living children), reasons for method discontinuation along with source of removal, switching behaviour, and client satisfaction the IUCD services. Data were double-entered in Visual FoxPro version 6.0 (Copyright © 1988–1998 Microsoft Corporation).

Out of 3,000 women, a total of 2,789 (93% response rate) women were successfully interviewed, of which 526 women had removed IUCD at some point in time before the survey due to any reason. We further eliminated cases where women discontinued the use of IUCD due to the desire for pregnancy and performed analysis on 333 cases for this paper.

The study protocol was reviewed and approved by the Research & Metrics Department of Marie Stopes International (MSI), London, UK.

4. Study Variables

The dependent variable was "method switching" where women coded "1" if they began to use another contraceptive method including traditional methods (within 1 month) after IUCD removal and "0" for women who stopped practicing contraception or became nonusers.

Some key independent variables included demographic characteristics (women's age, education, and number of living children), geographic region, type of IUCD, receiving IUCD through free vouchers, contraceptive status before the insertion of IUCD, experiencing method related side effects after IUCD insertion, reasons for IUCD insertion and removal, duration of IUCD use before discontinuation, time taken to travel to a *Suraj* facility, and the source of IUCD removal services.

5. Statistical Analysis

We analyzed data using Stata 11.2 (StataCorp. 2009, Stata Statistical Software: Release 11; StataCorp LP, College Station, TX). Simple frequencies and percentages were used to describe sample sociodemographic and health services characteristics. The association between explanatory variables and method switching was assessed using univariable and multivariable logistic regression techniques. A P value of ≤ 0.05 was taken to indicate statistical significance. The variables that showed a P value of >0.20 were not included in the multivariable modeling. Moreover, few satisfaction indicators ("recommendation of IUCD to friend" and "willingness to use IUCD in future") were excluded from the final model due to the issue of multicollinearity.

6. Results

Table 1 describes the characteristics of women who had removed IUCD due to any reason other than the desire for pregnancy. A majority (45.0%) of the respondents belonged to Southern Punjab, aged between 25 and 35 years (65.5%), and had no formal education (62.2%) and almost half had 5 or more children at the time of survey. Moreover, 62.8% had received IUCD through vouchers (for free), 76.6% had inserted the multiload, two-thirds were not using any form of contraception prior to IUCD insertion, and three-fourths had experienced method related side effects after IUCD insertion.

7. Switching Behaviors

The contraceptive status of women prior to IUCD insertion and after IUCD removal is presented in Table 2.

TABLE 1: Percentage distribution of women who removed IUCD due to any reason (other than pregnancy desire).

Characteristics	Women discontinued n (%)
Geographic region	
Sindh	59 (17.7)
Southern Punjab	150 (45.1)
Northern Punjab	124 (37.2)
Women received IUCD	
24 months ago	108 (32.4)
12 months ago	107 (32.1)
6 months ago	118 (35.4)
Age group of women	
≤25 years	21 (6.3)
>25–≤35 years	218 (65.5)
>35–49 years	94 (28.2)
Women's education	
No formal education	207 (62.2)
Primary	72 (21.6)
Secondary	45 (13.5)
Intermediate and post	9 (2.7)
Number of alive children	
1-2	47 (14.1)
3-4	120 (36.0)
5+	166 (49.9)
Type of client	
Referral (paid out of pocket)	124 (37.2)
Voucher (free)	209 (62.8)
Type of IUCD	
Multiload	255 (76.6)
Copper-T	78 (23.4)
Status of contraception before IUCD insertion	
Using a contraceptive method	113 (33.9)
Not using any method	220 (66.1)
Experience of side effects after IUCD insertion	
No	81 (24.3)
Yes	252 (75.7)
Number of cases	$N = 333$

7.1. Overall Switching Method. Overall, within one month after the removal of IUCD, 2 out of 5 women abandoned the usage of contraception altogether whereas 33.3% and 19.8% opted for short-term and traditional methods, respectively.

7.2. Switching among Nonusers. Among women who were not using any method prior to IUCD insertion, a majority (45.2%) did not switch to other contraceptive methods and became nonusers after the removal of IUCD; 29.0% switched to short-term methods and 17.6% started using traditional methods.

TABLE 2: Method switching behavior among women who had IUCD removal.

Contraceptive status after IUCD removal	Contraceptive status before IUCD insertion			Overall switching after IUCD removal
	Nonuser n (%)	Short-term[1] n (%)	Traditional[2] n (%)	
Nonuser	100 (45.2)	30 (30.6)	3 (21.4)	133 (39.9)
Short-term[1]	64 (29.0)	44 (44.9)	3 (21.4)	111 (33.3)
Permanent[2]	18 (8.1)	5 (5.1)	0 (0.0)	23 (3.9)
Traditional[3]	39 (17.6)	19 (19.4)	8 (57.1)	66 (19.8)
Total	221 (100.0)	98 (100.0)	14 (100.0)	333 (100.0)

[1]Condom, oral pill, and injection.
[2]Female sterilization.
[3]Withdrawal and periodic abstinence.

7.3. Switching among Short-Term Contraceptive Users. Similarly, amongst women who were using short-term methods prior to IUCD insertion, a majority (44.9%) returned to short-term methods, 30.6% became nonusers, and 19.4% opted for traditional methods.

7.4. Switching among Traditional Method Users. Among users of traditional methods prior to IUCD insertion, 57.1% ($n = 14$) had returned to the same while 21.4% of women switched to short-term methods and an equal proportion became nonusers.

8. Univariate Analyses

The association between risk factors and method switching is presented in Table 3 by means of unadjusted odds ratios. Women living in Southern Punjab had 3.35 times higher odds of switching to another contraceptive method compared to women from Northern Punjab. Among health services variables, women practicing contraception before IUCD insertion were more likely to switch to another method as compared to those who were not using any contraception (odds ratio, 2.02). Similarly, users of multiload had 2.10 times higher odds of switching as compared to users of Copper-T. Moreover, women who received IUCD services for free (through voucher scheme) were less likely to switch to another method after its removal as compared to women who paid out of pocket for IUCD insertion. We also found that women who discontinued the use of IUCD within 3 months or between 3 and 6 months were more likely to switch to another method as compared to women who discontinued after 6 months of usage. Interaction or meeting with community health workers after IUCD removal substantially increased the chances of switching (odds ratio, 3.39). A measure of satisfaction levels also showed significant association with method switching.

9. Multivariable Analyses

In multivariable analyses fewer variables remained significant at a 5% level of significance (Table 4). Prior use of contraceptive methods and postremoval follow-up with community health worker showed positive association with method switching. Women who received IUCD for free (through voucher scheme) were less likely to switch to another method.

Moreover, women who felt neutral or dissatisfied with IUCD were more likely to switch to another method. The women residing in Southern Punjab had 3.41 times higher odds of switching as compared to the women in Northern Punjab.

10. Discussion

The findings of this study reveal that only three-fifths of the women switched to another method after IUCD removal within one month, leaving others at right of unintended pregnancy at a given point in time [8–10]. Moreover, it is noteworthy to observe that women who were using any contraceptive method before the insertion of IUCD were more likely to switch back to the same (short-term) contraceptive methods after IUCD removal, which were less effective [27]. A possible reason for this may be attributed to the fact that the *Suraj* services providers were midlevel providers who are not allowed to provide implant that is another form of long-term contraceptive method or female sterilization (permanent method) as per national health policy. Yet, these services may have been available elsewhere.

The study also elicited higher chances of switching among women who were practicing contraception before the insertion of an IUCD. This behavior aligns with the aforementioned results (in Table 2) yielded from the study, depicting that women tend to revert to the original method that they were using before IUCD uptake. Also, keeping in view of the smaller difference between the proportion of ever and current use in Pakistan [23], it may be previous contraceptive exposure, experience, and henceforth knowledge that motivate women to switch to another method of their choice, instead of stopping usage altogether.

The study revealed that women who had received IUCD for free (through voucher scheme) were less likely to switch to another method, indicating that cost is a significant factor influencing method uptake after IUCD discontinuation [24]. It is also pertinent to note that the free voucher scheme only provided IUCD services whereas clients had to pay for the other modern contraceptive services irrespective of their economic status. Since vouchers were provided to clients that lacked affordability, they may have been restricted in terms of choice for alternate free modern contraceptive methods. Perhaps they would have preferred another method but were unable to afford it. However, there may be other influencing

TABLE 3: Unadjusted odds ratios of method switching versus method stopping, according to selected sociodemographic and reproductive health risk factors.

Characteristics	N	Method switched n (%)	OR (95% C.I.)
Geographic region			
Northern Punjab	124	58 (46.8)	1
Sindh	59	30 (50.8)	1.17 (0.63–2.18)
Southern Punjab	150	112 (74.7)	3.35 (2.01–5.58)**
Age of women			
≤25 years	21	11 (52.4)	1
>25–≤35 years	218	136 (62.4)	1.50 (0.61–3.70)
>35–49 years	94	53 (56.4)	1.17 (0.45–3.03)
Women education			
No formal education	207	119 (57.5)	1
Primary	72	42 (58.3)	1.03 (0.60–1.78)
≥Secondary	54	39 (72.2)	1.92 (0.99–3.70)
Number of children			
1-2	47	23 (48.9)	1
3-4	120	78 (65.0)	1.93 (0.97–3.84)
5+	166	99 (59.6)	1.54 (0.80–2.95)
Type of client			
Voucher (free)	209	117 (56.0)	1
Referral (paid out of pocket)	124	83 (66.9)	1.59 (1.00–2.52)*
Type of IUCD			
Copper-T	78	36 (46.2)	1
Multiload	255	164 (64.3)	2.10 (1.25–3.51)**
Status of contraception before IUCD insertion			
Not using any method	220	120 (54.5)	1
Using a contraceptive method	113	80 (70.8)	2.02 (1.24–3.27)**
Reason for choosing IUCD			
Encouraged by FWM	148	88 (59.5)	1
Any other reason	185	112 (60.5)	1.04 (0.67–1.62)
Meeting with community after IUCD insertion			
No	99	39 (39.4)	1
Yes	234	161 (68.8)	3.39 (2.08–5.53)***
Reason for IUCD discontinuation			
Nonhealth related	85	46 (54.1)	1
Method related side effects	248	154 (62.1)	1.39 (0.84–2.23)
Place of IUCD removal			
Government clinic	23	12 (52.2)	1
Private clinic	65	45 (69.2)	2.06 (0.78–5.46)
Expulsion	24	13 (54.2)	1.08 (0.34–3.41)
Suraj centre	221	130 (58.8)	1.30 (0.55–3.10)
Duration of IUCD use before discontinuation			
>6 to 24	165	83 (50.3)	1
>3 to 6	73	47 (64.4)	1.79 (1.01–3.15)*
≤3 months	95	70 (73.7)	2.77 (1.60–4.80)***
Time travel for removal services			
Less than 1 hour	305	183 (60.0)	1
≥1 hour	28	17 (60.7)	1.03 (0.46–2.28)
Satisfaction with IUCD services			
Satisfied or very satisfied	173	90 (52.0)	1
Neutral or unsatisfied	160	110 (68.8)	2.03 (1.29–3.18)**
Would use IUCD in future, if needed			
Yes, readily	119	60 (50.4)	1
No or not sure	214	140 (70.0)	1.86 (1.18–2.93)**
Would recommend IUCD to friend			
Yes	277	168 (60.6)	1
No	56	32 (57.1)	0.87 (0.48–1.55)

P value: *P < 0.05, **P < 0.01, and ***P < 0.001.

TABLE 4: Adjusted odds ratios of method switching versus method stopping, according to selected sociodemographic and reproductive health risk factors.

Characteristics	Method switched	
	AOR	(95% C.I.)
Region		
Northern Punjab	1	
Sindh	1.06	0.52–2.14
Southern Punjab	3.41	1.80–6.46***
Type of client		
Voucher (free)	1	
Referral (paid out of pocket)	2.01	1.18–3.43*
Status of contraception before IUCD insertion		
Not using any method	1	
Using a contraceptive method	2.26	1.31–3.87**
Meeting with community health worker after IUCD insertion		
No	1	1
Yes	2.00	1.11–3.60*
Satisfaction with IUCD related services		
Satisfied or very satisfied	1	1
Neutral or unsatisfied	1.72	1.04–2.82*

P value: *$P < 0.05$, **$P < 0.01$, and ***$P < 0.001$.

factors as poor clients can always switch to traditional methods. The findings warrant further investigation on this aspect for better understanding [28].

Moreover, women who met with community health workers after IUCD removal were more likely to adopt another contraceptive method. This is consistent with another study conducted in Bangladesh [1, 29]. It also emphasizes the need of repeated follow-ups and counseling to women after the removal of an IUCD, so that they may be better guided towards alternate contraceptive options.

We observed that users who were less satisfied with IUCD were more likely to switch to another method upon its removal which is consistent with earlier study where women who are less satisfied with quality of care often switch to another method [12]. This might have been due to higher satisfaction levels of women with previous contraceptive exposure that motivated women to revert to the same method.

Finally, our study also found different switching rates by geographic region. Though similar results were observed in other studies [17, 30], we suggest in-depth investigations to understand this phenomenon in our context. Interestingly enough, this study did not find association between method related side effects and method switching. This stands in stark opposition to the results from other studies conducted on the matter that depict IUCD side effects as one of the major reasons behind IUCD discontinuation [1, 3].

This study also has some limitations, common to all retrospective studies. A major limitation was the potential of recall bias, owing to the time lag between the client's IUCD discontinuation and when the survey was actually undertaken. The study only focused on women who discontinued the use of IUCD only whereas data regarding other contraceptive methods are beyond the scope of this study. Moreover, we did not capture data on partner-related factors which may influence the behaviour or practice of contraceptive use. Also, the data did not capture the continuation time of the new method uptake, post-IUCD discontinuation, among women who opted for an IUCD removal. This might have been a significant contribution in indicating whether new method was used for a day, a week, or few months and whether clients switched back to an IUCD after the new method uptake. Similarly, those who did not opt for a new method within a month of removal might have used any contraceptive method later on. Lastly, because the study is cross-sectional, deriving temporal associations is not possible. For example, it is assumed that the interaction/follow-up by a healthcare provider increases the likelihood of switching; the reverse may also be true; that is, the motive to switch causes the contact with healthcare provider. A comprehensive prospective study for a longer period of time could answer these questions.

Despite the aforementioned limitations, the insight generated from this study reveals interesting findings. To the best of authors' knowledge, this study is the first of its kind in Pakistan which specially focuses on contraceptive method switching behaviour and its determinants.

11. Conclusion

To promote method switching among IUCD discontinuers, this study emphasizes the need for effective counseling services and follow-up by community health workers. Immediate FP counseling and follow-up can significantly increase contraceptive uptake after IUCD removal especially among the women who discontinue a method for reasons other than the desire to get pregnant. Moreover, improved choices to a wider range of contraceptives for poor clients, quality services, and user satisfaction are crucial for promoting method switching in order to prevent the risk of unintended pregnancies. In addition, it will help dispelling myths and misconceptions regarding IUCD and may help in increasing the stagnated contraceptive use in the country. Yet, we recommend a rigorous prospective mix-method research to substantiate or endorse the determinants of method switching identified in our study.

Disclaimer

The present study protocol includes the collective views of an international group of experts and does not necessarily represent the decisions or the stated policy of the World Health Organization or Marie Stopes Society, Pakistan. The authors alone are responsible for the content and the writing of the paper.

Conflict of Interests

The authors report no conflict of interests in this work. The authors, though, are affiliated with the organization that implemented the program; they neither come under nor are part of program implementation team.

Authors' Contribution

Waqas Hameed conceptualized and designed the experiment, supervised the data analysis, and wrote the paper; Syed Khurram Azmat, Ghulam Mustafa, Safdar Ali, Moazzam Ali, and Marleen Temmerman reviewed the draft and provided critical feedback; and Aftab Ahmed, Muhammad Ishaque, and Wajahat Hussain supervised the data collection and assisted in the literature search, data cleaning, and analysis. All authors read and approved the final paper.

Acknowledgments

The authors are indebted to the participants of this study and all district and regional teams of Marie Stopes Society, Pakistan.

References

[1] J. Barden-O'Fallon and I. Speizer, "What differentiates method stoppers from switchers? contraceptive discontinuation and switching among honduran women," International Perspectives on Sexual and Reproductive Health, vol. 37, no. 1, pp. 16–23, 2011.

[2] J. Cleland and I. H. Shah, Causes and Consequences of Contraceptive Discontinuation: Evidence from 60 Demographic and Health Surveys, World Health Organization, Geneva, Switzerland, 2012.

[3] S. E. K. Bradley, H. M. Schwandt, and S. Khan, "Levels, trends, and reasons for contraceptive discontinuation," DHS Analytical Studies Report 20, ICF Macro, Calverton, Md, USA, 2009.

[4] M. M. Ali, R. K. Sadler, J. Cleland, T. D. Ngo, and I. H. Shah, Long-Term Contraceptive Protection, Discontinuation and Switching Behaviour: Intrauterine Device (IUD) Use Dynamics in 14 Developing Countries, World Health Organization and Marie Stopes International, London, UK, 2011.

[5] M. M. Ali and J. Cleland, "Oral contraceptive discontinuation and its aftermath in 19 developing countries," Contraception, vol. 81, no. 1, pp. 22–29, 2010.

[6] United Nations Department of Economic and Social Affairs, Levels and Trends of Contraceptive Use As Assessed in 2002, United Nations, New York, NY, USA, 2002.

[7] T. D. Ngo and G. Eva, MSI Mobile Outreach Services: Retrospective Evaluations from Ethiopia, Myanmar, Pakistan, Sierra Leone and Vietnam, Marie Stopes International, London, UK, 2010.

[8] J. L. Barden-O'Fallon, I. S. Speizer, and J. S. White, "Association between contraceptive discontinuation and pregnancy intentions in Guatemala," Revista Panamericana de Salud Publica, vol. 23, no. 6, pp. 410–417, 2008.

[9] A. K. Blanc, S. L. Curtis, and T. N. Croft, "Monitoring contraceptive continuation: links to fertility outcomes and quality of care," Studies in Family Planning, vol. 33, no. 2, pp. 127–140, 2002.

[10] S. L. Curtis, E. Evens, and W. Sambisa, "Contraceptive discontinuation and unintended pregnancy: an imperfect relationship," International Perspectives on Sexual and Reproductive Health, vol. 37, no. 2, pp. 58–66, 2011.

[11] J. Bongaarts and J. Bruce, "The causes of unmet need for contraception and the social content of services," Studies in Family Planning, vol. 26, no. 2, pp. 57–75, 1995.

[12] F. Steele and I. Diamond, "Contraceptive switching in Bangladesh," Studies in Family Planning, vol. 30, no. 4, pp. 315–328, 1999.

[13] W. R. Grady, J. O. G. Billy, and D. H. Klepinger, "Contraceptive method switching in the United States," Perspectives on Sexual and Reproductive Health, vol. 34, no. 3, pp. 135–145, 2002.

[14] D. N. Hamill, A. O. Tsui, and S. Thapa, "Determinants of contraceptive switching behavior in rural Sri Lanka," Demography, vol. 27, no. 4, pp. 559–578, 1990.

[15] S. K. Azmat, B. T. Shaikh, W. Hameed et al., "Rates of IUCD discontinuation and its associated factors among the clients of a social franchising network in Pakistan," BMC Women's Health, vol. 12, no. 1, article 8, 2012.

[16] J. Cleland, S. Bernstein, A. Ezeh, A. Faundes, A. Glasier, and J. Innis, "Family planning: the unfinished agenda," The Lancet, vol. 368, no. 9549, pp. 1810–1827, 2006.

[17] I. C. Leite and N. Gupta, "Assessing regional differences in contraceptive discontinuation, failure and switching in Brazil," Reproductive Health, vol. 4, article 6, 2007.

[18] Government of Pakistan, Pakistan Economic Survey, 2012-13, Finance Division, Economic Advisor's Wing, Islamabad, Pakistan, 2013.

[19] United Nations Department of Economic and Social Affaris Population Division, World Population Prospects: The 2008 Revision, 2008.

[20] WHO, UNICEF, UNFPA, and The World Bank Estimates, Trends in Maternal Mortality:1990 to 2010, World Health Organization, Geneva, Switzerland, 2012.

[21] Z. Sathar, S. Singh, G. Rashida, Z. Shah, and R. Niazi, "Induced abortions and unintended pregnancies in Pakistan," Studies in Family Planning, vol. 45, no. 4, pp. 471–491, 2014.

[22] Z. A. Sathar, S. Singh, and F. F. Fikree, "Estimating the incidence of abortion in Pakistan," Studies in Family Planning, vol. 38, no. 1, pp. 11–22, 2007.

[23] National Institute of Population Studies Pakistan and Macro International Inc, Pakistan Demographic and Health Survey 2006-7, Government of Pakistan, Islamabad, Pakistan, 2008.

[24] National Institute of Population Studies Pakistan and Macro International Inc, *Pakistan Demographic and Health Survey 2012-13*, Government of Pakistan, Islamabad, Pakistan, 2014.

[25] Marie Stopes Society, *Case Study: "Suraj"—A Private Provider Partnership*, Marie Stopes International, 2010.

[26] T. D. Ngo and V. L. Pernito, *Discontinuation of IUDs among Women Receiving Mobile Outreach Services in the Philippines, 2006–2008*, Marie Stopes International, London, UK, 2009.

[27] J. Trussell, "Contraceptive failure in the United States," *Contraception*, vol. 70, no. 2, pp. 89–96, 2004.

[28] S. L. Curtis and A. K. Blanc, "Determinants of contraceptive failure, switching, and discontinuation: an analysis of DHS contraceptive histories," Tech. Rep. 6, Macro International, Calverton, Md, USA, 1997.

[29] M. B. Hossain, "Analysing the relationship between family planning workers' contact and contraceptive switching in rural Bangladesh using multilevel modelling," *Journal of Biosocial Science*, vol. 37, no. 5, pp. 529–554, 2005.

[30] M. M. Ali, M. H. Park, and T. D. Ngo, "Levels and determinants of switching following intrauterine device discontinuation in 14 developing countries," *Contraception*, vol. 90, no. 1, pp. 47–53, 2014.

13

Foley Catheter versus Vaginal Misoprostol for Labour Induction

Nasreen Noor, Mehkat Ansari, S. Manazir Ali, and Shazia Parveen

Department of Obstetrics and Gynaecology and Department of Pediatrics, JNMCH, AMU, L-Block 107 Safina Apartment, Medical Road, Aligarh 202002, India

Correspondence should be addressed to Nasreen Noor; nasreen_71@rediffmail.com

Academic Editor: Hind A. Beydoun

Objectives. To compare the efficacy and safety of intravaginal misoprostol with transcervical Foley catheter for labour induction. *Material and Methods.* One hundred and four women with term gestation, with Bishop score < 4, and with various indications for labour induction were randomly divided into two groups. In Group I, 25 μg of misoprostol tablet was placed intravaginally, 4 hourly up to maximum 6 doses. In Group II, Foley catheter 16F was placed through the internal os of the cervix under aseptic condition and then inflated with 50 cc of sterile saline. Statistical analysis was done using SPSS software. *Results.* The induction to delivery interval was 14.03 ± 7.61 hours versus 18.40 ± 8.02 hours ($p < 0.01$). The rate of vaginal delivery was 76.7% versus 56.8% in misoprostol and transcervical Foley catheter group, respectively. Uterine hyperstimulation was more common with misoprostol. Neonatal outcome was similar in both the groups. *Conclusion.* Intravaginal misoprostol is associated with a shorter induction to delivery interval as compared to Foley's catheter and it increases the rate of vaginal delivery in cases of unripe cervix at term. Transcervical Foley catheter is associated with a lower incidence of uterine hyperstimulation during labour.

1. Introduction

In the recent decade, there has been a considerable increase in the rate of labour induction. Achievement of a vaginal delivery for a woman who requires induction of labour may be among the greatest challenges facing obstetricians today. Labour induction is usually performed when the risks of continuing a pregnancy are more than the benefits of delivery. Indications for induction of labour include immediate conditions such as severe preeclampsia or ruptured membranes with chorioamnionitis. The other common medical and obstetric indications include membrane rupture without labour, gestational hypertension, postdated pregnancy, oligohydramnios, nonreassuring fetal status, intrauterine growth restriction, chronic hypertension, and diabetes [1]. Undoubtedly, cervical ripening has a close relationship with the success rate of vaginal delivery. Different methods are used for labour induction but none of the available methods of induction of labour is free of associated medical risks; therefore, labour should only be induced when the risk of allowing the continuation of pregnancy outweighs the risk of induction. Ideally, agents used for induction should mimic spontaneous labour without causing excessive uterine

activity. The most common methods of labour induction when the status of cervix is unfavourable involve intravaginal use of misoprostol, transcervical insertion of Foley's catheter, and insertion of prostaglandin gel whereas with a ripe cervix oxytocin may be administered intravenously. Serum levels after vaginal absorption are more prolonged; irrespective of serum levels, vaginally absorbed misoprostol has locally mediated effects; thus there has been increasing interest in misoprostol for use as a pharmacological agent for labour induction. However, there remains some controversy concerning the dosage, the mode, and interval of administration of misoprostol. Although perhaps more effective, use of a high dose could be associated with an increased risk for hyperstimulation of the uterus; however there are ongoing trials regarding optimal dose, dosing regimen, and route of administration. In the case of women who have previously undergone a caesarean section and thereby run an increased risk for uterine rupture in connection with vaginal delivery, induction of labour with misoprostol may further enhance this risk and is not recommended. Another procedure adopted for routine induction of labour involves transcervical application of Foley's catheter. Such a catheter appears to induce labour not only through direct mechanical dilation of the cervix but also by stimulating endogenous release of prostaglandins. The aim of this study is the comparison of vaginal misoprostol and transcervical Foley's catheter for induction of labour.

2. Material and Methods

This randomized clinical study was conducted in the Department of Obstetrics and Gynaecology in collaboration with the Department of Paediatrics, JNMCH, AMU, Aligarh (UP), India, during May 2013–August 2014. The included criteria were singleton pregnancy cephalic presentation, gestation age >37 weeks on the basis of LMP or first trimester ultrasonography, intact membranes, unfavourable cervix (Bishop score ≤ 4), and imminent delivery for fetal or maternal indication. Women were excluded from the study if any of the following criteria were encountered: rupture of membranes, chorioamnionitis, antepartum haemorrhage, cervical dilation >2.5 cm, temperature >38°C, contracted pelvis, fetal distress, polyhydramnios, indication for immediate delivery, and previous caesarean section or other uterine surgeries (for Group I).

A total of one hundred and four (104) women requiring indicated induction of labour with an unfavourable cervix (Bishop score ≤ 4) were included in the study. They were randomly divided into two groups: 60 women induced with intravaginal misoprostol (Group I) and 44 women induced with transcervical Foley catheter (Group II). At first, the method of the study was completely explained to them; if the written consent was obtained, they were enrolled in the study. This study was approved by the Ethics Committee of Faculty of Medicine, Aligarh Muslim University. Cases were selected from antenatal clinic (ANC), outpatient department (OPD), and patients admitted in the hospital. The two groups were comparable with respect to maternal age, parity, and gestational and preinduction Bishop score. Demographic and clinical data were collected at routine antenatal visits. In Group I, 25 mcg of misoprostol tablet was placed intravaginally, 4 hourly for maximum 6 doses. In the presence of spontaneous and frequent contractions (>40–45 seconds every 3 minutes), the next dose was not administered. If there was no effective uterine contractions after the sixth dose, then it was considered as failure of induction by the concerned method. In Group II, 18 F Foley catheter was inserted into the endocervical canal under direct vision by doing a per-speculum examination. The catheter was advanced into the endocervical canal. Once past the internal os, the balloon was filled with 50 mL of sterile saline solution and the catheter was taped to the inner thigh to maintain traction. The catheter was checked for extrusion of the balloon from the cervix every 6 hours by cervical examination and the catheter remained in place until the balloon was expelled spontaneously and labour augmentation was done by artificial membrane rupture or oxytocin drip (2.5 or 5 IU in 500 mL of Ringer's lactate solution was started then and it was titrated according to frequency and intensity of uterine contractions) whichever is indicated. The primary outcome measures were induction to delivery interval and secondary outcome measures include

TABLE 1: Demographic profile and indication for induction.

Parameters	Group I (n = 60) (misoprostol)	Group II (n = 44) (Foley catheter)	"p" value
Age (years) (mean ± SD)	25.1 ± 2.8	25.6 ± 4.1	>0.05
Gravidity			
Primigravida	41.7%	31.8%	>0.05
Multigravida	58.3%	68.2%	>0.05
Gestational age (weeks) (mean ± SD)	39.1 ± 1.4	39.4 ± 1.2	>0.05
Indication for induction			
Oligohydramnios	11 (18.3)	08 (18.2)	>0.05
Preeclampsia	11 (18.3)	04 (09.1)	>0.05
Intrauterine growth rsestriction	07 (11.7)	04 (09.1)	>0.05
Gestational diabetes mellitus	02 (03.4)	01 (02.3)	>0.05

TABLE 2: Induction to delivery interval (mean ± SD).

Parameters	Group I (n = 60) (misoprostol)	Group II (n = 44) (Foley catheter)	"p" value
Induction to active phase interval (hrs) (mean ± SD)	11.6 ± 5.21	11.8 ± 5.82	>0.05
Induction to delivery interval (hrs) (mean ± SD)	14.03 ± 7.61	18.40 ± 8.02	<0.01

uterine contractile abnormalities like uterine tachysystole (6 contractions in a 10-minute period), uterine hypertonus (a single contraction lasting longer than 2 minutes) and uterine hyperstimulation is when either condition leads to a nonreassuring fetal heart rate pattern, meconium stained liquor, mode of delivery, maternal and neonatal outcome, neonatal birth weight, and Apgar score. Any maternal or fetal complications were also recorded.

3. Results

A total of one hundred and four (104) women were included in the study. They were randomly divided into two groups: Group I: women induced with intravaginal misoprostol (n = 60) and Group II: women induced with transcervical Foley catheter (n = 44). Maternal baseline characteristics were similar between the two groups in terms of age, parity, gestational age, preinduction Bishop score, and indications for induction (Table 1).

As shown in Table 2 the induction to delivery interval (mean ± SD) in women induced with intravaginal misoprostol was 14.03 ± 7.61 hours while that of women induced with transcervical Foley catheter was 18.40 ± 8.02 hours.

TABLE 3: Outcome in labour.

Augmentation required	Group I (Misoprostol)		Group II (Foley catheter)		X^2	p value
	n	%	n	%		
Oxytocin drip	29	48.3	34	77.2	8.9	<0.01
Artificial rupture of membrane	40	66.7	42	95.5	12.6	<0.001
Oxytocin + ARM	25	41.7	34	77.2	13.1	<0.001
Complications						
Hyperstimulation	07	11.7	00	00.0	—	—
Tachysystole	00	00.0	00	00.0	—	—
Uterine rupture	00	00.0	00	00.0	—	—

TABLE 4: Comparison of mode of delivery.

Mode of delivery	Group I (Misoprostol)		Group II (Foley catheter)		Total		"p" value
	n	%	n	%	n	%	
Vaginal delivery	46	76.7	25	56.8	71	68.3	<0.05
Caesarean delivery	14	23.3	19	43.2	33	31.7	<0.05
Total	60	100.0	44	100.0	104	100.0	

The induction to delivery interval in misoprostol group was significantly shorter than that in Foley catheter group ($p < 0.01$).

The use of oxytocin and ARM for labour augmentation was significantly higher in women induced with Foley catheter as compared to women induced with intravaginal misoprostol 77.2% versus 48.3% and 95.5% versus 66.7%, respectively. Combined use of oxytocin and ARM was 41.7% and 77.2% in misoprostol and Foley catheter group, respectively, and statistically it was very highly significant ($p < 0.001$). Uterine contractile abnormalities like hyperstimulation were reported in 11.7% of women while there was no case of hyperstimulation noted in Foley catheter group (Table 3).

As depicted in Table 4, the rate of vaginal delivery and caesarean section was 76.7% versus 56.8% and 23.3% versus 43.2% in misoprostol and Foley catheter group, respectively. The rate of vaginal delivery was significantly more in misoprostol group as compared to Foley catheter group ($p < 0.05$). In this study, there was a tendency towards more frequent caesarean section in response to fetal distress among women who were given misoprostol. This finding is in agreement with most of the studies that have demonstrated a higher incidence of hyperstimulation associated with fetal distress in women induced with misoprostol. In women induced with Foley catheter, nonprogression of labour and scar tenderness were seen in 20.5% and 9.1% women, respectively. Meconium amniotic fluid was seen in 5 women (8.3%) induced with misoprostol and 4 women (9.1%) induced with Foley catheter. Both the groups were comparable in terms of meconium amniotic fluid as an indication of caesarean section. The caesarean section rate was more in Foley catheter group as compared to misoprostol group and the results were statistically significant ($p < 0.05$).

The birth weight (mean ± SD) was 2.79 ± 0.43 kg and 2.91 ± 0.53 kg in misoprostol and Foley catheter group.

TABLE 5: Neonatal outcome in Group I and Group II.

Parameters	Group I (n = 60) (misoprostol)	Group II (n = 44) (Foley catheter)	"p" value
Birth weight (kg) (mean ± SD)	2.79 ± 0.43	2.91 ± 0.53	>0.05
Apgar score (at 1 min) Mean ± SD	7.80 ± 0.77	7.91 ± 0.33	>0.05
Apgar score (at 5 min) Mean ± SD	8.92 ± 0.38	8.98 ± 0.15	>0.05
Admission in neonatal intensive care unit	13.3%	13.6%	>0.05
Meconium aspiration syndrome	8.3%	9.1%	>0.05

The difference in the birth weight between the two study groups was statistically not significant ($p > 0.05$). The Apgar score at 1 minute and 5 minutes (mean ± SD) was 7.80 ± 0.77 versus 7.91 ± 0.33 and 8.92 ± 0.38 versus 8.98 ± 0.15 in misoprostol and Foley catheter group, respectively (Table 5). Statistically there was no significant difference in the Apgar score between the two groups at 1 minute and 5 minutes ($p > 0.05$).

4. Discussion

Induction of labour is an integral component of all maternity practice and is often taken up in the interest of the mother and the fetus. Labour induction in the presence of an unfavorable cervix is associated with an increased likelihood of prolonged labour and increased incidence of caesarean section. Hence, the use of cervical ripening agents prior to conventional methods of induction is now a standard practice. Until now different methods for labour induction are used. In literature, contradictory results are reported regarding efficacy and safety of the induction methods. Therefore in this study, we compared the efficacy and safety of 25 μg vaginal misoprostol with transcervical Foley catheter for induction of labour.

Our results on induction to delivery interval show that the interval was significantly shorter in misoprostol group as compared to Foley catheter group. Our findings were similar to Promila et al. [2], Sheikher et al. [3], Filho et al. [4], and Roudsari et al. [5], who also found significantly shorter induction to delivery interval in misoprostol group. Tuuli et al. [6] reported that the total duration of labour was not significantly different in women induced with misoprostol compared with the Foley catheter (median duration from 1 to 10 cm: 12 versus 14.2 hours, $p = 0.19$). Jindal et al. [7] also reported shorter interval for misoprostol compared to Foley's catheter (11.58 hours versus 19.45 hours). The shorter induction delivery interval in misoprostol group could be explained on the basis of greater oxytocic effect on uterus via vaginal route due to direct access to myometrium by cervical canal. In the study performed by Chung et al. [8] and Adeniji et al. [9], the induction to delivery interval did not differ significantly between the two groups. Our study is not in accordance with Prager et al. [10], who found that a induction to delivery interval was significantly shorter in Foley catheter group as compared to misoprostol and PGE2; the most important cause for this may be lower dose of misoprostol (25 μg) used in our study compared with their studies [10]. Use of oxytocin for labour augmentation was significantly higher in women induced with Foley catheter as compared to women induced with intravaginal misoprostol. Uterine contractile abnormalities were more common in women using misoprostol as compared to Foley's catheter. The finding that transcervical Foley catheter is associated with no risk of hyperstimulation may be particularly useful when inducing labour in woman with previous caesarean section who are at increased risk of uterine rupture. No case of tachysystole or uterine rupture was found in both the groups. Roudsari et al. [5] found hyperstimulation occurring more frequently in the misoprostol group. Chung et al. [8] in their study found that hyperstimulation occurred in 33.3% women in misoprostol group and 11.1% women in Foley catheter group. Mozurkewich et al. [1] found that contractile abnormalities were more frequent in the misoprostol group than the Foley catheter group and thus this finding is in agreement with the findings that have demonstrated a higher incidence of hyperstimulation associated with fetal distress in women induced with misoprostol. Both the groups were comparable in terms of meconium amniotic fluid as an indication of caesarean section. Statistically there was no significant difference in the Apgar score between the two groups at 1 minute and 5 minutes. Similar results were obtained by Filho et al. [4] and Roudsari et al. [5] and our present study supports these results.

5. Conclusion

The present study suggests intravaginal misoprostol is associated with a shorter induction to delivery interval as compared to Foley's catheter and it increases the rate of vaginal delivery in cases of unripe cervix at term. Transcervical Foley catheter is associated with a lower incidence of uterine hyperstimulation; thus Foley catheter may be a reasonable alternative for patients who are at risk of uterine rupture during labour.

Conflict of Interests

The authors declare that there is no conflict of interests regarding the publication of this paper.

References

[1] E. Mozurkewich, J. Chilimigras, E. Koepke, K. Keeton, and V. J. King, "Indications for induction of labour: a best-evidence review," *BJOG: An International Journal of Obstetrics and Gynaecology*, vol. 116, no. 5, pp. 626–636, 2009.

[2] J. Promila, G. B. Kaur, and T. Bala, "A comparison of vaginal misoprostol versus Foley's catheter with oxytocin for induction of labor," *The Journal of Obstetrics and Gynecology of India*, vol. 57, no. 1, pp. 42–47, 2007.

[3] C. Sheikher, N. Suri, and U. Kholi, "Comparative evaluation of oral misoprostol, vaginal misoprostol and intracervical Folley's catheter for induction of labour at term," *JK Science*, vol. 11, no. 2, pp. 75–77, 2009.

[4] O. B. M. Filho, R. M. Albuquerque, and J. G. Cecatti, "A randomized controlled trial comparing vaginal misoprostol versus foley catheter plus oxytocin for labor induction," *Acta Obstetricia et Gynecologica Scandinavica*, vol. 89, no. 8, pp. 1045–1052, 2010.

[5] F. V. Roudsari, S. Ayati, M. Ghasemi et al., "Comparison of vaginal misoprostol with Foley catheter for cervical ripening and induction of labor," *Iranian Journal of Pharmaceutical Research*, vol. 10, no. 1, pp. 149–154, 2011.

[6] M. G. Tuuli, M. B. Keegan, A. O. Odibo, K. Roehl, G. A. Macones, and A. G. Cahill, "Progress of labor in women induced with misoprostol versus the Foley catheter," *American Journal of Obstetrics and Gynecology*, vol. 209, no. 3, pp. 237.e1–237.e7, 2013.

[7] P. Jindal, B. K. Gill, and B. Tirath, "A comparison of vaginal misoprostol versus Foley's catheter with oxytocin for induction of labour," *The Journal of Obstetrics and Gynecology of India*, vol. 57, no. 1, pp. 42–47, 2007.

[8] J. H. Chung, W. H. Huang, P. J. Rumney, T. J. Garite, and M. P. Nageotte, "A prospective randomized controlled trial that compared misoprostol, foley catheter, and combination misoprostol-foley catheter for labor induction," *American Journal of Obstetrics and Gynecology*, vol. 189, no. 4, pp. 1031–1035, 2003.

[9] A. O. Adeniji, O. Olayemi, and A. A. Odukogbe, "Intravaginal misoprostol versus transcervical Foley catheter in pre-induction cervical ripening," *International Journal of Gynecology and Obstetrics*, vol. 92, no. 2, pp. 130–132, 2006.

[10] M. Prager, E. Eneroth-Grimfors, M. Edlund, and L. Marions, "A randomised controlled trial of intravaginal dinoprostone, intravaginal misoprostol and transcervical balloon catheter for labour induction," *BJOG: An International Journal of Obstetrics & Gynaecology*, vol. 115, no. 11, pp. 1443–1450, 2008.

14

The Role of Metformin in Metabolic Disturbances during Pregnancy: Polycystic Ovary Syndrome and Gestational Diabetes Mellitus

Joselyn Rojas, Mervin Chávez-Castillo, and Valmore Bermúdez

Endocrine and Metabolic Diseases Research Center, School of Medicine, University of Zulia, 20th Avenue, Maracaibo 4004, Venezuela

Correspondence should be addressed to Joselyn Rojas; rojas.joselyn@gmail.com

Academic Editor: Daniela Romualdi

Maintenance of gestation implicates complex function of multiple endocrine mechanisms, and disruptions of the global metabolic environment prompt profound consequences on fetomaternal well-being during pregnancy and postpartum. Polycystic Ovary Syndrome (PCOS) and gestational diabetes mellitus (GDM) are very frequent conditions which increase risk for pregnancy complications, including early pregnancy loss, pregnancy-induced hypertensive disorders, and preterm labor, among many others. Insulin resistance (IR) plays a pivotal role in the pathogenesis of both PCOS and GDM, representing an important therapeutic target, with metformin being the most widely prescribed insulin-sensitizing antidiabetic drug. Although traditional views neglect use of oral antidiabetic agents during pregnancy, increasing evidence of safety during gestation has led to metformin now being recognized as a valuable tool in prevention of IR-related pregnancy complications and management of GDM. Metformin has been demonstrated to reduce rates of early pregnancy loss and onset of GDM in women with PCOS, and it appears to offer better metabolic control than insulin and other oral antidiabetic drugs during pregnancy. This review aims to summarize key aspects of current evidence concerning molecular and epidemiological knowledge on metformin use during pregnancy in the setting of PCOS and GDM.

1. Introduction

Infertility currently affects approximately 48.5 million of women aged 20–44 years around the world [1], with severe implications in their physical and mental well-being [2]. Female fertility entails a complex array of endocrine mechanisms surrounding the integrity of the hypothalamus-pituitary-ovary (HPO) axis, which are especially important in maintenance of a healthy pregnancy, particularly due to the demands of the growing fetus [3]. Many conditions may disrupt this environment, and Polycystic Ovary Syndrome (PCOS)—an endocrine-metabolic disease that encompasses multiple hormonal alterations related to female infertility—stands out mainly due to its high prevalence, affecting 6-7% of women aged 12–45 years [4], with a worrisome 70% of women estimated to remain undiagnosed [5].

The hallmarks of this gynecoendocrine disease are disruption of ovarian steroidogenesis, giving rise to hyperandrogenemia and insulin resistance (IR) [6]. A complex IR-hyperinsulinemia-hyperandrogenemia cycle involved in the endocrine disruptions in PCOS [7] leads not only to the typical clinical picture of PCOS—featuring oligoanovulation and hyperandrogenic manifestations—but also to diverse cardiometabolic comorbidities, such as impaired glucose tolerance [8], dyslipidemia [9], hypertension [10], central obesity [11, 12], accelerated atherosclerosis [13], and metabolic syndrome [14], which can appear as a myriad of distinct metabolic phenotypes [15] including mild, moderate, and severe forms of PCOS.

Insulin resistance is an important component in the etiopathogenesis of PCOS, being associated with obesity, *acanthosis nigricans*, hirsutism [16], and early pregnancy loss [17] in these women. In addition, utilizing the HOMA-IR index as a surrogate for IR quantification, Huidobro et al. [18] reported this condition to be associated with gestational diabetes mellitus (GMD), which supports the notion that this pregnancy-related metabolic disorder may be part of

TABLE 1: Diagnostic criteria for Polycystic Ovary Syndrome.

	Clinical or biochemical hyperandrogenism	Oligo/anovulation	US finding of polycystic ovaries[*]
NIH, 1990 **BOTH** of the following:	+	+	
ESHARE/ASRM, 2003 **ONLY 2** of the following:	+	+	+
AES, 2006 **ALL 3** of the following:	+	+	+

NIH = National Institute of Health of the United States; ESHRE = European Society of Human Reproduction and Embryology; ASRM = American Society of Reproductive Medicine; AES = Androgen Excess and PCOS Society.

All sets of criteria require the exclusion of other etiologies such as congenital adrenal hyperplasia, androgen-secreting neoplasms, and Cushing's syndrome, among others.

[*]Ultrasound polycystic ovaries defined as the presence of ≥12 follicles of 2–9 mm width; or an increase in ovarian volume (>10 mL) in at least one ovary, in women not consuming oral contraceptives.

the insulin resistance syndrome [14, 19]. Moreover, GDM is observed in almost 50% of pregnancies in women with PCOS [10], which has been described as an independent predictor of the former [20]. Although the consequences of PCOS are not limited to reproductive dysfunction, these implications often represent the most critical aspect for both patients and clinicians, as it conveys an increase in the risk for pregnancy-induced hypertension, preeclampsia, and preterm birth [20].

Amidst the metabolic milieu generated by PCOS, GDM appears when pancreatic β-cell function is unable to compensate the converging increase of both PCOS-related IR and normal gravidic IR [21]. Given the profound influence IR exerts on reproduction, it has become an important pharmacological target, associated with improvement of ovulation induction [22], prevention of endocrine-metabolic gestational complications [23], and management of GDM [24]. To this end, oral antidiabetic agents such as metformin have been proposed as a valuable tool during pregnancy [25], albeit remaining an FDA Pregnancy Category B drug [26].

The purpose of this review is to describe the pharmacology of metformin during gestation and analyze its benefits in metabolically challenged pregnancies, such as in women with PCOS and/or GDM. We have compiled several peer-evaluated studies, both prospective and cross-sectional, which aid in the description and analysis of the role of metformin during pregnancy, including animal models, *in vitro* analyses, and clinical studies. These data were organized per the following reasoning: (a) the role of IR in the development of PCOS and GDM; (b) the impact of their endocrine-metabolic derangements in pregnancy; and (c) the use of metformin in regards to PCOS and pregnancy and in GDM.

2. Insulin Resistance as the Key Endocrine Disruption in Polycystic Ovary Syndrome

The etiology of PCOS is complex and multifactorial, including several endocrine disturbances, such as (a) increased pulsatile secretion of gonadotropin-releasing hormone (GnRH) and luteinizing hormone (LH), prompting theca cell hyperstimulation and androgen hypersecretion [27]; (b) nonselection of a dominant ovarian follicle, mediated by intrinsic and extrinsic ovary factors, with follicular cells hyperplasia [28];

(c) genetic predisposition to hyperandrogenemia, linked to abnormal *in utero* androgenic exposure [29]; and (d) genetic predisposition to hyperinsulinemia, also linked to prenatal androgen exposure and pancreatic β-cell dysfunction [30]. Although it is difficult to establish the relative importance or chronology of these and subsequent alterations, PCOS is characterized by an IR-hyperinsulinemia-hyperandrogenemia positive feedback circuit (Figure 1), where the latter component determines the majority of clinical manifestations and the diagnostic criteria for this condition (Table 1). Moreover, obesity is a very common feature in females with PCOS, which appears to magnify all previous pathophysiologic mechanisms [7].

Insulin resistance, defined as a decrease in cellular responsiveness to insulin signaling [31], triggers increased insulin secretion, a phenomenon termed "compensatory hyperinsulinemia" [32]. Although this mechanism attempts to maintain lipid, carbohydrate, and protein metabolism homeostasis, it contributes to multiple aggregate consequences, such as the cardiovascular PCOS comorbidities [33], and favors hyperandrogenemia through various pathways. In this respect, disruption of the HPO is particularly relevant: insulin has been shown to elevate GnRH and LH secretion both dose- and time-dependently [34, 35], potentially mediated through the MAPK pathway [36]. This results in increased frequency and amplitude of GnRH and LH pulse secretion, with increased LH/FSH ratio, potentiating ovarian steroidogenic alterations [6]. Other features frequently found in women with PCOS act in synergy with insulin towards enhancing LH release, including hyperleptinemia via AgRP/NPY neural pathways and kiss peptidergic signaling [37], and decreased opioidergic tone, which appears to sensitize pituitary LH-secreting cells to GnRH signaling [38]. Hyperinsulinemia has also been associated with diminished Sex Hormone-Binding Globulin (SHBG) levels, although insulin appears to be unable to directly inhibit *shbg* expression; instead, this effect depends on hyperglycemia-mediated Hepatocyte Nuclear Factor 4-α downregulation [39]. Lower SHBG synthesis results in increased sex hormone availability, exacerbating androgenic signaling [40].

Lastly, PCOS is also characterized by selective IR in ovarian tissue, wherein mitogenic pathways are favored while

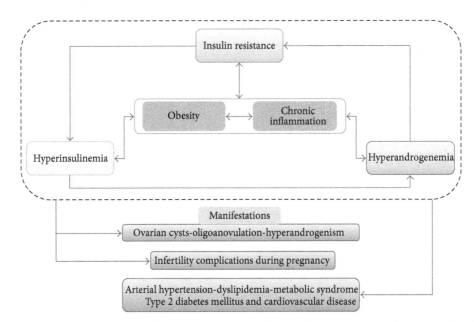

FIGURE 1: The insulin resistance-hyperinsulinemia-hyperandrogenemia cycle in Polycystic Ovary Syndrome. PCOS is dominated by three major endocrine disruptions: insulin resistance, hyperinsulinemia, and hyperandrogenemia. Although it is difficult to establish which disturbance develops first in any given case, these components are interconnected by many reinforcing mechanisms, constituting a positive feedback cycle. Furthermore, obesity and chronic inflammatory states—present in both obese and lean women with PCOS—amplify pathophysiologic pathways linked to all elements in this triad. The cycle leads to the manifestations of PCOS and infertility, complications during pregnancy, and chronic cardiometabolic comorbidities.

metabolic signaling is absent, yielding follicular cell hyperplasia and potentiation of steroidogenesis [41]. Several theories surround this concept, including cAMP-dependent activation of PKA with subsequent activation of Steroidogenic Acute Regulatory (StAR) protein [42], increased PI3K/Akt activity via serine phosphorylation by a hypothetical kinase in theca cells [43], and inositolphosphoglycan signaling, which appears to deviate from insulin-dependent pathways aside from being activated by the insulin receptor itself [44]. At any rate, IR-hyperinsulinemia activity leads to hyperandrogenemia, which in turn induces pro-IR structural and functional modifications in key insulin target tissues, including decreased amount of more oxidative, insulin-sensitive type I muscle fibers, and increased amount of more glycolytic, less sensitive type II fibers [40], as well as elevated lipolysis in adipocytes, favoring free fatty acid- (FFA-) mediated IR [45], perpetuating the IR-hyperinsulinemia-hyperandrogenemia feedback [7].

Although physical activity and lower caloric intake are considered fundamental lifestyle interventions [46], insulin-sensitizing agents are also a hallmark of PCOS management, with metformin being the most frequently used molecule [47]. Metformin has been described to offer significant improvement of several parameters, including Body Mass Index (BMI), LH, androstenedione, testosterone [48], DHEAS, blood pressure [49], menstrual cyclicity, fasting insulin [50], IR, dyslipidemia, oxidative stress, endothelial dysfunction [51], and several inflammatory markers [52]. This biguanide has also been reported to improve other features such as anovulation rate and acne [53] as well as BMI and LH [54] in non-IR women with PCOS. Moreover, it appears to

be beneficial in both obese and lean women with PCOS [53], which may explain the persistent benefits of metformin even with several different metabotypes.

The subset of lean women with PCOS is particularly interesting. Although all PCOS phenotypes tend towards a more "apple-like" adipose distribution [55], lean subjects usually have less visceral fat [56]. Likewise, in these individuals, IR and hyperandrogenemia are predominantly related to low SHBG levels [57], with increased risk for elevated inflammation markers [58] and early vascular disease [59]. Although both lean and obese PCOS women tend to exhibit higher oxidative stress [60], they appear to behave differently regarding aging and risk of developing type 2 diabetes mellitus (DM2), which seems to be less frequent in lean women with PCOS [61]. Indeed, women who are able to maintain normal weight with aging appear to boast a healthier metabolic profile than those who do not [62]. These differences may influence the impact of metformin in each group [63]: whereas reproductive benefits are observed in both obese and lean PCOS women [64], metabolic advantages, such as lowering of proinsulin and insulin levels, are seen predominantly in the obese and overweight subset [65].

Other antidiabetic drugs have been evaluated to be applied in PCOS, particularly thiazolidinediones (TZD). Despite reports indicating these agents to be more effective than metformin at reducing IR in subjects with PCOS [66], their use remains less widespread, due to concerns of increased cardiovascular risk [67]. Indeed, despite significantly ameliorating IR, glucose homeostasis, hyperandrogenic ovarian response, and systemic inflammation [68, 69], TZD appear to induce several deleterious modifications in

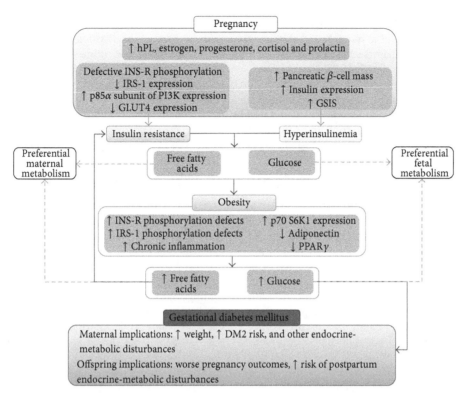

FIGURE 2: Mechanisms underlying insulin resistance in normal pregnancy physiology and gestational diabetes mellitus. Insulin resistance is a physiologic state which develops parallel to increased secretion of hPL, estrogen, progesterone, cortisol, and prolactin, principally. Although they favor IR by altering components of peripheral insulin signaling cascades, they also activate various mechanisms enhancing β-cell function. The result is an increased release of free fatty acids, which are predominantly metabolized by mothers, allowing for shunting of glucose towards fetal metabolism. In obesity several pathophysiologic mechanisms worsen IR in target tissues, leading to greater free fatty acid levels and dysregulation of glucose homeostasis. DM2: type 2 diabetes mellitus; GSIS: glucose-stimulated insulin secretion; hPL: human placental lactogen; INS-R: insulin receptor; IRS-1: insulin receptor substrate-1; PPARγ: peroxisome proliferator-activated receptor γ.

cardiac tissue transcriptomes, including upregulation of met-alloproteinases implicated in atheromatous plaque rupture, potassium channels required for action potential generation, and genes involved in sphingolipid and ceramide metabolism [70]. Beyond these molecular findings, the impact of TZD on cardiovascular risk is also reflected in epidemiologic findings, with a higher risk of congestive heart failure in prediabetic and diabetic subjects (RR = 1.72, 95% CI: 1.21–2.42, P = 0.002) [71].

3. Exacerbation of Physiologic Insulin Resistance as the Fundament of Gestational Diabetes Mellitus

Insulin resistance is a physiologic state during gestation, driven by several maternal hormones such as estrogen, progesterone, cortisol, and particularly human placental lactogen (hPL) [72]. Target cell modifications include defective tyrosine phosphorylation of the β subunit of the insulin receptor [73] and decreased expression of IRS-1 [74], whereas expression of the p85α subunit of phosphoinositol 3-kinase is increased, which interferes with heterodimeric conformation of this enzyme and thus prevents further insulin signaling [72]. Similarly, GLUT4 expression has been noted to be decreased in adipose tissue of pregnant females, significantly hindering insulin responsiveness [75]. Although the elevated serum levels of free fatty acids triggered by IR represent an important adaptive mechanism in order to increase the glucose offer for fetal metabolism, they also serve as a self-reinforcing pathway for IR (Figure 2) [76].

These pro-IR phenomena are counterbalanced by several pancreatic function-enhancing signals, which allow for the typical over twofold increase in insulin secretion during the second and third trimesters of gestation [77]. These signals include hPL, prolactin, and estrogens, all of which rise progressively and prominently throughout pregnancy [78], associated with increases in pancreatic β-cell mass and insulin transcription, and improve glucose-stimulated insulin secretion by promoting glucokinase and GLUT-2 expression, as well as raising glucose utilization and oxidation in pancreatic β cells [78]. These compensatory pathways are valuable, as they aim to maintain adequate glucose metabolism whilst allowing for increased FFA production [77]. Nonetheless, these mechanisms may be intrinsically defective or insufficient in some women, leading to the development of GDM, defined as glucose intolerance of onset or first recognition during pregnancy [79].

To this end, obesity is an important risk factor for GDM, with an OR = 2.6; 95% CI: 2.1–3.4; P < 0.05 [80]. Aside from enhancing all previously described pro-IR mechanisms [72], obesity favors the development of a systemic inflammatory state, with elevated levels of mediators such as TNF [81]. This cytokine is implicated in IR by allowing IRS-1 serine phosphorylation via activation of JNK and NF-κB pathways [82]. Likewise, states of nutrient excess have been linked to upregulation of p70 S6K1, an IRS-1 serine kinase which induces degradation of this protein and may contribute to IRS-1 deficiency in GDM [72]. Similarly, both obesity and PCOS are associated with decreased expression of GLUT4 [83].

Another important factor is adiponectin, a proteic hormone with insulin-sensitizing activity, whose levels are decreased in obesity [84]. Although adipocytes are the primary site for adiponectin synthesis, placental production of adiponectin appears to be a paramount regulator of metabolism homeostasis during gestation [85]. Moreover, cytokines such as TNF, IFNγ, IL-6, and leptin have been found to modulate adiponectin and adiponectin receptor expression in women with GDM [86], harmonizing with reports associating hypoadiponectinemia with postpartum IR, β-cell dysfunction, and dysglycemia [87]. Expression of PPARγ is also diminished, leading to subdued lipogenic pathways, favoring greater FFA release [88] and disturbance of proper lipid partition, which would enhance lipid deposition in nonprofessional tissues such as skeletal muscle, enhancing the IR cycle [7]. Other related metabolic markers have been independently associated with higher risk for GDM: the Coronary Artery Risk Development in Young Adults (CARDIA) Study [89] reported that impaired fasting glucose (OR = 4.74; 95% CI: 2.14–10.51; P < 0.01), hyperinsulinemia (OR = 2.36; 95% CI: 1.20–4.63; P < 0.01), and low levels of HDL-C (OR = 3.07; 95% CI: 1.62–5.84; P < 0.01) are associated with GDM risk after adjusting for race, age, parity, and birth order.

4. Implications of Gestational Diabetes Mellitus on Fetomaternal Health

Gestational diabetes mellitus has been noted to prevail in females with predisposition to metabolic disturbances, with pregnancy acting as stress test on endocrine physiology [90], reflected on both obesity and PCOS representing independent risk factors for GDM, as previously discussed [20, 80]. This condition entails several consequences on both mother and offspring well-being. Maternal implications consist principally of higher risk for development of DM2 after pregnancy, with approximately 10% of women diagnosed with DM2 shortly after delivery and up to 40% after 10-year follow-up [91]. Indeed, gestation may reveal or worsen preexisting defects in β-cell function, accelerating onset of DM2 and other related conditions [90]. This influence is present even in nonobese women with GDM, with findings of endothelial dysfunction and chronic inflammation markers—both associated with the pathogenesis of DM2, cardiovascular disease, and metabolic syndrome—in this population [92]. HOMA-IR assessment boasts promising results as predictor of postpartum β-cell dysfunction [93].

On the other hand, the Hyperglycemia and Adverse Pregnancy Outcome (HAPO) study [94] has demonstrated that hyperglycemia during pregnancy—even in nondiabetic ranges—is associated with increased birth weight and elevated cord blood C-peptide serum levels. GDM is related to greater risk of macrosomia, shoulder dystocia, birth injuries, neonatal hypoglycemia, hypocalcemia, hyperbilirrubinemia, respiratory distress syndrome, and polycythemia [95], as well as teratogenesis, particularly in obese subjects [96]. Furthermore, elevated cord-blood insulin concentrations are linked to glucose intolerance in offspring, and children exposed to GDM appear to display various metabolic disturbances well into childhood, including higher blood pressure and lower HDL-C [97].

These epidemiological data obey profound disruptions in embryonic and fetal metabolism, and numerous hypotheses attempt to explain this panorama. The theory of fuel-induced teratogenesis was first outlined by Freinkel [98], who proposed fuel excess and overgrowth to be the pathogenic basis of maternal hyperglycemia. This notion is founded on findings of maternal hyperglycemia-induced enhancing fetal insulin secretion, potentiating tissue growth—macrosomia—via fetal IGF-1 [99]. Alternatively, Hales and Barker [100] have propelled the thrifty phenotype theory, suggesting *in utero* malnutrition to bear a strong influence on postnatal risk of obesity, cardiovascular disease, and DM2, and even risk of PCOS and future pregnancy complications [101]. These premises are complemented by the concept of metabolic memory, related to endocrine-metabolic reprogramming of offspring amidst the diabetic environment during pregnancy [102]. This notion encompasses fetal inflammation, blunted myogenesis, oxidative stress, and disruption of immune system tolerance, among various other alterations [103]. Likewise, fetal exposure to diabetes appears to modify hypothalamic functionality in animal models, associated with hyperphagic behavior and obesity-proneness after birth [104].

AMP-dependent kinase (AMPK), a classic target of metformin action, may be an important mediator in this context [105], as it intervenes in processes such as lipogenesis via inhibition of acetyl-CoA carboxylase [106], myogenesis through the modulation of myocyte enhancer factor 2 [107], cell cycle [108], and appetite pathways [109]. Animal models have shown that metformin-induced AMPK activation yields beneficial effects over embryonic implantation [110], fetal inflammation [111], maternal liver function [112], and pregnancy outcomes [113]. Notwithstanding that these and other molecular pathways remain under research and certain aspects require further characterization, metformin has proven to beat the test of time, standing as a promising recourse in many circumstances, including GDM.

5. Metformin Pharmacokinetics during Pregnancy

Uptake and distribution of metformin towards the circulatory system requires the participation of bidirectional transporters located in the intestine and liver [114, 115]; see Figure 3. In the apical membrane of enterocytes, PMAT (Plasma Membrane Monoamine Transporter) and OCT3 (Organic Cation Transporters) mediate absorption. Mobilization of the drug

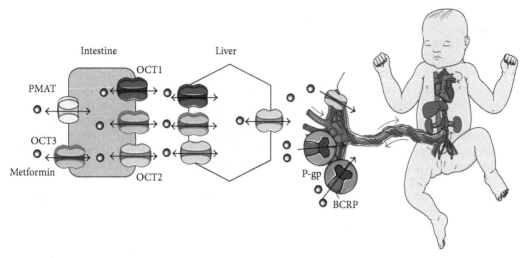

FIGURE 3: Absorption and distribution of metformin during pregnancy.

towards the liver requires OCT1, OCT2, and OCT3, while OCT2 is needed in order to reach the bloodstream, kidneys, and excretion [116]. Renal clearance of metformin increases during mid (723 ± 243 mL/min, $P < 0.01$) and late pregnancy (625 ± 130 mL/min, $P < 0.01$) [116], relating to a concentration of the drug in umbilical cord blood at time of birth between undetectable levels and 1263 ng/mL. Placental tissue expresses OCT2 transporter, yet under strict epigenetic control [117, 118], underlying ample interindividual differences in this aspect. However, other transporters are also involved in drug efflux through the placenta. Reflecting the high protectiveness of the human syncytiotrophoblast regarding the fetus, this tissue has been described to express a series of transporters in the apical membrane, such as P-glycoprotein (P-gp), Multidrug Resistance-Associated Protein 1 (MRP1), and Breast Cancer Resistance Protein (BCRP) [119–122], with metformin being transported mainly via P-gp ($58\% \pm 20\%$) and BCRP ($25\% \pm 14\%$) [119]. Competition between this biguanide and other drugs can also limit the exposure of the fetus, further limiting the presence of toxic concentrations during pregnancy.

Animal studies using dosages up to 600 mg/kg daily have failed to report evidence of teratogenic effects [123] and extremely high dosages between 900 and 1500 mg/kg daily failed to induce carcinogenicity [124]. Furthermore, in 2003 Gutzin et al. [125] reported their results concerning first trimester exposure, ascertaining no higher rates of major malformations with an OR of 1.05 (95% CI: 0.65–1.70), while neonatal death rendered an OR of 1.16 (95% CI: 0.67–2.00). Likewise, Gilbert et al. [126] conducted a meta-analysis on 8 studies concerning fetal malformations associated with metformin use during pregnancy, indicating this drug to yield an OR of 0.50 (95% CI: 0.15–1.60)—rendering a minor protective effect. Finally, the pooling analysis showed that the control group had a malformation rate of 7.2%, compared to 1.7% in the metformin group [126], strongly supporting metformin's safety during pregnancy.

Concerning breast milk-related exposure [127], it has been confirmed that metformin can be detected at ranges between 0.13 and 0.28 mg/mL, equivalent to <0.5% of the mother's weight-adjusted dosage [106]. Other reports have quantified metformin in breast milk at 0.28–1.08% [128] and 0.18–0.21% [129] of maternal dose. Placental partition coefficient for metformin has been calculated at 36.3%, with a cord plasma concentration of 0.1–2.9 mg/L during labor [130]. Such findings confirm that neonatal exposure to metformin is actually quite insignificant, and it is not related to glucose abnormality in infants, granting safe use before, during, and after pregnancy [128–130].

6. Metformin Use in Pregnant Women with Polycystic Ovary Syndrome: Different Outcomes, Different Efficacy

Because infertility is one of the main consequences of female reproduction in patients with PCOS [4, 5], ovulation induction remains the most common intervention during fertility counseling. Current guidelines heavily promote lifestyle modifications and support clomiphene as the first-line agent for ovulation induction, while recognizing that complementation with metformin improves ovulation and pregnancy success [131], as reported by Lord et al. [22] in their meta-analysis concerning effectiveness of this antidiabetic drug in achievement of ovulation in 15 trials involving 543 participants. This yielded an OR of 3.88 (95% CI: 2.25–6.69) for metformin alone and 4.41 (95% CI: 2.37–8.22) for metformin combined with clomiphene. In addition, the results from Khorram et al. [132] showed that two-week treatment with insulin reduced insulin levels and IR while improving SHBG levels and clomiphene-induced ovulation. In regards to metformin and gonadotropin use, Palomba et al. [133] reported that the biguanide improved live birth rates (OR = 1.95; 95% CI: 1.10–3.44; $P = 0.020$) and pregnancy success (OR = 2.25; 95% CI: 1.50–3.38; $P < 0.0001$).

Early pregnancy loss (EPL) is defined as the interruption of pregnancy before the 20th week of gestation [134]. Although chromosomal abnormalities are the principal cause of EPL [135], they are uncommonly reported in women with PCOS [136]. It has been proposed that endocrine disruptions may play a role in EPL, with elevated androgens being associated with EPL in women with PCOS, and with recurrent EPL in women with and without PCOS [21]. Additionally, several endometrial molecular alterations have been described during implantation in PCOS: (a) androgen-dependent suppression of glycodelin [137], a cell-adhesion molecule involved in endometrial receptivity [138]; (b) IR-hyperinsulinemia can also diminish glycodelin expression, alongside IGFBP-1, key molecules for endometrial preimplantation maturation [139]; and (c) a hypofibrinolytic state due to increased synthesis of plasminogen activator inhibitor-1 (PAI-1), which has been found to be an independent risk factor for EPL in PCOS [140]. In this context, PCOS patients prescribed with metformin have lower pooled odds ratios for EPL (OR = 0.32, 95% CI: 0.19–0.55) and preterm birth (OR = 0.30, 95% CI: 0.13–0.68) [141], suggesting that this treatment can reverse the impact of PCOS on implantation success observed in this gynecoendocrine disease.

Other benefits have been attributed to metformin throughout gestation in women with PCOS, but perhaps one of the most important ones, is the 40% reduction of new-onset diabetes in high risk individuals as reported by Salpeter et al. [142]. In their meta-analysis using 31 trials and 4,570 subjects, the resulting pooled OR was 0.6 (95% CI: 0.5–0.8), with an absolute risk reduction of 6% (95% CI: 4–8) during a period of treatment of 1.8 years [142]. On the other hand, Nawaz et al. [143] have described decreased prevalence of fetal growth restriction and increased live birth rates, as well as an absence of intrauterine deaths or stillbirths, in women taking metformin during pregnancy, in line with claims of metformin being unrelated to teratogenicity [144].

Nevertheless, metformin during pregnancy appears unable to significantly reduce rates of preeclampsia and preterm birth in subjects with PCOS. A randomized, placebo-controlled, double-blind, multicenter study by Vanky et al. [145] found that preeclampsia prevalence was 7.4% in the metformin group and 3.7% in the placebo group (3.7%; 95% CI: −1.7–9.2; $P = 0.18$), whereas preterm birth prevalence was 3.7% in the metformin group and 8.2% in the placebo group (−4.4%; 95% CI: −10.1–1.2; $P = 0.12$); the inefficacy of metformin at preventing preeclampsia may be due to the complex etiopathogenesis of this disease. Data from Stridsklev et al. [146] support this phenomenon, in which reporting metformin treatment did not affect uterine artery flow during gestation, while also describing an association between uterine artery flow and androgens, highlighting the complexity of the mechanisms underlying placentation, conservation of uterine artery flow, and vessel compliance [147, 148].

Indeed, despite several mechanisms related to IR-hyperinsulinemia being involved in the etiopathogenesis of preeclampsia—chronic systemic inflammation, increased sympathetic tone, and vascular smooth muscle growth [149]—metformin may be unable to effectively modify the pathogenic root of this disease, which is faulty placentation [150]. Similarly, although metformin's effects may aid in prevention of preterm birth by ameliorating oxidative stress and chronic inflammation [151], various elements underlying preterm labor may escape the reach of metformin's activity, including the most common factors associated with this condition—defective placentation, intrauterine infection, and maternal immunologic receptivity [152].

Still, metformin seems to offer other benefits to offspring of women with PCOS even in the postnatal period. In this scenario, metformin throughout pregnancy has been associated with diminished neonatal hypoglycemia [153], as well as normal growth and motor-social development in the first 18 months of life [154]. Likewise, the growth and motor-social skills of breast-fed children of women with PCOS taking metformin have been demonstrated to be similar to those of formula-fed infants, with no abnormalities [155].

7. Metformin in Pregnant Women with Gestational Diabetes Mellitus: Challenging Insulin as the Go-To Therapy

Although insulin therapy has been considered the best management option for GDM, recent evidence diverges from this precept. The first major trial concerning the use of metformin and/or insulin during pregnancies complicated with GDM was the metformin in gestational diabetes (MiG) [156], whose goal was to determine the effects of either drug on prevention of fetal hyperinsulinemia and promotion of lower maternal glycemia. This research group ascertained metformin (500–2500 mg/day) with or without supplemental insulin not to be associated with higher perinatal complications, in comparison to insulin alone [157], findings later corroborated by Silva et al. [158]. Furthermore, patients tend to prefer metformin over insulin as treatment schemes and would rather be prescribed such drug if possible [156]. Likewise, metformin use during pregnancy failed to adversely affect maternal lipid parameters, C-reactive protein levels, or birth weight [159].

After this emblematic trial, several other studies have supported the effectiveness of metformin in GDM. Niromanesh et al. [160] conducted a randomized controlled trial with 160 pregnant patients with GDM, 80 of them treated with metformin (500–2500 mg) and the rest with insulin NPH (0.2 U/kg bedtime) and regular (1 U per 10 mg/dL over). Results revealed metformin to reduce rates of macrosomia and maternal weight gain. Additionally, Rowan et al. [161] also ascertained a decline in macrosomia and preeclampsia rates and suggested glycemic goals in GDM should be more rigorous. Metformin in GDM has also been described to lower incidence of surgical delivery [162]. Notably, these effects are observed even in spite of lowering of vitamin B12 [163], a recognized side effect of the drug [164].

Although various oral hypoglycemic agents—aside from metformin—are known to confer adequate metabolic control during pregnancy compared to insulin [165], metformin seems to be the superior choice, offering better control than glyburide, as reported by Silva et al. [158]. This research group has also reported newborns from mothers treated with metformin to obtain lower weight (3193 g versus 3387 g; $P = 0.01$) and ponderal index results (2.87 versus 2.96; $P = 0.05$) as well as less maternal weight gain, in women with GDM, when compared to those treated with glyburide (10.3 kg versus 7.6 kg; $P = 0.02$) [166], possibly reducing probabilities of other weight-related complications, such as preeclampsia. On the other hand, data on TZD use during GDM is relatively scarce, and trials conducted to date are considered insufficient to definitively establish these drugs as safe during pregnancy [25]. In this context, PPARγ has been noted to be key in embryonic development [167], and TZD administration during pregnancy has been associated with impaired fetal development [168], with this drug class remaining within the FDA Pregnancy Category C [169]. Therefore, further research is needed to explore the role of TZD in pregnancy and GDM.

Beyond evidence supporting metformin use in GDM, a key issue regarding pharmacological management of this disease is the prediction and selection of the best suited alternative (insulin alone, metformin alone, or both combined) for each specific patient. Insulin remains the most recommended option in mild cases of GDM [170] and in women with elevated BMI [171]. Indeed, in women with GDM, HOMA-IR values 1.29–2.89—interpreted as decreased insulin secretion—have been proposed to indicate a requirement of insulin therapy, whereas values >2.89 are thought to underline insufficient compensation of IR, rendering insulin-sensitizing agents more adequate [172]. Likewise, women with GDM and a fasting glucose result from oral glucose tolerance test below 93.3 mg/dL have displayed a probability of favorable pharmacological response of 93% to metformin [173]. On the other hand, early detection of GDM is a predictor for supplemental insulin treatment in women initially treated with metformin [174], as well as older age and elevated serum fructosamine concentration [175].

8. Concluding Remarks

Pregnancies complicated with GDM or with history of PCOS are a challenge for both obstetricians and endocrinologists, representing a halfway point where these specialties merge and highlighting the importance of multidisciplinary prenatal management. In our experience, we have observed that patients with PCOS who continue with metformin treatment throughout pregnancy and those who receive this drug as a pharmacological intervention in GDM yield better pregnancy outcomes and a better postpartum metabolic prognosis for both mothers and their offspring.

Nevertheless, further studies are needed to uncover and elucidate the benefits and shortcomings of metformin in this context, in both molecular and epidemiological fields. Ongoing studies concerning these issues include the Metformin to Prevent Late Miscarriage and Preterm Delivery in Women With Polycystic Ovary Syndrome Trial (PregMet2) [176] and the Metformin Treatment in Gestational Diabetes and Noninsulin Dependent Diabetes in Pregnancy in a Developing Country Trial (migdm&t2dm) [177] as well as additional data from the MiG trial, among many others. Indeed, the future appears compelling and exciting in this aspect, with these sources promising valuable information which may reshape and refine views on metformin use during pregnancy.

Conflict of Interests

There are no financial or other contractual agreements that might cause conflict of interests.

Acknowledgments

This work was supported by Research Grant no. CC-0437-10-21-09-10 from CONDES, University of Zulia, and Research Grant no. FZ-0058-2007 from Fundacite-Zulia.

References

[1] H. Teede, A. Deeks, and L. Moran, "Polycystic ovary syndrome: a complex condition with psychological, reproductive and metabolic manifestations that impacts on health across the lifespan," *BMC Medicine*, vol. 8, article 41, 2010.

[2] M. T. Sheehan, "Polycystic ovarian syndrome: diagnosis and management," *Clinical Medicine & Research*, vol. 2, no. 1, pp. 13–27, 2004.

[3] C. B. Kallen, "Steroid hormone synthesis in pregnancy," *Obstetrics and Gynecology Clinics of North America*, vol. 31, no. 4, pp. 795–816, 2004.

[4] J. Vrbikova and V. Hainer, "Obesity and polycystic ovary syndrome," *Obesity Facts*, vol. 2, no. 1, pp. 26–35, 2009.

[5] M. N. Mascarenhas, S. R. Flaxman, T. Boerma, S. Vanderpoel, and G. A. Stevens, "National, regional, and global trends in infertility prevalence since 1990: a systematic analysis of 277 health surveys," *PLoS Medicine*, vol. 9, no. 12, Article ID e1001356, 2012.

[6] E. Diamanti-Kandarakis, "Polycystic ovarian syndrome: pathophysiology, molecular aspects and clinical implications," *Expert Reviews in Molecular Medicine*, vol. 10, p. e3, 2008.

[7] J. Rojas, M. Chávez, L. Olivar et al., "Polycystic ovary syndrome, insulin resistance, and obesity: navigating the pathophysiologic labyrinth," *International Journal of Reproductive Medicine*, vol. 2014, Article ID 719050, 17 pages, 2014.

[8] S. A. Arslanian, V. D. Lewy, and K. Danadian, "Glucose intolerance in obese adolescents with polycystic ovary syndrome: roles of insulin resistance and β-cell dysfunction and risk of cardiovascular disease," *The Journal of Clinical Endocrinology and Metabolism*, vol. 86, no. 1, pp. 66–71, 2001.

[9] S. Robinson, A. D. Henderson, S. V. Gelding et al., "Dyslipidaemia is associated with insulin resistance in women with polycystic ovaries," *Clinical Endocrinology*, vol. 44, no. 3, pp. 277–284, 1996.

[10] M. W. Elting, T. J. M. Korsen, P. D. Bezemer, and J. Schoemaker, "Prevalence of diabetes mellitus, hypertension and cardiac complaints in a follow-up study of a Dutch PCOS population," *Human Reproduction*, vol. 16, no. 3, pp. 556–560, 2001.

[11] Z. H. Huang, B. Manickam, V. Ryvkin et al., "PCOS is associated with increased CD11c expression and crown-like structures in adipose tissue and increased central abdominal fat depots independent of obesity," *The Journal of Clinical Endocrinology & Metabolism*, vol. 98, no. 1, pp. E17–E24, 2013.

[12] S. Borruel, E. Fernández-Durán, M. Alpañés et al., "Global adiposity and thickness of intraperitoneal and mesenteric adipose tissue depots are increased in women with polycystic ovary syndrome (PCOS)," *Journal of Clinical Endocrinology and Metabolism*, vol. 98, no. 3, pp. 1254–1263, 2013.

[13] R. Shroff, A. Kerchner, M. Maifeld, E. J. R. van Beek, D. Jagasia, and A. Dokras, "Young obese women with polycystic ovary

syndrome have evidence of early coronary atherosclerosis," *The Journal of Clinical Endocrinology & Metabolism*, vol. 92, no. 12, pp. 4609–4614, 2007.

[14] A. J. Cussons, B. G. A. Stuckey, and G. F. Watts, "Metabolic syndrome and cardiometabolic risk in PCOS," *Current Diabetes Reports*, vol. 7, no. 1, pp. 66–73, 2007.

[15] M. C. Amato, V. Guarnotta, D. Forti, M. Donatelli, S. Dolcimascolo, and C. Giordano, "Metabolically healthy polycystic ovary syndrome (MH-PCOS) and metabolically unhealthy polycystic ovary syndrome (MU-PCOS): a comparative analysis of four simple methods useful for metabolic assessment," *Human Reproduction*, vol. 28, no. 7, pp. 1919–1928, 2013.

[16] E. Mor, A. Zograbyan, P. Saadat et al., "The insulin resistant subphenotype of polycystic ovary syndrome: clinical parameters and pathogenesis," *The American Journal of Obstetrics and Gynecology*, vol. 190, no. 6, pp. 1654–1660, 2004.

[17] L. B. Craig, R. W. Ke, and W. H. Kutteh, "Increased prevalence of insulin resistance in women with a history of recurrent pregnancy loss," *Fertility and Sterility*, vol. 78, no. 3, pp. 487–490, 2002.

[18] A. Huidobro, A. M. Prentice, A. J. C. Fulford, and J. Rozowski, "Antropometría como predictor de diabetes gestacional: estudio de cohorte," *Revista Médica de Chile*, vol. 138, pp. 1373–1377, 2010.

[19] C. M. Clark Jr., C. Qiu, B. Amerman et al., "Gestational diabetes: should it be added to the syndrome of insulin resistance?" *Diabetes Care*, vol. 20, no. 5, pp. 867–871, 1997.

[20] C. M. Boomsma, M. J. C. Eijkemans, E. G. Hughes, G. H. A. Visser, B. C. J. M. Fauser, and N. S. Macklon, "A meta-analysis of pregnancy outcomes in women with polycystic ovary syndrome," *Human Reproduction Update*, vol. 12, no. 6, pp. 673–683, 2006.

[21] S. Kamalanathan, J. P. Sahoo, and T. Sathyapalan, "Pregnancy in polycystic ovary syndrome," *Indian Journal of Endocrinology and Metabolism*, vol. 17, pp. 37–43, 2013.

[22] J. M. Lord, I. H. Flight, and R. J. Norman, "Insulin-sensitising drugs (metformin, troglitazone, rosiglitazone, pioglitazone, D-chiro-inositol) for polycystic ovary syndrome," *Cochrane Database of Systematic Reviews*, vol. 3, Article ID CD003053, 2003.

[23] H. C. Zisser, "Polycystic ovary syndrome and pregnancy: is metformin the magic bullet?" *Diabetes Spectrum*, vol. 20, no. 2, pp. 85–89, 2007.

[24] M.-E. Lautatzis, D. G. Goulis, and M. Vrontakis, "Efficacy and safety of metformin during pregnancy in women with gestational diabetes mellitus or polycystic ovary syndrome: a systematic review," *Metabolism: Clinical and Experimental*, vol. 62, no. 11, pp. 1522–1534, 2013.

[25] D. S. Feig, G. G. Briggs, and G. Koren, "Oral antidiabetic agents in pregnancy and lactation: a paradigm shift?" *Annals of Pharmacotherapy*, vol. 41, no. 7-8, pp. 1174–1180, 2007.

[26] Package Insert for Glucophage, http://www.glucophagexr.com/pages/default.aspx.

[27] C. R. McCartney, C. A. Eagleson, and J. C. Marshall, "Regulation of gonadotropin secretion: implications for polycystic ovary syndrome," *Seminars in Reproductive Medicine*, vol. 20, no. 4, pp. 317–325, 2002.

[28] M. Karoshi and S. O. Okolo, "Commentary: Polycystic ovarian disease (PCOD): a misnomer, looking for a new name," *International Journal of Fertility and Women's Medicine*, vol. 49, no. 4, pp. 191–192, 2004.

[29] D. H. Abbott, D. A. Dumesic, and S. Franks, "Developmental origin of polycystic ovary syndrome—a hypothesis," *Journal of Endocrinology*, vol. 174, no. 1, pp. 1–5, 2002.

[30] D. A. Dumesic, D. H. Abbott, and V. Padmanabhan, "Polycystic ovary syndrome and its developmental origins," *Reviews in Endocrine and Metabolic Disorders*, vol. 8, no. 2, pp. 127–141, 2007.

[31] M. H. Shanik, Y. Xu, J. Skrha, R. Dankner, Y. Zick, and J. Roth, "Insulin resistance and hyperinsulinemia: is hyperinsulinemia the cart or the horse?" *Diabetes Care*, vol. 31, supplement 2, pp. S262–S268, 2008.

[32] G. M. Reaven, "Compensatory hyperinsulinemia and the development of an atherogenic lipoprotein profile: the price paid to maintain glucose homeostasis in insulin-resistant individuals," *Endocrinology and Metabolism Clinics of North America*, vol. 34, no. 1, pp. 49–62, 2005.

[33] J. Rojas, V. Bermúdez, E. Leal et al., "Insulinorresistencia e hiperinsulinemia como factores de riesgo para enfermedad cardiovascular," *AVFT*, vol. 27, pp. 29–39, 2008.

[34] N. Sekar, J. C. Garmey, and J. D. Veldhuis, "Mechanisms underlying the steroidogenic synergy of insulin and luteinizing hormone in porcine granulosa cells: joint amplification of pivotal sterol-regulatory genes encoding the low-density lipoprotein (LDL) receptor, steroidogenic acute regulatory (stAR) protein and cytochrome P450 side-chain cleavage (P450scc) enzyme," *Molecular and Cellular Endocrinology*, vol. 159, no. 1-2, pp. 25–35, 2000.

[35] E. Y. Adashi, A. J. W. Hsueh, and S. S. C. Yen, "Insulin enhancement of luteinizing hormone and follicle-stimulating hormone release by cultured pituitary cells," *Endocrinology*, vol. 108, no. 4, pp. 1441–1449, 1981.

[36] R. Salvi, E. Castillo, M.-J. Voirol et al., "Gonadotropin-releasing hormone-expressing neurons immortalized conditionally are activated by insulin: implication of the mitogen-activated protein kinase pathway," *Endocrinology*, vol. 147, no. 2, pp. 816–826, 2006.

[37] J. W. Hill, J. K. Elmquist, and C. F. Elias, "Hypothalamic pathways linking energy balance and reproduction," *American Journal of Physiology: Endocrinology and Metabolism*, vol. 294, no. 5, pp. E827–E832, 2008.

[38] A. D. Eyvazzadeh, K. P. Pennington, R. Pop-Busui, M. Sowers, J.-K. Zubieta, and Y. R. Smith, "The role of the endogenous opioid system in polycystic ovary syndrome," *Fertility and Sterility*, vol. 92, no. 1, pp. 1–12, 2009.

[39] D. M. Selva, K. N. Hogeveen, S. M. Innis, and G. L. Hammond, "Monosaccharide-induced lipogenesis regulates the human hepatic sex hormone-binding globulin gene," *Journal of Clinical Investigation*, vol. 117, no. 12, pp. 3979–3987, 2007.

[40] A. Gambineri, C. Pelusi, V. Vicennati, U. Pagotto, and R. Pasquali, "Obesity and the polycystic ovary syndrome," *International Journal of Obesity*, vol. 26, no. 7, pp. 883–896, 2002.

[41] C.-B. Book and A. Dunaif, "Selective insulin resistance in the polycystic ovary syndrome," *Journal of Clinical Endocrinology and Metabolism*, vol. 84, no. 9, pp. 3110–3116, 1999.

[42] E. Méndez, N. Montserrat, and J. V. Planas, "Modulation of the steroidogenic activity of luteinizing hormone by insulin and insulin-like growth factor-I through interaction with the cAMP-dependent protein kinase signaling pathway in the trout ovary," *Molecular and Cellular Endocrinology*, vol. 229, no. 1-2, pp. 49–56, 2005.

[43] A. Dunaif, J. Xia, C.-B. Book, E. Schenker, and Z. Tang, "Excessive insulin receptor serine phosphorylation in cultured

fibroblasts and in skeletal muscle: a potential mechanism for insulin resistance in the polycystic ovary syndrome," *Journal of Clinical Investigation*, vol. 96, no. 2, pp. 801–810, 1995.

[44] J. E. Nestler, D. J. Jakubowicz, and M. J. Iuorno, "Role of inositolphosphoglycan mediators of insulin action in the polycystic ovary syndrome," *Journal of Pediatric Endocrinology & Metabolism*, vol. 13, supplement 5, pp. 1295–1298, 2000.

[45] P. Arner, "Effects of testosterone on fat cell lipolysis. Species differences and possible role in polycystic ovarian syndrome," *Biochimie*, vol. 87, no. 1, pp. 39–43, 2005.

[46] L. J. Moran, R. Pasquali, H. J. Teede, K. M. Hoeger, and R. J. Norman, "Treatment of obesity in polycystic ovary syndrome: a position statement of the Androgen Excess and Polycystic Ovary Syndrome Society," *Fertility and Sterility*, vol. 92, no. 6, pp. 1966–1982, 2009.

[47] L. Radosh, "Drug treatments for polycystic ovary syndrome," *American Family Physician*, vol. 79, no. 8, pp. 671–676, 2009.

[48] A. D. Genazzani, E. Chierchia, E. Rattighieri et al., "Metformin administration restores allopregnanolone response to adrenocorticotropic hormone (ACTH) stimulation in overweight hyperinsulinemic patients with PCOS," *Gynecological Endocrinology*, vol. 26, no. 9, pp. 684–689, 2010.

[49] E. M. Velazquez, S. Mendoza, T. Hamer, F. Sosa, and C. J. Glueck, "Metformin therapy in polycystic ovary syndrome reduces hyperinsulinemia, insulin resistance, hyperandrogenemia, and systolic blood pressure, while facilitating normal menses and pregnancy," *Metabolism: Clinical and Experimental*, vol. 43, no. 5, pp. 647–654, 1994.

[50] A. Kriplani and N. Agarwal, "Effects of metformin on clinical and biochemical parameters in polycystic ovary syndrome," *The Journal of Reproductive Medicine*, vol. 49, no. 5, pp. 361–367, 2004.

[51] D. Kocer, F. Bayram, and H. Diri, "The effects of metformin on endothelial dysfunction, lipid metabolism and oxidative stress in women with polycystic ovary syndrome," *Gynecological Endocrinology*, vol. 30, no. 5, pp. 367–371, 2014.

[52] E. Diamanti-Kandarakis, T. Paterakis, and H. A. Kandarakis, "Indices of low-grade inflammation in polycystic ovary syndrome," *Annals of the New York Academy of Sciences*, vol. 1092, pp. 175–186, 2006.

[53] S. Tan, S. Hahn, S. Benson et al., "Metformin improves polycystic ovary syndrome symptoms irrespective of pre-treatment insulin resistance," *European Journal of Endocrinology*, vol. 157, no. 5, pp. 669–676, 2007.

[54] J. Nawrocka and A. Starczewski, "Effects of metformin treatment in women with polycystic ovary syndrome depends on insulin resistance," *Gynecological Endocrinology*, vol. 23, no. 4, pp. 231–237, 2007.

[55] R. Horejsi, R. Möller, S. Rackl et al., "Android subcutaneous adipose tissue topography in lean and obese women suffering from PCOS: comparison with type 2 diabetic women," *The American Journal of Physical Anthropology*, vol. 124, no. 3, pp. 275–281, 2004.

[56] J. G. Dolfing, C. M. Stassen, P. M. M. Van Haard, B. H. R. Wolfenbuttel, and D. H. Schweitzer, "Comparison of MRI-assessed body fat content between lean women with polycystic ovary syndrome (PCOS) and matched controls: less visceral fat with PCOS," *Human Reproduction*, vol. 26, no. 6, pp. 1495–1500, 2011.

[57] J.-P. Baillargeon and A. Carpentier, "Role of insulin in the hyperandrogenemia of lean women with polycystic ovary syndrome and normal insulin sensitivity," *Fertility and Sterility*, vol. 88, no. 4, pp. 886–893, 2007.

[58] R. Keskin Kurt, A. G. Okyay, A. U. Hakverdi et al., "The effect of obesity on inflammatory markers in patients with PCOS: a BMI-matched case-control study," *Archives of Gynecology and Obstetrics*, vol. 290, no. 2, pp. 315–319, 2014.

[59] C. Celik, E. Bastu, R. Abali et al., "The relationship between copper, homocysteine and early vascular disease in lean women with polycystic ovary syndrome," *Gynecological Endocrinology*, vol. 29, no. 5, pp. 488–491, 2013.

[60] S. A. Blair, T. Kyaw-Tun, I. S. Young, N. A. Phelan, J. Gibney, and J. McEneny, "Oxidative stress and inflammation in lean and obese subjects with polycystic ovary syndrome," *Journal of Reproductive Medicine*, vol. 58, no. 3-4, pp. 107–114, 2013.

[61] D. W. Stovall, A. P. Bailey, and L. M. Pastore, "Assessment of insulin resistance and impaired glucose tolerance in lean women with polycystic ovary syndrome," *Journal of Women's Health*, vol. 20, no. 1, pp. 37–43, 2011.

[62] S. Livadas, A. Kollias, D. Panidis, and E. Diamanti-Kandarakis, "Diverse impacts of aging on insulin resistance in lean and obese women with polycystic ovary syndrome: evidence from 1345 women with the syndrome," *European Journal of Endocrinology*, vol. 171, no. 3, pp. 301–309, 2014.

[63] G. Önalan, U. Goktolga, T. Ceyhan, T. Bagis, R. Onalan, and R. Pabuçcu, "Predictive value of glucose—insulin ratio in PCOS and profile of women who will benefit from metformin therapy: obese, lean, hyper or normoinsulinemic?" *European Journal of Obstetrics Gynecology and Reproductive Biology*, vol. 123, no. 2, pp. 204–211, 2005.

[64] A. S. Kumari, A. Haq, R. Jayasundaram, L. O. Abdel-Wareth, S. A. al Haija, and M. Alvares, "Metformin monotherapy in lean women with polycystic ovary syndrome," *Reproductive BioMedicine Online*, vol. 10, no. 1, pp. 100–104, 2005.

[65] A. Kruszyńska, J. Słowińska-Srzednicka, W. Jeske, and W. Zgliczyński, "Proinsulin, adiponectin and hsCRP in reproductive age women with polycystic ovary syndrome (PCOS)—the effect of metformin treatment," *Endokrynologia Polska*, vol. 65, no. 1, pp. 2–10, 2014.

[66] Q. Du, Y. J. Wang, S. Yang, B. Wu, P. Han, and Y. Y. Zhao, "A systematic review and meta-analysis of randomized controlled trials comparing pioglitazone versus the treatment of polycystic ovary syndrome," *Current Medical Research and Opinion*, vol. 28, pp. 723–730, 2012.

[67] A. Ziaee, S. Oveisi, A. Abedini, S. Hashemipour, T. Karimzadeh, and A. Ghorbani, "Effect of metformin and pioglitazone treatment on cardiovascular risk profile in polycystic ovary syndrome," *Acta Medica Indonesiana*, vol. 44, no. 1, pp. 16–22, 2012.

[68] V. R. Aroda, T. P. Ciaraldi, P. Burke et al., "Metabolic and hormonal changes induced by pioglitazone in polycystic ovary syndrome: a randomized, placebo-controlled clinical trial," *Journal of Clinical Endocrinology and Metabolism*, vol. 94, no. 2, pp. 469–476, 2009.

[69] T. P. Ciaraldi, V. Aroda, S. R. Mudaliar, and R. R. Henry, "Inflammatory cytokines and chemokines, skeletal muscle and polycystic ovary syndrome: effects of pioglitazone and metformin treatment," *Metabolism: Clinical and Experimental*, vol. 62, no. 11, pp. 1587–1596, 2013.

[70] K. D. Wilson, Z. Li, R. Wagner et al., "Transcriptome alteration in the diabetic heart by rosiglitazone: implications for cardiovascular mortality," *PLoS ONE*, vol. 3, no. 7, Article ID e2609, 2008.

[71] R. M. Lago, P. P. Singh, and R. W. Nesto, "Congestive heart failure and cardiovascular death in patients with prediabetes and type 2 diabetes given thiazolidinediones: a meta-analysis

of randomised clinical trials," *The Lancet*, vol. 370, no. 9593, pp. 1129–1136, 2007.

[72] L. A. Barbour, C. E. McCurdy, T. L. Hernandez, J. P. Kirwan, P. M. Catalano, and J. E. Friedman, "Cellular mechanisms for insulin resistance in normal pregnancy and gestational diabetes," *Diabetes Care*, vol. 30, no. 2, pp. S112–S119, 2007.

[73] J. Shao, P. M. Catalano, H. Yamashita et al., "Decreased insulin receptor tyrosine kinase activity and plasma cell membrane glycoprotein-1 overexpression in skeletal muscle from obese women with gestational diabetes mellitus (GDM): evidence for increased serine/threonine phosphorylation in pregnancy and GDM," *Diabetes*, vol. 49, no. 4, pp. 603–610, 2000.

[74] P. M. Catalano, S. E. Nizielski, J. Shao, L. Preston, L. Qiao, and J. E. Friedman, "Downregulated IRS-1 and PPARγ in obese women with gestational diabetes: relationship to FFA during pregnancy," *American Journal of Physiology: Endocrinology and Metabolism*, vol. 282, no. 3, pp. E522–E533, 2002.

[75] S. Okuno, S. Akazawa, I. Yasuhi et al., "Decreased expression of the GLUT4 glucose transporter protein in adipose tissue during pregnancy," *Hormone and Metabolic Research*, vol. 27, no. 5, pp. 231–234, 1995.

[76] E. Sivan and G. Boden, "Free fatty acids, insulin resistance, and pregnancy," *Current Diabetes Reports*, vol. 3, no. 4, pp. 319–322, 2003.

[77] P. M. Catalano, L. Huston, S. B. Amini, and S. C. Kalhan, "Longitudinal changes in glucose metabolism during pregnancy in obese women with normal glucose tolerance and gestational diabetes mellitus," *The American Journal of Obstetrics and Gynecology*, vol. 180, no. 4, pp. 903–916, 1999.

[78] A. Nadal, P. Alonso-Magdalena, S. Soriano, A. B. Ropero, and I. Quesada, "The role of oestrogens in the adaptation of islets to insulin resistance," *The Journal of Physiology*, vol. 587, no. 21, pp. 5031–5037, 2009.

[79] R. Kaaja and T. Rönnemaa, "Gestational diabetes: pathogenesis and consequences to mother and offspring," *Review of Diabetic Studies*, vol. 5, no. 4, pp. 194–202, 2008.

[80] J. L. Weiss, F. D. Malone, D. Emig et al., "Obesity, obstetric complications and cesarean delivery rate—a population-based screening study," *American Journal of Obstetrics & Gynecology*, vol. 190, no. 4, pp. 1091–1097, 2004.

[81] T. Tzanavari, P. Giannogonas, and K. P. Karalis, "TNF-α and obesity," *Current Directions in Autoimmunity*, vol. 11, pp. 145–156, 2010.

[82] S. E. Shoelson, J. Lee, and A. B. Goldfine, "Inflammation and insulin resistance," *The Journal of Clinical Investigation*, vol. 116, no. 7, pp. 1793–1801, 2006.

[83] D. Rosenbaum, R. S. Haber, and A. Dunaif, "Insulin resistance in polycystic ovary syndrome: decreased expression of GLUT-4 glucose transporters in adipocytes," *The American Journal of Physiology—Endocrinology and Metabolism*, vol. 264, no. 2, pp. E197–E202, 1993.

[84] J. Kawano and R. Arora, "The role of adiponectin in obesity, diabetes, and cardiovascular disease," *Journal of the CardioMetabolic Syndrome*, vol. 4, no. 1, pp. 44–49, 2009.

[85] I. L. M. H. Aye, T. L. Powell, and T. Jansson, "Review: adiponectin—the missing link between maternal adiposity, placental transport and fetal growth?" *Placenta*, vol. 34, pp. S40–S45, 2013.

[86] J. Chen, B. Tan, E. Karteris et al., "Secretion of adiponectin by human placenta: differential modulation of adiponectin and its receptors by cytokines," *Diabetologia*, vol. 49, no. 6, pp. 1292–1302, 2006.

[87] R. Retnakaran, Y. Qi, P. W. Connelly, M. Sermer, A. J. Hanley, and B. Zinman, "Low adiponectin concentration during pregnancy predicts postpartum insulin resistance, beta cell dysfunction and fasting glycaemia," *Diabetologia*, vol. 53, no. 2, pp. 268–276, 2010.

[88] T. A. Buchanan and A. H. Xiang, "Gestational diabetes mellitus," *The Journal of Clinical Investigation*, vol. 115, no. 3, pp. 485–491, 2005.

[89] E. P. Gunderson, C. P. Quesenberry Jr., D. R. Jacobs Jr., J. Feng, C. E. Lewis, and S. Sidney, "Longitudinal study of prepregnancy cardiometabolic risk factors and subsequent risk of gestational diabetes mellitus," *The American Journal of Epidemiology*, vol. 172, no. 10, pp. 1131–1143, 2010.

[90] D. Williams, "Pregnancy: a stress test for life," *Current Opinion in Obstetrics and Gynecology*, vol. 15, no. 6, pp. 465–471, 2003.

[91] J. Lauenborg, T. Hansen, D. M. Jensen et al., "Increasing incidence of diabetes after gestational diabetes: a long-term follow-up in a Danish population," *Diabetes Care*, vol. 27, no. 5, pp. 1194–1199, 2004.

[92] I. Mrizak, A. Arfa, M. Fekih et al., "Inflammation and impaired endothelium-dependant vasodilatation in non obese women with gestational diabetes mellitus: preliminary results," *Lipids in Health and Disease*, vol. 12, article 93, 2013.

[93] R. Retnakaran, Y. Qi, C. Ye et al., "Hepatic insulin resistance is an early determinant of declining β-cell function in the first year postpartum after glucose intolerance in pregnancy," *Diabetes Care*, vol. 34, no. 11, pp. 2431–2434, 2011.

[94] The HAPO Study Cooperative Research Group, B. E. Metzger, L. P. Lowe et al., "Hyperglycemia and adverse pregnancy outcomes," *The New England Journal of Medicine*, vol. 358, pp. 1991–2002, 2008.

[95] J. M. Perkins, J. P. Dunn, and S. M. Jagasia, "Perspectives in gestational diabetes mellitus: a review of screening, diagnosis, and treatment," *Clinical Diabetes*, vol. 25, no. 2, pp. 57–62, 2007.

[96] HAPO Study Cooperative Research Group, "Hyperglycemia and Adverse Pregnancy Outcome (HAPO) Study: associations with neonatal anthropometrics," *Diabetes*, vol. 58, pp. 453–459, 2009.

[97] W. H. Tam, R. C. W. Ma, X. Yang et al., "Glucose intolerance and cardiometabolic risk in children exposed to maternal gestational diabetes mellitus in utero," *Pediatrics*, vol. 122, no. 6, pp. 1229–1234, 2008.

[98] N. Freinkel, "Of pregnancy and progeny," *Diabetes*, vol. 29, no. 12, pp. 1023–1035, 1980.

[99] J. Jakšić, F. Mikulandra, M. Periša et al., "Effect of insulin and insulin-like growth factor I on fetal macrosomia in healthy women," *Collegium Antropologicum*, vol. 25, no. 2, pp. 535–543, 2001.

[100] C. N. Hales and D. J. P. Barker, "The thrifty phenotype hypothesis," *British Medical Bulletin*, vol. 60, pp. 5–20, 2001.

[101] T. J. Wilkin and L. D. Voss, "Metabolic syndrome: maladaptation to a modern world," *Journal of the Royal Society of Medicine*, vol. 97, no. 11, pp. 511–520, 2004.

[102] A. Yessoufou and K. Moutairou, "Maternal diabetes in pregnancy: early and long-term outcomes on the offspring and the concept of 'metabolic memory'," *Experimental Diabetes Research*, vol. 2011, Article ID 218598, 12 pages, 2011.

[103] M. Du, X. Yan, J. F. Tong, J. Zhao, and M. J. Zhu, "Maternal obesity, inflammation, and fetal skeletal muscle development," *Biology of Reproduction*, vol. 82, no. 1, pp. 4–12, 2010.

[104] K. Franke, T. Harder, L. Aerts et al., ""Programming" of orexigenic and anorexigenic hypothalamic neurons in offspring of treated and untreated diabetic mother rats," *Brain Research*, vol. 1031, no. 2, pp. 276–283, 2005.

[105] J. Rojas, N. Arraiz, M. Aguirre, M. Velasco, and V. Bermúdez, "AMPK as target for intervention in childhood and adolescent obesity," *Journal of Obesity*, vol. 2011, Article ID 252817, 19 pages, 2011.

[106] R. W. Brownsey, A. N. Boone, J. E. Elliott, J. E. Kulpa, and W. M. Lee, "Regulation of acetyl-CoA carboxylase," *Biochemical Society Transactions*, vol. 34, no. 2, pp. 223–227, 2006.

[107] L. Al-Khalili, A. V. Chibalin, M. Yu et al., "MEF2 activation in differentiated primary human skeletal muscle cultures requires coordinated involvement of parallel pathways," *The American Journal of Physiology—Cell Physiology*, vol. 286, no. 6, pp. C1410–C1416, 2004.

[108] M. M. Mihaylova and R. J. Shaw, "The AMPK signalling pathway coordinates cell growth, autophagy and metabolism," *Nature Cell Biology*, vol. 13, no. 9, pp. 1016–1023, 2011.

[109] R. Stark, S. E. Ashley, and Z. B. Andrews, "AMPK and the neuroendocrine regulation of appetite and energy expenditure," *Molecular and Cellular Endocrinology*, vol. 366, no. 2, pp. 215–223, 2013.

[110] P. Banerjee, R. R. Bhonde, and R. Pal, "Diverse roles of metformin during peri-implantation development: revisiting novel molecular mechanisms underlying clinical implications," *Stem Cells and Development*, vol. 22, no. 22, pp. 2927–2934, 2013.

[111] N. Desai, A. Roman, B. Rochelson et al., "Maternal metformin treatment decreases fetal inflammation in a rat model of obesity and metabolic syndrome," *American Journal of Obstetrics and Gynecology*, vol. 209, no. 2, pp. 136-e1–136-e9, 2013.

[112] H.-Y. Lee, D. Wei, and M. R. Loeken, "Lack of metformin effect on mouse embryo AMPK activity: implications for metformin treatment during pregnancy," *Diabetes/Metabolism Research and Reviews*, vol. 30, no. 1, pp. 23–30, 2014.

[113] G. S. Eng, R. A. Sheridan, A. Wyman et al., "AMP kinase activation increases glucose uptake, decreases apoptosis, and improves pregnancy outcome in embryos exposed to high IGF-I concentrations," *Diabetes*, vol. 56, no. 9, pp. 2228–2234, 2007.

[114] J. J. Marin, "Plasma membrane transporters in modern liver pharmacology," *Scientifica*, vol. 2012, Article ID 428139, 15 pages, 2012.

[115] L. Gong, S. Goswami, K. M. Giacomini, R. B. Altman, and T. E. Klein, "Metformin pathways: pharmacokinetics and pharmacodynamics," *Pharmacogenetics and Genomics*, vol. 22, no. 11, pp. 820–827, 2012.

[116] J. W. Jonker and A. H. Schinkel, "Pharmacological and physiological functions of the polyspecific organic cation transporters: OCT1, 2, and 3 (SLC22A1-3)," *Journal of Pharmacology and Experimental Therapeutics*, vol. 308, no. 1, pp. 2–9, 2004.

[117] S. Eyal, T. R. Easterling, D. Carr et al., "Pharmacokinetics of metformin during pregnancy," *Drug Metabolism and Disposition*, vol. 38, no. 5, pp. 833–840, 2010.

[118] J. Saito, T. Hirota, N. Kikunaga, K. Otsubo, and I. Ieiri, "Interindividual differences in placental expression of the *SLC22A2* (*OCT2*) gene: relationship to epigenetic variations in the 5*t*-upstream regulatory region," *Journal of Pharmaceutical Sciences*, vol. 100, no. 9, pp. 3875–3883, 2011.

[119] M. Kovo, N. Kogman, O. Ovadia, I. Nakash, A. Golan, and A. Hoffman, "Carrier-mediated transport of metformin across the human placenta determined by using the ex vivo perfusion of the placental cotyledon model," *Prenatal Diagnosis*, vol. 28, no. 6, pp. 544–548, 2008.

[120] M. Maliepaard, G. L. Scheffer, I. F. Faneyte et al., "Subcellular localization and distribution of the breast cancer resistance protein transporter in normal human tissues," *Cancer Research*, vol. 61, no. 8, pp. 3458–3464, 2001.

[121] M. V. St.-Pierre, M. A. Serrano, R. I. R. Macias et al., "Expression of members of the multidrug resistance protein family in human term placenta," *The American Journal of Physiology—Regulatory Integrative and Comparative Physiology*, vol. 279, no. 4, pp. R1495–R1503, 2000.

[122] V. Ganapathy, P. D. Prasad, M. E. Ganapathy, and F. H. Leibach, "Placental transporters relevant to drug distribution across the maternal-fetal interface," *Journal of Pharmacology and Experimental Therapeutics*, vol. 294, no. 2, pp. 413–420, 2000.

[123] G. G. Briggs, R. K. Freeman, and S. J. Yaffe, *Drugs in Pregnancy and Lactation*, Lippincott Williams & Wilkins, Philadelphia, Pa, USA, 2002.

[124] *Package Insert: Metformin Hydrochloride*, Bristol-Myers Squibb, New York, NY, USA, 2009.

[125] S. J. Gutzin, E. Kozer, L. A. Magee, D. S. Feig, and G. Koren, "The safety of oral hypoglycemic agents in the first trimester of pregnancy: a meta-analysis," *Canadian Journal of Clinical Pharmacology*, vol. 10, no. 4, pp. 179–183, 2003.

[126] C. Gilbert, M. Valois, and G. Koren, "Pregnancy outcome after first-trimester exposure to metformin: a meta-analysis," *Fertility and Sterility*, vol. 86, no. 3, pp. 658–663, 2006.

[127] G. G. Briggs, P. J. Ambrose, M. P. Nageotte, G. Padilla, and S. Wan, "Excretion of metformin into breast milk and the effect on nursing infants," *Obstetrics and Gynecology*, vol. 105, no. 6, pp. 1437–1441, 2005.

[128] C. J. Glueck and P. Wang, "Metformin before and during pregnancy and lactation in polycystic ovary syndrome," *Expert Opinion on Drug Safety*, vol. 6, no. 2, pp. 191–198, 2007.

[129] S. J. Gardiner, C. M. J. Kirkpatrick, E. J. Begg, M. Zhang, M. Peter Moore, and D. J. Saville, "Transfer of metformin into human milk," *Clinical Pharmacology and Therapeutics*, vol. 73, no. 1, pp. 71–77, 2003.

[130] B. Charles, R. Norris, X. Xiao, and W. Hague, "Population pharmacokinetics of metformin in late pregnancy," *Therapeutic Drug Monitoring*, vol. 28, no. 1, pp. 67–72, 2006.

[131] T. D. R. Vause, A. P. Cheung, S. Sierra et al., "Ovulation induction in polycystic ovary syndrome," *Journal of Obstetrics and Gynaecology Canada*, vol. 32, no. 5, pp. 495–502, 2010.

[132] O. Khorram, J. P. Helliwell, S. Katz, C. M. Bonpane, and L. Jaramillo, "Two weeks of metformin improves clomiphene citrate-induced ovulation and metabolic profiles in women with polycystic ovary syndrome," *Fertility and Sterility*, vol. 85, no. 5, pp. 1448–1451, 2006.

[133] S. Palomba, A. Falbo, and G. B. La Sala, "Metformin and gonadotropins for ovulation induction in patients with polycystic ovary syndrome: a systematic review with meta-analysis of randomized controlled trials," *Reproductive Biology and Endocrinology*, vol. 12, article 3, 2014.

[134] R. G. Farquharson, E. Jauniaux, and N. Exalto, "Updated and revised nomenclature for description of early pregnancy events," *Human Reproduction*, vol. 20, no. 11, pp. 3008–3011, 2005.

[135] H. B. Ford and D. J. Schust, "Recurrent pregnancy loss: etiology, diagnosis, and therapy," *Reviews in Obstetrics and Gynecology*, vol. 2, pp. 76–83, 2009.

[136] P. A. Essah, K. I. Cheang, and J. E. Nestler, "The pathophysiology of miscarriage in women with polycystic ovary syndrome. Review and proposed hypothesis of mechanisms involved," *Hormones*, vol. 3, pp. 221–227, 2004.

[137] E. M. Tuckerman, M. A. Okon, T.-C. Li, and S. M. Laird, "Do androgens have a direct effect on endometrial function? An in vitro study," *Fertility and Sterility*, vol. 74, no. 4, pp. 771–779, 2000.

[138] N. C. Douglas, M. H. Thornton, S. K. Nurudeen, M. Bucur, R. A. Lobo, and M. V. Sauer, "Differential expression of serum glycodelin and insulin-like growth factor binding protein 1 in early pregnancy," *Reproductive Sciences*, vol. 20, no. 11, pp. 1376–1381, 2013.

[139] D. J. Jakubowicz, P. A. Essah, M. Seppälä et al., "Reduced serum glycodelin and insulin-like growth factor-binding protein-1 in women with polycystic ovary syndrome during first trimester of pregnancy," *The Journal of Clinical Endocrinology & Metabolism*, vol. 89, no. 2, pp. 833–839, 2004.

[140] K. A. Toulis, D. G. Goulis, G. Mintziori et al., "Meta-analysis of cardiovascular disease risk markers in women with polycystic ovary syndrome," *Human Reproduction Update*, vol. 17, no. 6, Article ID dmr025, pp. 741–760, 2011.

[141] J. Zheng, P. F. Shan, and W. Gu, "The efficacy of metformin in pregnant women with polycystic ovary syndrome: a meta-analysis of clinical trials," *Journal of Endocrinological Investigation*, vol. 36, no. 10, pp. 797–802, 2013.

[142] S. R. Salpeter, N. S. Buckley, J. A. Kahn, and E. E. Salpeter, "Meta-analysis: metformin treatment in persons at risk for diabetes mellitus," *The American Journal of Medicine*, vol. 121, no. 2, pp. 149.e2–157.e2, 2008.

[143] F. H. Nawaz, R. Khalid, T. Naru, and J. Rizvi, "Does continuous use of metformin throughout pregnancy improve pregnancy outcomes in women with polycystic ovarian syndrome?" *Journal of Obstetrics and Gynaecology Research*, vol. 34, no. 5, pp. 832–837, 2008.

[144] G. Koren, C. Gilbert, and M. Valois, "Metformin use during the first trimester of pregnancy: is it safe?" *Canadian Family Physician*, vol. 52, pp. 171–172, 2006.

[145] E. Vanky, S. Stridsklev, R. Heimstad et al., "Metformin *Versus* placebo from first trimester to delivery in polycystic ovary syndrome: a randomized, controlled multicenter study," *Journal of Clinical Endocrinology and Metabolism*, vol. 95, no. 12, pp. E448–E455, 2010.

[146] S. Stridsklev, S. M. Carlsen, Ø. Salvesen, I. Clemens, and E. Vanky, "Midpregnancy Doppler ultrasound of the uterine artery in metformin- versus placebo-treated PCOS women: a randomized trial," *The Journal of Clinical Endocrinology & Metabolism*, vol. 99, pp. 972–977, 2014.

[147] F. Sharifzadeh, M. Kashanian, and F. Fatemi, "A comparison of serum androgens in pre-eclamptic and normotensive pregnant women during the third trimester of pregnancy," *Gynecological Endocrinology*, vol. 28, no. 10, pp. 834–836, 2012.

[148] T.-Y. Hsu, K.-C. Lan, C.-C. Tsai et al., "Expression of androgen receptor in human placentas from normal and preeclamptic pregnancies," *Taiwanese Journal of Obstetrics and Gynecology*, vol. 48, no. 3, pp. 262–267, 2009.

[149] J. M. Roberts and H. Gammill, "Insulin resistance in preeclampsia," *Hypertension*, vol. 47, no. 3, pp. 341–342, 2006.

[150] J. Uzan, M. Carbonnel, O. Piconne, R. Asmar, and J.-M. Ayoubi, "Pre-eclampsia: pathophysiology, diagnosis, and management," *Vascular Health and Risk Management*, vol. 7, no. 1, pp. 467–474, 2011.

[151] R. Menon, "Spontaneous preterm birth, a clinical dilemma: etiologic, pathophysiologic and genetic heterogeneities and racial disparity," *Acta Obstetricia et Gynecologica Scandinavica*, vol. 87, no. 6, pp. 590–600, 2008.

[152] L. Lettieri, A. M. Vintzileos, J. F. Rodis, S. M. Albini, and C. M. Salafia, "Does "idiopathic" preterm labor resulting in preterm birth exist?" *American Journal of Obstetrics and Gynecology*, vol. 168, no. 5, pp. 1480–1485, 1993.

[153] S. Bolton, B. Cleary, J. Walsh, E. Dempsey, and M. J. Turner, "Continuation of metformin in the first trimester of women with polycystic ovarian syndrome is not associated with increased perinatal morbidity," *European Journal of Pediatrics*, vol. 168, no. 2, pp. 203–206, 2009.

[154] C. J. Glueck, N. Goldenberg, J. Pranicoff, M. Loftspring, L. Sieve, and P. Wang, "Height, weight, and motor-social development during the first 18 months of life in 126 infants born to 109 mothers with polycystic ovary syndrome who conceived on and continued metformin through pregnancy," *Human Reproduction*, vol. 19, no. 6, pp. 1323–1330, 2004.

[155] C. J. Glueck, M. Salehi, L. Sieve, and P. Wang, "Growth, motor, and social development in breast- and formula-fed infants of metformin-treated women with polycystic ovary syndrome," *Journal of Pediatrics*, vol. 148, no. 5, pp. 628.e2–632.e2, 2006.

[156] J. A. Rowan and MiG Investigators, "A trial in progress: gestational diabetes. Treatment with metformin compared with insulin (the Metformin in Gestational Diabetes [MiG] trial)," *Diabetes Care*, vol. 30, supplement 2, pp. S214–S219, 2007.

[157] J. A. Rowan, W. M. Hague, W. Gao, M. R. Battin, M. P. Moore, and MiG Trial Investigators, "Metformin versus insulin for the treatment of gestational diabetes," *The New England Journal of Medicine*, vol. 358, no. 19, pp. 2003–2015, 2008.

[158] J. C. Silva, D. R. R. N. Fachin, M. L. Coral, and A. M. Bertini, "Perinatal impact of the use of metformin and glyburide for the treatment of gestational diabetes mellitus," *Journal of Perinatal Medicine*, vol. 40, no. 3, pp. 225–228, 2012.

[159] H. L. Barrett, K. L. Gatford, C. M. Houda et al., "Maternal and neonatal circulating markers ofmetabolic and cardiovascular risk in themetformin in gestational diabetes (MiG) trial," *Diabetes Care*, vol. 36, no. 3, pp. 529–536, 2013.

[160] S. Niromanesh, A. Alavi, F. R. Sharbaf, N. Amjadi, S. Moosavi, and S. Akbari, "Metformin compared with insulin in the management of gestational diabetes mellitus: a randomized clinical trial," *Diabetes Research and Clinical Practice*, vol. 98, no. 3, pp. 422–429, 2012.

[161] J. A. Rowan, W. Gao, W. M. Hague, and H. D. McIntyre, "Glycemia and its relationship to outcomes in the metformin in gestational diabetes trial," *Diabetes Care*, vol. 33, no. 1, pp. 9–16, 2010.

[162] H. Ijäs, M. Vääräsmäki, L. Morin-Papunen et al., "Metformin should be considered in the treatment of gestational diabetes: a prospective randomised study," *An International Journal of Obstetrics and Gynaecology*, vol. 118, no. 7, pp. 880–885, 2011.

[163] K. L. Gatford, C. M. Houda, Z. X. Lu et al., "Vitamin B_{12} and homocysteine status during pregnancy in the metformin in gestational diabetes trial: responses to maternal metformin compared with insulin treatment," *Diabetes, Obesity and Metabolism*, vol. 15, no. 7, pp. 660–667, 2013.

[164] R. Obeid, "Metformin causing vitamin b12 deficiency: a guilty verdict without sufficient evidence," *Diabetes Care*, vol. 37, no. 2, pp. e22–e23, 2014.

[165] J. S. Dhulkotia, B. Ola, R. Fraser, and T. Farrell, "Oral hypoglycemic agents vs insulin in management of gestational diabetes: a systematic review and metaanalysis," *American Journal of Obstetrics & Gynecology*, vol. 203, no. 5, pp. 457.e1–457.e9, 2010.

[166] J. C. Silva, C. Pacheco, J. Bizato, B. V. De Souza, T. E. Ribeiro, and A. M. Bertini, "Metformin compared with glyburide for the management of gestational diabetes," *International Journal of Gynecology and Obstetrics*, vol. 111, no. 1, pp. 37–40, 2010.

[167] Y. Barak, M. C. Nelson, E. S. Ong et al., "PPARγ is required for placental, cardiac, and adipose tissue development," *Molecular Cell*, vol. 4, no. 4, pp. 585–595, 1999.

[168] J. Sevillano, I. C. López-Pérez, E. Herrera, M. Del Pilar Ramos, and C. Bocos, "Englitazone administration to late pregnant rats produces delayed body growth and insulin resistance in their fetuses and neonates," *Biochemical Journal*, vol. 389, no. 3, pp. 913–918, 2005.

[169] P. Froment and P. Touraine, "Thiazolidinediones and fertility in polycystic ovary syndrome (PCOS)," *PPAR Research*, vol. 2006, Article ID 73986, 8 pages, 2006.

[170] J. Gui, Q. Liu, and L. Feng, "Metformin vs insulin in the management of gestational diabetes: a meta-analysis," *PLoS ONE*, vol. 8, no. 5, Article ID e64585, 2013.

[171] V. W. Wong and B. Jalaludin, "Gestational diabetes mellitus: who requires insulin therapy?" *Australian and New Zealand Journal of Obstetrics and Gynaecology*, vol. 51, no. 5, pp. 432–436, 2011.

[172] A. Sokup, B. Ruszkowska-Ciastek, K. Góralczyk, M. Walentowicz, M. Szymański, and D. Rość, "Insulin resistance as estimated by the homeostatic method at diagnosis of gestational diabetes: estimation of disease severity and therapeutic needs in a population-based study," *BMC Endocrine Disorders*, vol. 13, article 21, 2013.

[173] A. Corbould, F. Swinton, A. Radford, J. Campbell, S. McBeath, and A. Dennis, "Fasting blood glucose predicts response to extended-release metformin in gestational diabetes mellitus," *Australian and New Zealand Journal of Obstetrics and Gynaecology*, vol. 53, pp. 125–129, 2013.

[174] C. P. Spaulonci, L. S. Bernardes, T. C. Trindade, M. Zugaib, and R. P. Francisco, "Randomized trial of metformin vs insulin in the management of gestational diabetes," *American Journal of Obstetrics & Gynecology*, vol. 209, no. 1, pp. 34.e1–34.e7, 2013.

[175] K. Tertti, U. Ekblad, P. Koskinen, T. Vahlberg, and T. Rönnemaa, "Metformin vs. insulin in gestational diabetes. A randomized study characterizing metformin patients needing additional insulin," *Diabetes, Obesity and Metabolism*, vol. 15, no. 3, pp. 246–251, 2013.

[176] Identifier NCT01587378, Metformin to Prevent Late Miscarriage and Preterm Delivery in Women with Polycystic Ovary Syndrome Trial (PregMet2), ClinicalTrials.gov, Bethesda, Md, USA, National Library of Medicine, 2012, http://clinicaltrials.gov/show/NCT01855763.

[177] National Library of Medicine, "Metformin treatment in gestational diabetes and noninsulin dependent diabetes in pregnancy in a developing country (migdm&t2dm)," ClinicalTrials.gov NCT01855763, National Library of Medicine, Bethesda, Md, USA, 2013, http://clinicaltrials.gov/show/NCT01855763.

15

Incidence and Correlates of Maternal Near Miss in Southeast Iran

Tayebeh Naderi,[1] **Shohreh Foroodnia,**[2] **Samaneh Omidi,**[1]
Faezeh Samadani,[2] **and Nouzar Nakhaee**[3]

[1]*Research Center for Health Services Management, Institute of Futures Studies in Health, Kerman University of Medical Sciences, Kerman 76175-113, Iran*
[2]*Research Center for Social Determinants of Health, Institute of Futures Studies in Health, Kerman University of Medical Sciences, Kerman 76175-113, Iran*
[3]*Neuroscience Research Center, Institute of Neuropharmacology, Kerman University of Medical Sciences, Kerman 76175-113, Iran*

Correspondence should be addressed to Nouzar Nakhaee; nakhaeen@kmu.ac.ir

Academic Editor: Hind A. Beydoun

This prospective study aimed to estimate the incidence and associated factors of severe maternal morbidity in southeast Iran. During a 9-month period in 2013, all women referring to eight hospitals for termination of pregnancy as well as women admitted during 42 days after the termination of pregnancy were enrolled into the study. Maternal near miss conditions were defined based on Say et al.'s recommendations. Five hundred and one cases of maternal near miss and 19,908 live births occurred in the study period, yielding a maternal near miss ratio of 25.2 per 1000 live births. This rate was 7.5 and 105 per 1000 in private and tertiary care settings, respectively. The rate of maternal death in near miss cases was 0.40% with a case:fatality ratio of 250 : 1. The most prevalent causes of near miss were severe preeclampsia (27.3%), ectopic pregnancy (18.4%), and abruptio placentae (16.2%). Higher age, higher education, and being primiparous were associated with a higher risk of near miss. Considering the high rate of maternal near miss in referral hospitals, maternal near miss surveillance system should be set up in these hospitals to identify cases of severe maternal morbidity as soon as possible.

1. Introduction

There are approximately 287,000 preventable maternal deaths annually, of which 99% occur in developing countries [1]. As a sentinel event, maternal death is also a prime indicator in evaluating the quality of a nation's health care delivery systems [2, 3]. Mothers are pivotal to the social, economic, and cultural development of a community [2]; maintaining their health elevates the physical, psychological, and social well-being of their children and families and, by extension, society as a whole [4]. For this reason, improving maternal health has been proposed by the World Health Organization (WHO) as one of their eight Millennium Development Goals (MDG) [1].

Traditionally, maternal death evaluation has been viewed as key to maternal death prevention [5]. However, in countries with few maternal deaths, this approach fails to provide comprehensive information, leaving policy makers to react based on current rather than past statistics. To facilitate the development of precautionary measures and safer environments that minimize maternal deaths, it is essential that near miss data are recorded and analyzed [6]. The WHO defines an individual having experienced severe acute maternal morbidity (SAMM) (i.e., near miss) as "a woman who nearly died but survived a complication that occurred during pregnancy, childbirth or within 42 days of termination of pregnancy" [7].

In fact, maternal near miss includes those cases in which a woman nearly died but survived during pregnancy or during 42 days after the delivery [8]. Using near miss data in maternal death prevention planning has several advantages. First, because the number of near miss cases exceeds maternal death cases, near miss is a better predicate for preventive planning. Second, because the mother survives a near miss, she can provide valuable details on what she experienced. Lastly, because near miss is one step removed from death, obtaining any information about the event could prove useful in preventing maternal death [8–10].

The prevalence of maternal near miss varies among different countries based on health care quality and availability. Nevertheless, in a systematic review using disease-specific criteria, near miss rates have been reported to be between 0.6% and 14.98% [11].

From a global perspective, Iran has been notably successful in reducing maternal mortality. Between 1990 and 2008, Iran has managed to decrease its maternal mortality rate by 80% [1], which, at present, translates to about 25 deaths in 100,000 [12]. The availability of emergency obstetrical care, improvements in women's education [13], and the expansion of family planning services have all contributed to the decrease in maternal mortality [14]. In Iran, a national maternal mortality surveillance system examines maternal death cases by reviewing files and interviewing key parties to determine the cause of death [15]. Although some studies have been carried out in Iran and the Middle East regarding the causes of maternal death and risk factors of pregnancy [12–17], the authors know of no published study on severe maternal morbidities and near miss occurrences from Iran or other Middle Eastern countries. The present study aimed to establish a profile of severe maternal morbidities in Iran and their relationship with other underlying factors.

2. Method

This prospective study encompassed eight hospitals with maternity facilities located in the two large cities of Kerman and Jiroft in southeast Iran. The study was performed in 2013 for a period of nine months. The study protocol was approved by the Ethical Committee of Kerman University of Medical Sciences (E.C./90/518). After explaining the study's nature and aims, oral consent was obtained from the participants who all were ensured that their information would remain confidential. First, a list of maternal near miss conditions was prepared based on Say et al.'s recommendations for prospective surveillance of maternal near miss cases [8]. This list included four major groups of haemorrhagic disorders, hypertensive disorders, severe management indicators, and other systemic disorders. Moreover, a category including other conditions was also considered so as not to miss any other life-threatening illness [8]. All women admitted during the nine-month study period for delivery or completion of pregnancy as well as women admitted within 42 days after the termination of pregnancy were enrolled into the study. After the participating hospitals' maternity, labour, general ICU, emergency, and admission departments were fully coordinated, our case survey was implemented. A check list was completed for cases with potentially life-threatening conditions by a team consisting of a midwife and gynaecologist. The check list was composed of two parts. The first part included demographic and clinical data such as age, educational level, place of residency, gravidity, parity, type of delivery, and gestational age. The second part comprised the list of potentially life-threatening conditions. Next, a

TABLE 1: Maternal near miss ratio according to hospital type.

Hospital type	Number of near miss cases	Number of live births	Ratio (CI 95%)
Referral	345	3293	104.8 (94.8–115.7)
Public	128	2877	9.9 (8.3–11.8)
Private	28	3738	7.5 (5.2–10.8)
Total	501	9908	25.2 (23.1–27.5)

woman admitted to the delivery room at the same hospital was randomly selected from the list of patients as the control, and the first part of the check list was completed for her. In all stages, an experienced expert supervised completion of the check lists. According to the WHO definition maternal near miss ratio was defined as "the number of maternal near-miss cases per 1000 live births" [18].

Chi-square and independent t-tests were used to compare the qualitative and quantitative variables between near miss and control groups. A stepwise logistic regression model was used to determine the relationship between underlying variables and near miss ratio. The logistic regression model's goodness of fit was evaluated by the Hosmer-Lemeshow test.

3. Results

During the study period, there were 501 cases of near miss in 19,908 live births (a near miss ratio of 25.2 per 1000 live births). The highest near miss ratio (104.8 in 1000) was observed in the referral (educational) hospital (Table 1). The mean age of near miss cases was 28.3 ± 6.1 years versus the control group's 26.0 ± 5.8 years ($P < 0.001$). University degrees were seen more among near miss women (Table 2). In the near miss group, 208 women (41.5%) were primiparous, whereas, in the control group, the number was 225 (45.2%; $P = 0.243$). The frequency of abortion in the near miss and control groups was 18.6% and 1.6%, respectively ($P < 0.001$). The frequency of caesarean section in the near miss and control groups was 24.7% and 54.2%, respectively ($P < 0.001$).

In our study group, there were two cases of maternal death. One was a 19-year-old woman diagnosed with intracerebral haemorrhage (ICH); the other was a 28-year-old woman who had undergone curettage due to a failed abortion and died from sepsis because of perforations in the uterus and intestine.

The rate of maternal death in near miss cases was 0.40% with a case : fatality ratio of 250 : 1.

As shown in Table 3, the most prevalent causes of near miss were severe preeclampsia (27.3%), ectopic pregnancy (18.4%), and abruptio placentae (16.2%). In all, 15.2% had at least one systemic disease, and 43 women in the near miss group were hospitalised in the ICU (Table 3). The majority of the near miss cases were observed in the haemorrhagic disorders group (Table 3). Logistic regression analysis showed that four variables had significant relationship with near miss

TABLE 2: Baseline and clinical characteristics in near miss and control groups.

Variable	Total	Near miss ($n = 501$)	Control ($n = 498$)	P value
Age group* (yrs)				
<18	22	4 (18.2)	18 (81.8)	<0.001
18–35	978	432 (49.1)	447 (50.9)	
>35	98	65 (66.3)	33 (33.7)	
Education*				
≤Primary	251	127 (50.6)	124 (49.4)	<0.001
Secondary	576	260 (45.1)	316 (54.9)	
College	172	114 (66.3)	58 (33.7)	
Residence				
Urban	789	402 (51.0)	387 (49.0)	0.327
Rural	210	99 (47.1)	111 (52.9)	
Type of delivery*				
Normal vaginal delivery	501	134 (26.7)	367 (73.3)	<0.001
First cesarean delivery	254	189 (74.4)	65 (25.6)	
Repeat cesarean delivery	142	84 (59.2)	58 (40.8)	
Vaginal birth after cesarean delivery	1	1 (100)	0 (0)	
Type of abortion*				
Medical	54	51 (94.4)	3 (5.6)	0.545
Surgical	45	40 (88.9)	5 (11.1)	
Criminal	2	2 (100)	0 (0)	
Gravidity (mean ± SE)	—	2.3 (0.06)	2.1 (0.06)	0.012
Parity (mean ± SE)	—	1.1 (0.06)	1.0 (0.06)	0.048
Abortion (mean ± SE)	—	1.2 (0.08)	1.2 (0.07)	0.460
Living (mean ± SE)	—	2.3 (0.3)	1.7 (0.09)	0.058
Birth interval (mean ± SE)	—	5.3 (0.2)	4.7 (0.2)	0.055
Gestational age (mean ± SE)	—	27.7 (0.6)	34.8 (0.4)	<0.001
Number of prenatal care (mean ± SE)	—	6.4 (0.2)	6.9 (0.2)	0.028

*Numbers in parentheses are percents.

occurrence (Table 4). Of the 377 near miss cases (75.2%), the major problem was discerned at or during the first six hours of admission.

4. Discussion

In the present study, the near miss ratio was 25.2 per 1000 live births. In the private setting, this rate was 7.5 per 1000, and, in the tertiary care hospital, it was approximately 105 per 1000. The main advantages of this study were its prospective nature and its use of standard criteria for determining near miss cases. Because more than 97% of deliveries in Iran occur in hospitals [16], the present report may be considered as a population-based study. Because of the differences among patients and health care delivery systems, generalizing the results of this study on a countrywide basis should be done with caution.

The literature shows that maternal near miss ratios vary greatly depending on the population studied, how near miss is defined, and how the study is conducted (prospective versus retrospective) [11, 19]. Near miss ratios have been reported as 44.3 per 1000 in Brazil [9], 33 per 1000 in India [20], 3.83 per 1000 in Scotland [21], and 34 per 1000 in a WHO survey [10]. A recent systematic review using a unique definition for near miss showed SAMM rates in high-income countries to be significantly lower compared with those of low- and middle-income countries [11].

In this study, like some other studies [19, 20], the rate of near miss was significantly higher in the tertiary care setting (Table 1). The reason might be that, because of the limited facilities at private hospitals, women with complicated pregnancies are not usually referred to these centres.

In the present study, we found a higher rate of near miss and consequently a lower fatality rate (0.4%). These findings may be derived from our broader definition for near miss events, which combined disease-specific criteria with management-based criteria [8]. In Netherland, with a near miss ratio of 7.1 per 1000, the rate was 1.9% [22]. In Brazil, with a near miss ratio of 42 per 1000, the rate was 1.6% [19]. It should be mentioned that the maternal death rate shows a decreasing trend in Iran [12].

In our study, haemorrhagic disorders (46.1%) and hypertensive disorders (31.9%) were the most common causes of near miss (Table 3). These rates are similar to those reported

TABLE 3: Frequency of near miss criteria in 501 cases of severe maternal morbidity.

Type of near miss	Frequency (%)
Hemorrhagic disorders	
Abruptio placentae	81 (16.2)
Accreta/increta/percreta placenta	12 (2.4)
Ectopic pregnancy	92 (18.4)
Postpartum haemorrhage	50 (10)
Ruptured uterus	3 (0.6)
At least one type	231 (46.1)
Hypertensive disorders	
Severe preeclampsia	137 (27.3)
Eclampsia	11 (2.2)
Severe hypertension (>170/110)	35 (7.0)
Hypertensive encephalopathy	0 (0)
HELLP syndrome	10 (2.0)
At least one type	160 (31.9)
Other systemic disorders	
Endometritis	12 (2.4)
Pulmonary edema	0 (0)
Respiratory failure	7 (1.4)
Seizures	12 (2.4)
Sepsis	4 (0.8)
Shock	5 (1.0)
Thrombocytopenia < 100000	39 (7.8)
Thyroid crisis	0 (0)
At least one type	76 (15.2)
Severe management indicators	
Blood transfusion ≥ 5 units	17 (3.4)
Central venous access	2 (0.4)
Hysterectomy	10 (2.0)
ICU admission	43 (8.6)
Prolonged hospital stay (>7 postpartum days)	28 (5.6)
Nonanesthetic intubation	5 (1.0)
Return to operating room	7 (1.4)
Surgical intervention (other than cesarean section & hysterectomy)	10 (2.0)
Dialysis for acute renal failure	1 (0.2)
Cardiopulmonary resuscitation (CPR)	2 (0.4)
Others (please specify)	12 (2.4)
At least one type	91 (18.2)

TABLE 4: Baseline characteristics associated with near miss cases.

Baseline variables	Adjusted odds ratio	CI 95%	P value
Age	1.08	1.05–1.11	<0.001
Education			
College	1.97	1.35–2.88	<0.001
Others	1	—	—
Primiparous			
Yes	1.41	1.03–1.95	0.033
No	1	—	—
Number of prenatal care	0.94	0.91–0.98	0.003

According to our logistic regression model, four variables had a relationship with near miss (Table 4). In older women with university degrees, the near miss ratio was higher. In fact, most studies demonstrate a proportional relationship between higher near miss ratio and advancing age (particularly over 35 years) [22, 23]. In the WHO's global survey, the near miss ratio was significantly associated with higher educational levels. This finding has been attributed to the tendency among women with higher educational levels to undergo caesarean section, which increases the probability of near miss events [22]. The present study, as in previous studies, shows that being a primipara increases the probability of near miss ratio by 1.2%–1.4% [22, 23].

Although pregnancy complications are to a great extent unpredictable and unpreventable, early awareness of near miss cases can prevent the progress of disease and maternal death [19]. In this study, the feasibility of using WHO-recommended near miss criteria was recognized. However, because of inadequate health care services, it is necessary that the auditing of near miss cases be considered as important as the implementation of near miss surveillance systems [15, 23].

The present study showed that using data related to near miss cases can provide more comprehensive information when reviewing maternal death cases; therefore, establishing near miss surveillance systems in Iranian hospitals is highly recommended.

Conflict of Interests

The authors declare that there is no conflict of interests regarding the publication of this paper.

References

[1] WHO, UNICEF, UNFPA, and The World Bank, *Trends in Maternal Mortality: 1990 to 2010*, WHO, Geneva, Switzerland, 2012.

[2] T. Godal and L. Quam, "Accelerating the global response to reduce maternal mortality," *The Lancet*, vol. 379, no. 9831, pp. 2025–2026, 2012.

[3] J. Milliez, "Rights to safe motherhood and newborn health: ethical issues," *International Journal of Gynecology and Obstetrics*, vol. 106, no. 2, pp. 110–111, 2009.

from Scotland [21] and Indonesia [23]. In India, the two most common causes of near miss have been preeclampsia and haemorrhage [20]. In a study on 64 cases of maternal death in Kerman, Iran, the same two factors were the most prevalent causes of maternal mortality [15]. In our study, 43 cases required intensive care; that is, for every 1000 live births, 2.2 mothers are hospitalized in an ICU, which is nearly similar to the ICU admission rate in Netherland [22].

[4] M. Berer, "Maternal mortality or women's health: time for action," *Reproductive Health Matters*, vol. 20, no. 39, pp. 5–10, 2012.

[5] S. L. Clark, "Strategies for reducing maternal mortality," *Seminars in Perinatology*, vol. 36, no. 1, pp. 42–47, 2012.

[6] P. Stone, R. G. Hughes, and M. Dailey, "Creating a safe and high-quality health care environment," in *Patient Safety and Quality: An Evidence-Based Handbook for Nurses*, R. G. Hughes, Ed., vol. 2 of *AHRQ Publication No. 08-0043*, pp. 57–72, Agency for Healthcare Research and Quality, Rockville, Md, USA, 2008.

[7] R. Pattinson, L. Say, J. P. Souza, N. van den Broek, and C. Rooney, "WHO maternal death and near-miss classifications," *Bulletin of the World Health Organization*, vol. 87, no. 10, p. 734, 2009.

[8] L. Say, J. P. Souza, and R. C. Pattinson, "Maternal near miss—towards a standard tool for monitoring quality of maternal health care," *Best Practice and Research: Clinical Obstetrics and Gynaecology*, vol. 23, no. 3, pp. 287–296, 2009.

[9] M. H. Sousa, J. G. Cecatti, E. E. Hardy, and S. J. Serruya, "Severe maternal morbidity (near miss) as a sentinel event of maternal death. An attempt to use routine data for surveillance," *Reproductive Health*, vol. 5, no. 1, article 6, 2008.

[10] J. P. Souza, J. G. Cecatti, A. Faundes et al., "Maternal near miss and maternal death in the World Health Organization's 2005 global survey on maternal and perinatal health," *Bulletin of the World Health Organization*, vol. 88, no. 2, pp. 113–119, 2010.

[11] Ö. Tunçalp, M. J. Hindin, J. P. Souza, D. Chou, and L. Say, "The prevalence of maternal near miss: a systematic review," *BJOG*, vol. 119, no. 6, pp. 653–661, 2012.

[12] P. Tajik, S. Nedjat, N. E. Afshar et al., "Inequality in Maternal mortality in Iran: an ecologic study," *International Journal of Preventive Medicine*, vol. 3, no. 2, pp. 116–121, 2012.

[13] M. S. Moazzeni, "Maternal mortality in the Islamic Republic of Iran: on track and in transition," *Maternal and Child Health Journal*, vol. 17, no. 4, pp. 577–580, 2013.

[14] M. E. Motlaq, M. Eslami, M. Yazdanpanah, and N. Nakhaee, "Contraceptive use and unmet need for family planning in Iran," *International Journal of Gynecology and Obstetrics*, vol. 121, no. 2, pp. 157–161, 2013.

[15] R. Eftekhar-Vaghefi, S. Foroodnia, and N. Nakhaee, "Gaining insight into the prevention of maternal death using narrative analysis: an experience from Kerman, Iran," *International Journal of Health Policy and Management*, vol. 1, no. 4, pp. 255–259, 2013.

[16] M. Eslami, M. Yazdanpanah, R. Taheripanah, P. Andalib, A. Rahimi, and N. Nakhaee, "Importance of pre-pregnancy counseling in Iran: results from the high risk pregnancy survey 2012," *International Journal of Health Policy and Management*, vol. 1, no. 3, pp. 213–218, 2013.

[17] R. Mahaini and H. Mahmoud, "Reducing maternal mortality in the Eastern Mediterranean region," *Eastern Mediterranean Health Journal*, vol. 11, no. 4, pp. 539–544, 2005.

[18] WHO, *Evaluating the Quality of Care for Severe Pregnancy Complications. The WHO Near Miss Approach for Maternal Health*, World Health Organization, Geneva, Switzerland, 2011.

[19] J. P. Souza, J. G. Cecatti, M. A. Parpinelli, S. J. Serruya, and E. Amaral, "Appropriate criteria for identification of near-miss maternal morbidity in tertiary care facilities: a cross sectional study," *BMC Pregnancy and Childbirth*, vol. 7, article 20, 2007.

[20] P. Chhabra, K. Guleria, N. K. Saini, K. T. Anjur, and N. B. Vaid, "Pattern of severe maternal morbidity in a tertiary hospital of Delhi, India: a pilot study," *Tropical Doctor*, vol. 38, no. 4, pp. 201–204, 2008.

[21] V. Brace, G. Penney, and M. Hall, "Quantifying severe maternal morbidity: a Scottish population study," *BJOG*, vol. 111, no. 5, pp. 481–484, 2004.

[22] J. J. Zwart, J. M. Richters, F. Öry, J. I. P. de Vries, K. W. M. Bloemenkamp, and J. van Roosmalen, "Severe maternal morbidity during pregnancy, delivery and puerperium in the Netherlands: a nationwide population-based study of 371 000 pregnancies," *BJOG*, vol. 115, no. 7, pp. 842–850, 2008.

[23] A. Adisasmita, P. E. Deviany, F. Nandiaty, C. Stanton, and C. Ronsmans, "Obstetric near miss and deaths in public and private hospitals in Indonesia," *BMC Pregnancy and Childbirth*, vol. 8, article 10, 2008.

16

Theories on the Pathogenesis of Endometriosis

Samer Sourial,[1] Nicola Tempest,[1,2] and Dharani K. Hapangama[1,2]

[1] *Department of Women's and Children's Health, Institute of Translational Medicine, University of Liverpool, Liverpool L69 3BX, UK*
[2] *Centre for Women's Health Research, Liverpool Women's Hospital NHS Foundation Trust, Liverpool L8 7SS, UK*

Correspondence should be addressed to Dharani K. Hapangama; dharani.hapangama@liverpool.ac.uk

Academic Editor: Dimitris Loutradis

Endometriosis is a common, chronic inflammatory disease defined by the presence of extrauterine endometrial tissue. The aetiology of endometriosis is complex and multifactorial, where several not fully confirmed theories describe its pathogenesis. This review examines existing theories on the initiation and propagation of different types of endometriotic lesions, as well as critically appraises the myriad of biologically relevant evidence that support or oppose each of the proposed theories. The current literature suggests that stem cells, dysfunctional immune response, genetic predisposition, and aberrant peritoneal environment may all be involved in the establishment and propagation of endometriotic lesions. An orchestrated scientific and clinical effort is needed to consider all factors involved in the pathogenesis of this multifaceted disease and to propose novel therapeutic targets to reach effective treatments for this distressing condition.

1. Introduction

Endometriosis is a chronic, benign, oestrogen-dependent inflammatory disease affecting approximately 10% of reproductive age women and 35–50% of women with pelvic pain and infertility [1]. It can be a debilitating disease with symptoms of dysmenorrhoea, dyspareunia, and chronic pelvic pain [2].

The definition of endometriosis is histological and it requires the identification of the presence of endometrial gland and stroma-like tissue outside (ectopic) the uterus. These ectopic lesions are commonly located on the pelvic organs and peritoneum [3]. Occasionally, ectopic endometriotic lesions can be found in other parts of the body such as kidney, bladder, lungs, and even in the brain [4]. The clinical presentation of endometriosis is varied and conclusive diagnosis requires laparoscopy [5]. There has been efforts to standardize the surgical staging of endometriosis and histopathological changes with updated modified American Fertility Society scoring [6]. However this objective surgical staging does not necessarily correlate with the clinical symptoms [7]. Furthermore, there is a severe lack of knowledge on the natural progression of the disease in women since the severity measurement will require repeated invasive surgery. There

are reports of endometriosis associated with spontaneous regression, no progression [8], and progressing to ovarian carcinomas [9, 10]. At the present time no methods exist to predict future prognosis of the disease stage from initial surgical diagnosis. Endometriosis has estimated annual costs of US $12 419 per woman (approximately €9579), comprising one-third of the direct health care costs with two-thirds attributed to loss of productivity [11]. For obvious and above mentioned reasons, despite being the causal basis for over 30% of new referrals to gynaecology clinics (local data), the management of endometriosis remains difficult.

Currently, there is no curative treatment for endometriosis and clinical management of symptoms such as pain is through medical and/or surgical measures. Medical management follows the basic principle of reducing inflammation, suppressing ovarian cycles and inhibiting the effect of oestrogen. Surgical management attempts to either remove only the identified endometriotic lesions or complete excision of pelvic organs [1]. Controversies exist regarding the best method of treatment; for example, some authors have suggested that surgical excision promotes disease recurrence whilst others consider surgical excision as a way to reduce the risk of progression to severe disease or future ovarian cancer [10, 12]. Neither medical nor surgical options provide long term or universally acceptable relief for patients. Improving our current knowledge on the pathogenesis of endometriosis therefore helps the clinical and basic science researchers to identify novel more suitable targets for formulating more effective therapeutic and diagnostic means.

Many theories have been proposed to explain the pathogenesis of endometriosis and to date they all remain to be conclusively confirmed. In this review, the predisposing factors in developing endometriosis, as well as the interplay between the pathological mechanisms involved in the initiation and propagation of different endometriotic lesions, will be discussed.

2. Methods

2.1. Search Strategy and Selection Criteria. We initially searched "Pubmed" for relevant literature using the terms "endometriosis" and "pathogenesis" or "classification" for studies published from 2000 to 2013 and identified 872 manuscripts. Although those papers provided the basis for this review, for detailed understanding of the topic we extended our search to much older yet frequently referred articles. Studies that were deemed suitable by the authors included those that examined the pathophysiology of human endometriosis: from in vitro basic science (molecular, genetical and functional) studies, studies employing animal (rodent/primate) models, gene expression, and epidemiological studies.

3. Results

3.1. Classification of Endometriosis. Interrogation of pathogenesis of endometriosis highlights the current drawbacks associated with the classification of this disease. The revised American fertility society classifies endometriosis according to multiple criteria including histopathological as well as anatomical features, distinguishing superficial endometriosis from deep lesions of the peritoneum and ovaries [13]. Deep endometriosis is defined arbitrarily as adenomyosis externa, infiltrating the peritoneum by >5 mm [14]. It is noteworthy that the current classification system is limited by observer error as well as reproducibility and this may explain the poor correlation between extent of the disease and its clinical presentation [7]. Furthermore, histological information of endometriosis is limited by the technical efficiency in endometriotic biopsy sampling and processing, particularly when the lesions are located close to organs such as ureters, bowel and bladder [5]. A separate classification system (ENZIAN score) has been recently introduced for deep infiltrating endometriosis. It is a helpful aid in describing this type of endometriosis but it needs further refinement [15]. Clinical differences between superficial and deep endometriosis have been described, where severe pain is associated with >95% of deep endometriosis as compared with superficial endometriosis [16]. Progression of superficial endometriosis has been compared to that of a benign tumour, whereas the recurrence and progression of deep endometriosis has been reported to be rare [8, 17]. Superficial and

deep endometriosis has been categorised by some authors as two different diseases with different pathogeneses whereas others regard them as different manifestations of the same disease [7]. Naturally this lack of consensus with disease classification creates another ambiguity around much of the available literature on pathogenesis.

3.2. Retrograde Menstruation. Retrograde menstruation theory is the oldest principle explaining the aetiology of endometriosis. This theory proposes that endometriosis occurs due to the retrograde flow of sloughed endometrial cells/debris via the fallopian tubes into the pelvic cavity during menstruation [18]. However, retrograde menstruation occurs in 76%–90% of women with patent fallopian tubes and not all of these women have endometriosis [19]. The larger volume of retrograde menstrual fluid found in the pelvises of patients with endometriosis as compared with healthy women may increase the risk of endometriotic lesions implantation [20]. In non-human primate models, it is possible to induce endometriosis by inoculating autologous menstrual products simulating retrograde menstruation in the peritoneal cavity of baboons and macaques [12]. With a single inoculation of menstrual endometrial tissue directly in to the pelvic cavity, up to 46% of the animals have shown development of endometriotic lesions in the pelvic cavity [21], whereas 100% of animals developed peritoneal endometriotic lesions after two consecutive cycles of inoculations of curetted menstrual endometrium. These lesions were histologically and clinically similar to human ectopic endometriotic lesions [22]. Furthermore, in a recent study deep nodular endometriosis was generated by ectopic implantation of full thickness endometrium including the basalis layer, highlighting the involvement of the endometrial basalis layer in development of ectopic lesions [23]. However, only the well-differentiated cells from the superficial functionalis layer are shed normally with the menstrual flow, the deep endometrial basalis layer remains intact throughout the woman's life. The regeneration of endometrial functionalis after menstrual shedding is thought to originate from this basalis [24]. Therefore by placing this basalis tissue with the ability to generate endometrial functional layer in the pelvis, the non-human primate models may not completely mimic the events of spontaneous retrograde menstruation. Further evidence to support Sampson's theory come from the observation that factors obstructing menstruation, such as congenital abnormalities including imperforate hymen and iatrogenic cervical stenosis, increase retrograde menstruation and the risk of developing of endometriosis [3]. Increased retrograde menstruation through experimentally induced cervical stenosis also caused endometriosis in non-human primate models [21]. The location of superficial endometriotic lesions in the posterior aspect and left side of the pelvis may be due to the effects of gravity on regurgitated menstrual product and the anatomical position of the sigmoid colon [25]. However, this theory has been disputed in the past since it cannot explain the occurrence of endometriosis in pre-pubertal girls, newborns, or males. Neonatal uterine bleeding, occurs in the immediate postnatal period in most girls following the withdrawal of (maternal) ovarian hormones, similar to menstrual bleeding and retrograde flow of this uterine bleeding has been proposed as the reason for prepubertal endometriosis [26].

3.3. Metaplasia. Other theories have proposed that endometriosis originates from extrauterine cells that abnormally transdifferentiate or transform into endometrial cells. The Coelomic metaplasia theory postulates that endo-metriosis originates from the metaplasia of specialised cells that are present in the mesothelial lining of the visceral and abdominal peritoneum [27]. Hormonal or immunological factors are thought to stimulate the transformation of normal peritoneal tissue/cells into endometrium-like tissue [3]. The coelomic metaplasia theory may explain the occurrence of endometriosis in prepubertal girls [28]. However, the usual driving force for endometrial growth, oestrogen, is not present in the pre-pubertal girls and therefore this condition may be different from endometriosis that is found in women of reproductive age. Ectopic endometrial tissue has also been detected in female foetuses and it has been suggested that endometriosis may be the result of defective embryogenesis. According to this theory, residual embryonic cells of the Wolffian or Mullerian ducts persist and develop into endometriotic lesions that respond to oestrogen [3]. Furthermore, recent theories that are put forward suggest coelomic metaplasia to be the origin of adolescent variant of severe and progressive form of endometriosis [29]. However, this theory is imperfect due to endometriotic lesions being found in areas outside of the course of Mullerian duct. Others have also proposed that endogenous biochemical or immunological factors induce resident undifferentiated cells to differentiate into endometrial-like tissue in ectopic sites resulting in endometriosis [30]. This suggestion is supported by the studies describing hormone-dependent transformation of peritoneal cells into Mullerian-type cells [31].

3.4. Hormones. Steroid hormones should play a central role in the aetiology of endometriosis since it is a disease of women in reproductive age and not usually seen in postmenopausal women who are not on hormonal treatment [32]. Similar to the eutopic endometrium, the growth of ectopic lesions are thought to be regulated by ovarian steroid hormones. Oestrogen is the driving force of endometrial proliferation and ectopic lesions may have an increased responsiveness to oestrogen, thus enhancing the development of endometriosis [31]. Environmental toxins, such as dioxin, are implicated in the aetiology of endometriosis, which may mimic oestrogen via interacting with oestrogen receptors [32]. Furthermore, there may be a higher bioavailability of oestradiol in endometriotic tissue due to the local aromatisation of circulating androgens to oestradiol by endometriotic stromal cells and also there may be reduced conversion of oestradiol to the less potent oestrone due to the ectopic endometriotic tissue expressing decreased 17β-hydroxysteroid enzymes [3]. These factors may explain the proliferative promoting phenotype described in the ectopic endometriotic tissue [31]. Progesterone generally counteracts the proliferation promoting action of oestrogen in the eutopic healthy endometrium. Many authors believe that endometriosis is associated with resistance of the endometrium to progesterone which plays a pivotal role in the pathogenesis [33, 34]. The harnessing of the oestrogen-driven mitotic/proliferative action on the endometrium by progesterone during the secretory phase of the cycle does not occur in the endometriotic lesions and sustained proliferative activity is seen in the eutopic endometrium of women with endometriosis in the secretory phase [35, 36]. The progesterone resistance may be due to the endometriotic lesion having a lower expression of progesterone receptors or as a result of a functional abnormality of the existing progesterone receptors [37].

3.5. Oxidative Stress and Inflammation. Increased oxidation of lipoproteins has been associated with the pathogenesis of endometriosis, where reactive oxygen species (ROS) cause lipid peroxidation that leads to DNA damage in endometrial cells [38]. The presence of water and electrolytes in the increased peritoneal fluid volume in patients with endometriosis harbours the source of ROS [39]. These patients also have iron overload in their peritoneal cavities from the breakdown of haemoglobin, which in turn causes redox reactions [40]. The release of the proinflammatory heam products and the oxidative stress signals generated from the ROS cause inflammation which leads to the recruitment of lymphocytes and activated macrophages producing cytokines that induce oxidizing of enzymes and promotes endothelial growth [30]. The excess production of ROS is also accompanied by a decreased level of antioxidants that usually eliminates these molecules [38, 41]. Resulting accumulation of ROS may contribute to the propagation and maintenance of endometriosis and associated symptoms.

3.6. Immune Dysfunction. The observation that autoimmune diseases to be more common in women with endometriosis support the possibility that pathogenesis of endometriosis may involve a defective immune response in these patients [42]. Women with endometriosis have a higher concentration of activated macrophages, decreased cellular immunity, and a repressed NK cell function [43, 44]. The regurgitation of endometrial cells into the peritoneum triggers an inflammatory response, recruiting activated macrophages and leukocytes locally [45]. This inflammatory response may cause a defective "immune-surveillance" that prevents elimination of the menstrual debris and promotes the implantation and growth of endometrial cells in the ectopic sites [46]. Furthermore, there are suggestions that during the evolutionary process the peritoneal immune clearance that occurs in non-human primates has been lost in humans, and this may contribute to the persistence of the menstrual debris in the pelvic cavity and subsequent development of endometriosis in women [23]. The survival and resistance to immune-cell-mediated lyses of endometriotic cells are ensured by masking these ectopic cells to the immune system, where, for example, ectopic endometrial cells modulate the expression of HLA class I molecules [43, 47]. Both immune and endometrial cells secrete cytokines and growth factors, which induce cell proliferation and angiogenesis; thereby promoting implantation and growth of ectopic lesions [48]. Possibly as a consequence, women with endometriosis have higher expression of cytokines and vascular endothelial growth factors in their peritoneal fluid, which promote proliferation of endometrial cells and angiogenesis [49, 50].

3.7. Apoptosis Suppression and Alteration of Endometrial Cell Fate. Alteration of the endometrial cell fate to favour antiapoptotic and proproliferative phenotype is paramount for the survival of the endometrial cells in the peritoneal cavity to initiate ectopic deposits and for the maintenance of the established lesions [51]. By examining matched eutopic endometrium and ectopic lesions from women with endometriosis and in baboon with induced disease, we have recently shown that telomerase enzyme may play a central role in this altered endometrial cell phenotype [36, 51].

There is plethora of evidence suggesting an upregulation of antiapoptotic and prosurvival genes and reciprocal downregulation of the genes regulating the apoptosis pathway in ectopic endometrial cells [52]. In addition to the decreased scavenger activity, the endometrium in patients with endometriosis expresses higher levels of antiapoptotic factors [53]. The inhibition of the apoptosis of endometrial cells may also be mediated by the transcriptional activation of genes that normally promotes inflammation, angiogenesis, and cell proliferation [54].

3.8. Genetics. A genetic basis for the development of endometriosis is suggested by the reports of familial aggregation, the high risk of endometriosis in those with an affected first-degree relative [55], and the observations of concordance of endometriosis in twins [56]. A great number of studies have related genetic polymorphisms as a factor that contributes to the development of endometriosis. Endometriosis has a polygenic mode of inheritance that is likely to involve multiple loci and some chromosomal regions were reported to be associated with the corresponding endometriosis phenotype [57]. Inherited as well as acquired genetic factors may predispose women to the attachment of ectopic endometrial cells to the peritoneal epithelium and the evasion of these lesions from immune clearance [3]. Differences in genes and protein expression between patients with and without endometriosis have been reported [58]. Genes that have been implicated in the pathogenesis of endometriosis include those encoding detoxification enzymes, polymorphism in oestrogen receptor, and genes involved in the innate immune system [31]. Genetic predisposition can increase the frequency of cellular damage. Genetic mutations that cause cell damage are implemented in the progression of endometriosis, since women with endometriosis show altered endometrial cell behaviour, favouring extrauterine adhesion and growth [16]. Over the past decade several authors have employed gene arrays to identify endometriosis related genes. Using laser capture microdissection and high throughput and high resolution comparative genomic hybridization (CGH) arrays, considerable genomic alterations in both eutopic and ectopic

endometria of women with endometriosis have been identified [59, 60]. Recent genomewide association studies have also identified new loci to endometriosis [57]. Collectively this data suggests that different types of endometriosis may be associated with altering different gene clusters that regulate specific cellular functional aberrations.

3.9. Stem Cells. The monthly regeneration of the endometrium after menstrual shedding, reepithelialisation of the endometrium after parturition or surgical curettage, supports the existence of a stem cell pool [61]. Since the basalis layer of the endometrium is not shed with the monthly menstrual shedding of the functional layer, the stem cells are thought to reside in the basalis layer of the endometrium [62]. Recently, clonogenic cells, which are thought to represent the stem cell population in the human endometrium have been identified and proposed to be involved in the formation of ectopic endometrial lesions [63].

Stem cells are undifferentiated cells, characterized by their ability to self-renew and differentiate into one or several types of specialized cells [64]. Differentiation is defined as a change in cell phenotype secondary to alteration in the cell's gene expression, enabling the cell to have a specific function [28]. Endometrial self-generation may occur through stem cells in specific niches of the endometrium [65]. The undifferentiated endometrial stem cells may be less responsive to ovarian steroids than the terminally differentiated progeny due to lack of expression of hormone receptor [66]. In addition to the resident endometrial stem cells, incorporation of circulating bone marrow-derived stem cells may contribute to the cyclic regeneration of the endometrium [67].

The involvement of stem cells in the formation of endometriotic deposits could be as a result of abnormal translocation of normal endometrial basalis via retrograde menstruation [68]. Brosens et al. postulated that the uterine bleeding in neonatal girls contains a high amount of endometrial progenitor cells [29]. Some of these cells may deposit and survive in the peritoneal cavity after retrograde flow and may reactivate in the adolescents in response to ovarian hormones [29]. However, there is no current data on the amount of endometrial stem/progenitor cells in neonatal period when compared to the adult endometrium. Furthermore, since even the aging postmenopausal endometrium seem to have adequate amount of progenitor cells to generate a competent normal functionalis with the essential hormonal stimulation, it seems unlikely that there are significant differences in the progenitor activity between the premenopausal and postmenopausal endometrium. Leyendecker et al. [69] proposed that women with endometriosis abnormally shed the endometrial basalis tissue, which initiate endometriotic deposits after retrograde menstruation. The observation in the baboon model of endometriosis induction, where placement of the stem cell rich endometrial basalis in the pelvic cavity resulting in 100% induction of endometriosis in all animals, may further support Leyendeckers theory. If the basalis contains the stem/progenitor cells, they are likely to survive and initiate endometriotic deposits in the pelvis than the differentiated endometrial cells from the functionalis.

Due to their natural ability to regenerate, these stem cells may give rise to new endometriotic deposits. The fact that women with endometriosis possibly shed significantly more of the stem-cell rich basalis layer as compared to healthy women [69], together with the similarity observed between ectopic lesions and the basalis layer [24], may support the possibility of retrograde menstruation providing an access for the endometrial stem cells to extrauterine structures [63, 69]. Alternatively, these stem cells may be transported via the lymphatic or vascular pathways to ectopic sites [70]. The fact that some of the endometrial stem cells have bone marrow origin further supports the haematogenous dissemination theory of these cells [71]. Recent studies have further suggested that mobile stem cells may be involved in endometriosis progression, where cells derived from ectopic lesions in induced endometriosis migrated to the eutopic endometrium [71]. However, since stem cells are normally expected to differentiate into mature cells in concordance with the environmental niche, the supposedly multipotential endometrial stem cells in the peritoneal cavity should differentiate in to peritoneal-type cells. It is possible that the deposition of endometrial tissue fragments containing both endometrial stem cells and their niche cells in the peritoneal cavity promote regeneration of endometrium-like tissue, due to the signal received by the stem cells from the surrounding endometrial niche cells. On the other hand, the relocation of an aberrant or committed stem cell from the endometrium to an ectopic site may also generate endometrium-like lesions. Endometrial tissue produces several chemokines and angiogenic cytokines; therefore, neovascularisation in the ectopic sites can presumably follow, thus ensuring the establishment of these lesions [72].

A further possibility of stem cell involvement in endometriosis is the transdifferentiation of the peritoneal, haematopoietic, or ovarian stem cells into endometrium like tissue. Peritoneal cavity connects directly with the uterine cavity and there is a free flow of the cytokine/chemokine rich fluid between the two environments. This direct connection may regulate the endometrium-like differentiation of resident stem cell population in the peritoneal cavity. Although possible, the reasons for such specific differentiation of the peritoneal stem cells in to endometrium-like tissue in only up to 10% of the female population remain unexplained.

4. Discussion

The different theories implicated in the pathogenesis of endometriosis indicate that the aetiology of endometriosis is complex and multifactorial, involving hormonal, genetic, immune, and environmental components. Table 1 summarizes the role of each theory in the pathogenesis of endometriosis. While retrograde menstruation may be one of the initiating steps in the pathogenesis of superficial endometriosis, genetic and microenvironmental factors that prevent clearance of ectopic lesions and allows remodelling of peritoneum are essential for the propagation of endometriotic lesions [73, 74]. Pathogenesis of endometriosis is propagated by an altered peritoneal fluid composition as a result

Table 1: Role of the different theories in the pathogenesis of endometriosis.

Theory	Mechanism
Retrograde menstruation	Flow of endometrial content into pelvis, allowing implantation of endometrial lesions
Metaplasia	Transformation of peritoneal tissue/cells into endometrial tissue through hormonal and/or immunological factors
Hormones	Oestrogen-driven proliferation of endometrial lesions. Resistance to progesterone-mediated control of endometrial proliferation
Oxidative stress and inflammation	Recruitment of immune cells and their production of cytokines that promote endometrial growth
Immune dysfunction	Prevention of eliminating menstrual debris and promotion of implantation and growth of endometrial lesions
Apoptosis suppression	Promoting survival of endometrial cells and downregulation of apoptotic pathways
Genetic	Alteration of cellular function that increases attachment of endometrial cells and evasion of these cells from immune clearance
Stem cells	Initiation of endometriotic deposits by undifferentiated cells with natural ability to regenerate

of genetic, hormonal, and environmental factors [75, 76]. Figure 1 depicts the interplay between the different factors that may be involved in the pathogenesis of endometriosis.

Differences are present in the pathogenesis of deep versus superficial endometriosis. Retrograde menstruation may not explain the pathogenesis of deep endometriosis, where no deep endometrial lesions could be induced in animal models through peritoneal instillation after endocervical removal of menstrual endometrium [22]. However, deep nodular lesions, which is not usually shed at menstruation, could be readily induced with the transplantation of endometrial basalis tissue in a baboon model [23]. Other theories such as the coelomic metaplasia, induction of cellular transformation into endometrial cells, and the embryonic remnant theory may better explain the aetiology behind deep endometriosis.

5. Conclusion

Ectopically placed stem cells that are of endometrial or haematopoietic origin or abnormal endometrial differentiation of a resident tissue stem cell may be the first step in the establishment of an ectopic endometrial lesion. The subsequent proliferation and propagation of such lesions may also be dependent on mobile, endometrial progenitor-type cells in these ectopic lesions that are involved in initiating further lesion and also in maintaining the disease. A dysfunctional immune clearance and a genetic predisposition that allow these ectopic lesions to grow in an aberrant microenvironment may also contribute to the development of the disease. The current therapeutic regimens for endometriosis are usually based on manipulating the ovarian steroid hormones that

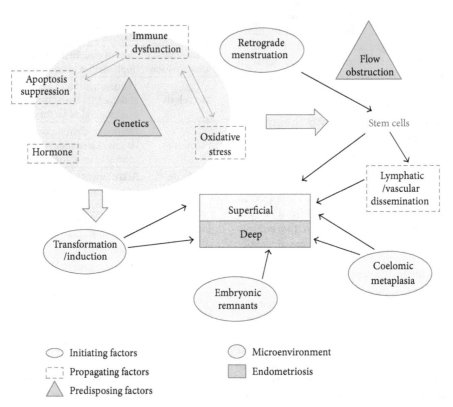

FIGURE 1: Summary of the proposed interplay between the different factors reported in the pathogenesis of superficial versus deep endometriosis. The different initiating, propagating, and predisposing factors are indicated through different shapes, respectively. The arrows indicate the interplay between the different factors. As indicated by the bold pink arrows, some of the labelled propagating factors create a microenvironment that impacts the differentiation of stem cells and/or the transdifferentiation of peritoneal cells into endometrial cells.

may preferentially target terminally-differentiated ectopic endometriotic cells which would normally die off via apoptosis, while the stem cells that propagate the disease may not be affected. Improving our understanding of the pathogenesis of endometriosis will direct further future work on more appropriate therapeutic targets that can provide the much needed curative and universally acceptable treatments for endometriosis.

Conflict of Interests

The authors declare that there is no conflict of interests regarding the publication of this paper.

Acknowledgments

The support from the Centre for Women's Health Research at Liverpool Women's Hospital, Department of Women's Health at University of Liverpool; Wellbeing of Women project Grant RG1073 to Dharani K. Hapangama and Wellbeing of Women's Entry Level Clinical Research Training Fellowship to Nicola Tempest (supervisor Dharani K. Hapangama) are gratefully acknowledged.

References

[1] L. C. Giudice, "Endometriosis," *The New England Journal of Medicine*, vol. 362, no. 25, pp. 2389–2398, 2010.

[2] M. M. Carneiro, I. D. D. S. Filogônio, L. M. P. Costa, I. De Ávila, and M. C. Ferreira, "Accuracy of clinical signs and symptoms in the diagnosis of endometriosis," *Journal of Endometriosis*, vol. 2, no. 2, pp. 63–70, 2010.

[3] R. O. Burney and L. Giudice, "Pathogenesis and pathophysiology of endometriosis," *Fertility and Sterility*, vol. 98, pp. 511–519, 2012.

[4] E. A. Pritts and R. N. Taylor, "An evidence-based evaluation of endometriosis-associated infertility," *Endocrinology and Metabolism Clinics of North America*, vol. 32, no. 3, pp. 653–667, 2003.

[5] K. L. Sharpe-Timms, "Defining endometrial cells: the need for improved identification at ectopic sites and characterization in eutopic sites for developing novel methods of management for endometriosis," *Fertility and Sterility*, vol. 84, no. 1, pp. 35–37, 2005.

[6] M. Canis, J. G. Donnez, D. S. Guzick et al., "Revised American Society for reproductive medicine classification of endometriosis: 1996," *Fertility and Sterility*, vol. 67, no. 5, pp. 817–821, 1997.

[7] G. D. Adamson, "Endometriosis classification: an update," *Current Opinion in Obstetrics and Gynecology*, vol. 23, no. 4, pp. 213–220, 2011.

[8] L. Fedele, S. Bianchi, G. Zanconato, R. Raffaelli, and N. Berlanda, "Is rectovaginal endometriosis a progressive disease?" *American Journal of Obstetrics and Gynecology*, vol. 191, no. 5, pp. 1539–1542, 2004.

[9] J. Nassif, S. Mattar, A. Abu Musa, and A. Eid, "Endometriosis and cancer: what do we know?" *Minerva Ginecologica*, vol. 65, pp. 167–179, 2013.

[10] A. Melin, C. Lundholm, N. Malki, M.-L. Swahn, P. Sparen, and A. Bergqvist, "Endometriosis as a prognostic factor for cancer survival," *International Journal of Cancer*, vol. 129, no. 4, pp. 948–955, 2011.

[11] P. A. Rogers, T. M. D'Hooghe, A. Fazleabas et al., "Defining future directions for endometriosis research: workshop report from the 2011 world congress of endometriosis in Montpellier, France," *Reproductive Science*, vol. 20, pp. 483–499, 2013.

[12] P. Harirchian, I. Gashaw, S. T. Lipskind et al., "Lesion kinetics in a non-human primate model of endometriosis," *Human Reproduction*, vol. 27, pp. 2341–2351, 2012.

[13] L. Aghajanova and L. C. Giudice, "Molecular evidence for differences in endometrium in severe versus mild endometriosis," *Reproductive Sciences*, vol. 18, no. 3, pp. 229–251, 2011.

[14] F. J. Cornillie, D. Oosterlynck, J. M. Lauweryns, and P. R. Koninckx, "Deeply infiltrating pelvic endometriosis: histology and clinical significance," *Fertility and Sterility*, vol. 53, no. 6, pp. 978–983, 1990.

[15] F. Tuttlies, J. Keckstein, U. Ulrich et al., "ENZIAN-Score, a classification of deep infiltrating endometriosis," *Zentralblatt für Gynäkologie*, vol. 127, no. 5, pp. 275–281, 2005.

[16] P. R. Koninckx, D. Barlow, and S. Kennedy, "Implantation versus infiltration: the sampson versus the endometriotic disease theory," *Gynecologic and Obstetric Investigation*, vol. 47, no. 1, pp. 3–10, 1999.

[17] P. R. Koninckx, A. Ussia, L. Adamyan, A. Wattiez, and J. Donnez, "Deep endometriosis: definition, diagnosis, and treatment," *Fertility and Sterility*, vol. 98, pp. 564–571, 2012.

[18] J. A. Sampson, "Heterotopic or misplaced endometrial tissue," *American Journal of Obstetrics and Gynecology*, vol. 10, no. 5, pp. 649–664, 1925.

[19] I. E. Sasson and H. S. Taylor, "Stem cells and the pathogenesis of endometriosis," *Annals of the New York Academy of Sciences*, vol. 1127, pp. 106–115, 2008.

[20] P. R. Koninckx, S. H. Kennedy, and D. H. Barlow, "Endometriotic disease: the role of peritoneal fluid," *Human Reproduction Update*, vol. 4, no. 5, pp. 741–751, 1998.

[21] T. M. D'Hooghe, C. S. Bambra, M. A. Suleman, G. A. Dunselman, H. L. Evers, and P. R. Koninckx, "Development of a model of retrograde menstruation in baboons (Papio anubis)," *Fertility and Sterility*, vol. 62, no. 3, pp. 635–638, 1994.

[22] J.-P. Dehoux, S. Defrre, J. Squifflet et al., "Is the baboon model appropriate for endometriosis studies?" *Fertility and Sterility*, vol. 96, no. 3, pp. 728–e3, 2011.

[23] O. Donnez, A. Van Langendonckt, S. Defrere et al., "Induction of endometriotic nodules in an experimental baboon model mimicking human deep nodular lesions," *Fertility and Sterility*, vol. 99, pp. 783–789, 2013.

[24] A. Valentijn, H. Al-Lamee, K. Palial et al., "SSEA-1 Isolates human endometrial basal glandular epithelial cells: phenotypic and functional characterisation and implications in pathogenesis of endometriosis," *Human Reproduction*, vol. 28, pp. 2695–2708, 2013.

[25] W. P. Dmowski and E. Radwanska, "Current concepts on pathology, histogenesis and etiology of endometriosis," *Acta Obstetricia et Gynecologica Scandinavica*, vol. 63, no. 123, pp. 29–33, 1984.

[26] I. Brosens and G. Benagiano, "Is neonatal uterine bleeding involved in the pathogenesis of endometriosis as a source of stem cells?" *Fertility and Sterility*, vol. 100, pp. 622–623, 2013.

[27] P. Gruenwald, "Origin of endometriosis from the mesenchyme of the celomic walls," *American Journal of Obstetrics and Gynecology*, vol. 44, no. 3, pp. 470–474, 1942.

[28] P. G. M. Figueira, M. S. Abrão, G. Krikun, and H. Taylor, "Stem cells in endometrium and their role in the pathogenesis of endometriosis," *Annals of the New York Academy of Sciences*, vol. 1221, no. 1, pp. 10–17, 2011.

[29] I. Brosens, S. Gordts, and G. Benagiano, "Endometriosis in adolescents is a hidden, progressive and severe disease that deserves attention, not just compassion," *Human Reproduction*, vol. 28, pp. 2026–2031, 2013.

[30] S. Gupta, A. Agarwal, N. Krajcir, and J. G. Alvarez, "Role of oxidative stress in endometriosis," *Reproductive BioMedicine Online*, vol. 13, no. 1, article 2291, pp. 126–134, 2006.

[31] A. Augoulea, A. Alexandrou, M. Creatsa, N. Vrachnis, and I. Lambrinoudaki, "Pathogenesis of endometriosis: the role of genetics, inflammation and oxidative stress," *Archives of Gynecology and Obstetrics*, pp. 1–5, 2012.

[32] C. Parente Barbosa, A. M. Bentes De Souza, B. Bianco, and D. M. Christofolini, "The effect of hormones on endometriosis development," *Minerva Ginecologica*, vol. 63, no. 4, pp. 375–386, 2011.

[33] J. J. Kim, T. Kurita, and S. E. Bulun, "Progesterone action in endometrial cancer, endometriosis, uterine fibroids, and breast cancer," *Endocrine Reviews*, vol. 34, pp. 130–162, 2013.

[34] L. Aghajanova, K. Tatsumi, J. A. Horcajadas et al., "Unique transcriptome, pathways, and networks in the human endometrial fibroblast response to progesterone in endometriosis," *Biology of Reproduction*, vol. 84, no. 4, pp. 801–815, 2011.

[35] S. E. Bulun, Y.-H. Cheng, P. Yin et al., "Progesterone resistance in endometriosis: link to failure to metabolize estradiol," *Molecular and Cellular Endocrinology*, vol. 248, no. 1-2, pp. 94–103, 2006.

[36] D. K. Hapangama, M. A. Turner, J. A. Drury et al., "Sustained replication in endometrium of women with endometriosis occurs without evoking a DNA damage response," *Human Reproduction*, vol. 24, no. 3, pp. 687–696, 2009.

[37] G. R. Attia, K. Zeitoun, D. Edwards, A. Johns, B. R. Carr, and S. E. Bulun, "Progesterone receptor isoform A but not B is expressed in endometriosis," *Journal of Clinical Endocrinology and Metabolism*, vol. 85, no. 8, pp. 2897–2902, 2000.

[38] A. A. Murphy, W. Palinski, S. Rankin, A. J. Morales, and S. Parthasarathy, "Evidence for oxidatively modified lipid-protein complexes in endometrium and endometriosis," *Fertility and Sterility*, vol. 69, no. 6, pp. 1092–1094, 1998.

[39] Y. Wang, J. Goldberg, R. K. Sharma, A. Agarwal, and T. Falcone, "Importance of reactive oxygen species in the peritoneal fluid of women with endometriosis or idiopathic infertility," *Fertility and Sterility*, vol. 68, no. 5, pp. 826–830, 1997.

[40] S. Kumar and U. Bandyopadhyay, "Free heme toxicity and its detoxification systems in human," *Toxicology Letters*, vol. 157, no. 3, pp. 175–188, 2005.

[41] A. A. Murphy, N. Santanam, A. J. Morales, and S. Parthasarathy, "Lysophosphatidyl choline, a chemotactic factor for

monocytes/T-lymphocytes is elevated in endometriosis," *Journal of Clinical Endocrinology and Metabolism*, vol. 83, no. 6, pp. 2110–2113, 1998.

[42] N. Sinaii, S. D. Cleary, M. L. Ballweg, L. K. Nieman, and P. Stratton, "High rates of autoimmune and endocrine disorders, fibromyalgia, chronic fatigue syndrome and atopic diseases among women with endometriosis: a survey analysis," *Human Reproduction*, vol. 17, no. 10, pp. 2715–2724, 2002.

[43] J. Sikora, A. Mielczarek-Palacz, and Z. Kondera-Anasz, "Role of Natural Killer cell activity in the pathogenesis of endometriosis," *Current Medicinal Chemistry*, vol. 18, no. 2, pp. 200–208, 2011.

[44] Y. Osuga, K. Koga, Y. Hirota, T. Hirata, O. Yoshino, and Y. Taketani, "Lymphocytes in Endometriosis," *American Journal of Reproductive Immunology*, vol. 65, no. 1, pp. 1–10, 2011.

[45] C. M. Kyama, A. Mihalyi, P. Simsa et al., "Role of cytokines in the endometrial-peritoneal cross-talk and development of endometriosis," *Frontiers in Bioscience*, vol. 1, pp. 444–454, 2009.

[46] G. Christodoulakos, A. Augoulea, I. Lambrinoudaki, V. Sioulas, and G. Creatsas, "Pathogenesis of endometriosis: the role of defective 'immunosurveillance'," *European Journal of Contraception and Reproductive Health Care*, vol. 12, no. 3, pp. 194–202, 2007.

[47] C. Semino, A. Semino, G. Pietra et al., "Role of major histocompatibility complex class I expression and natural killer-like T cells in the genetic control of endometriosis," *Fertility and Sterility*, vol. 64, no. 5, pp. 909–916, 1995.

[48] M. Ulukus and A. Arici, "Immunology of endometriosis," *Minerva Ginecologica*, vol. 57, no. 3, pp. 237–248, 2005.

[49] M. W. Laschke, C. Giebels, and M. D. Menger, "Vasculogenesis: a new piece of the endometriosis puzzle," *Human Reproduction Update*, vol. 17, no. 5, pp. 628–636, 2011.

[50] J. McLaren, A. Prentice, D. S. Charnock-Jones, and S. K. Smith, "Vascular endothelial growth factor (VEGF) concentrations are elevated in peritoneal fluid of women with endometriosis," *Human Reproduction*, vol. 11, no. 1, pp. 220–223, 1996.

[51] D. K. Hapangama, M. A. Turner, J. Drury et al., "Aberrant expression of regulators of cell-fate found in eutopic endometrium is found in matched ectopic endometrium among women and in a baboon model of endometriosis," *Human Reproduction*, vol. 25, no. 11, pp. 2840–2850, 2010.

[52] S. R. Ferryman and T. P. Rollason, "Pathology of the uterine body," *Current Opinion in Obstetrics and Gynecology*, vol. 6, no. 4, pp. 344–350, 1994.

[53] F. Taniguchi, A. Kaponis, M. Izawa et al., "Apoptosis and endometriosis," *Frontiers in Bioscience*, vol. 3, pp. 648–662, 2011.

[54] R. González-Ramos, A. Van Langendonckt, S. Defrere et al., "Involvement of the nuclear factor-κB pathway in the pathogenesis of endometriosis," *Fertility and Sterility*, vol. 94, no. 6, pp. 1985–1994, 2010.

[55] E. Seli, M. Berkkanoglu, and A. Arici, "Pathogenesis of endometriosis," *Obstetrics and Gynecology Clinics of North America*, vol. 30, no. 1, pp. 41–61, 2003.

[56] R. M. Hadfield, H. J. Mardon, D. H. Barlow, and S. H. Kennedy, "Endometriosis in monozygotic twins," *Fertility and Sterility*, vol. 68, no. 5, pp. 941–942, 1997.

[57] H. M. Albertsen, R. Chettier, P. Farrington, and K. Ward, "Genome-wide association study link novel loci to endometriosis," *PLOS ONE*, vol. 8, Article ID e58257, 2013.

[58] K. E. May, J. Villar, S. Kirtley, S. H. Kennedy, and C. M. Becker, "Endometrial alterations in endometriosis: a systematic review

of putative biomarkers," *Human Reproduction Update*, vol. 17, no. 5, pp. 637–653, 2011.

[59] Y. Afshar, J. Hastings, D. Roqueiro, J. W. Jeong, L. C. Giudice, and A. T. Fazlebas, "Changes in eutopic endometrial gene expression during the progression of experimental endometriosis in the baboon, papio Anubis," *Biology of Reproduction*, vol. 88, p. 44, 2013.

[60] M. A. Khan, J. Sengupta, S. Mittal, and D. Ghosh, "Genome-wide expressions in autologous eutopic and ectopic endometrium of fertile women with endoemtriosis," *Reproductive Biology and Endocrinology*, vol. 10, p. 84, 2012.

[61] S. Tsuji, M. Yoshimoto, K. Takahashi, Y. Noda, T. Nakahata, and T. Heike, "Side population cells contribute to the genesis of human endometrium," *Fertility and Sterility*, vol. 90, no. 4, pp. 1528–1537, 2008.

[62] H. A. Padykula, "Regeneration in the primate uterus: the role of stem cells," *Annals of the New York Academy of Sciences*, vol. 622, pp. 47–56, 1991.

[63] J. A. Deane, R. C. Gualano, and C. E. Gargett, "Regenerating endometrium from stem/progenitor cells; is it abnormal in endometriosis, Asherman's syndrome and infertility?" *Current Opinion in Obstetrics and Gynecology*, vol. 25, pp. 193–200, 2013.

[64] K. Kato, "Stem cells in human normal endometrium and endometrial cancer cells: characterization of side population cells," *Kaohsiung Journal of Medical Sciences*, vol. 28, no. 2, pp. 63–71, 2012.

[65] F. R. Oliveira, C. D. Cruz, H. L. del Puerto, Q. T. M. F. Vilamil, F. M. Reis, and A. F. Camargos, "Stem cells: are they the answer to the puzzling etiology of endometriosis?" *Histology and Histopathology*, vol. 27, no. 1, pp. 23–29, 2012.

[66] C. E. Gargett, R. W. S. Chan, and K. E. Schwab, "Hormone and growth factor signaling in endometrial renewal: role of stem/progenitor cells," *Molecular and Cellular Endocrinology*, vol. 288, no. 1-2, pp. 22–29, 2008.

[67] H. S. Taylor, "Endometrial cells derived from donor stem cells in bone marrow transplant recipients," *Journal of the American Medical Association*, vol. 292, no. 1, pp. 81–85, 2004.

[68] H. Masuda, Y. Matsuzaki, E. Hiratsu et al., "Stem cell-like properties of the endometrial side population: implication in endometrial regeneration," *PLoS ONE*, vol. 5, no. 4, Article ID e10387, 2010.

[69] G. Leyendecker, G. Kunz, M. Herbertz et al., "Uterine peristaltic activity and the development of endometriosis," *Annals of the New York Academy of Sciences*, vol. 1034, pp. 338–355, 2004.

[70] T. Maruyama, H. Masuda, M. Ono, T. Kajitani, and Y. Yoshimura, "Stem cell theory for the pathogenesis of endometriosis," *Frontier in Bioscience*, vol. 4, pp. 2854–2863, 2012.

[71] T. Maruyama, H. Masuda, M. Ono, T. Kajitani, and Y. Yoshimura, "Human uterine stem/progenitor cells: their possible role in uterine physiology and pathology," *Reproduction*, vol. 140, no. 1, pp. 11–22, 2010.

[72] X. Santamaria, E. E. Massasa, and H. S. Taylor, "Migration of cells from experimental endometriosis to the uterine endometrium," *Endocrinology*, vol. 153, pp. 5566–5574, 2012.

[73] H. Du and H. S. Taylor, "Reviews: stem cells and female reproduction," *Reproductive Sciences*, vol. 16, no. 2, pp. 126–139, 2009.

[74] K. Nasu, A. Yuge, A. Tsuno, M. Nishida, and H. Narahara, "Involvement of resistance to apoptosis in the pathogenesis of endometriosis," *Histology and Histopathology*, vol. 24, no. 9, pp. 1181–1192, 2009.

[75] J. Gilabert-Estelles, L. A. Ramon, F. España, J. Gilabert, R. Castello, and A. Estelles, "Expression of fibrinolytic components in endometriosis," *Pathophysiology of Haemostasis and Thrombosis*, vol. 35, no. 1-2, pp. P136–P140, 2006.

[76] M. Szczepańska, J. Koźlik, J. Skrzypczak, and M. Mikołajczyk, "Oxidative stress may be a piece in the endometriosis puzzle," *Fertility and Sterility*, vol. 79, no. 6, pp. 1288–1293, 2003.

17

Normal Pregnancy Is Associated with Changes in Central Hemodynamics and Enhanced Recruitable, but Not Resting, Endothelial Function

Juan Torrado,[1] Yanina Zócalo,[1] Ignacio Farro,[1] Federico Farro,[1] Claudio Sosa,[2] Santiago Scasso,[2] Justo Alonso,[2] and Daniel Bia[1]

[1]Centro Universitario de Investigación, Innovación y Diagnóstico Arterial (CUiiDARTE), Physiology Department, Faculty of Medicine, Republic University, General Flores 2125, 11800 Montevideo, Uruguay
[2]Department of Obstetrics and Gynecology "C", Pereira-Rossell Hospital, Faculty of Medicine, Republic University, Br. Artigas 1550, 11600 Montevideo, Uruguay

Correspondence should be addressed to Daniel Bia; dbia@fmed.edu.uy

Academic Editor: Padma Murthi

Introduction. Flow-mediated dilation (FMD), low flow-mediated constriction (L-FMC), and reactive hyperemia-related changes in carotid-to-radial pulse wave velocity (ΔPWVcr%) could offer complementary information about both "recruitability" and "resting" endothelial function (EF). Carotid-to-femoral pulse wave velocity (PWVcf) and pulse wave analysis-derived parameters (i.e., AIx@75) are the gold standard methods for noninvasive evaluation of aortic stiffness and central hemodynamics. If healthy pregnancy is associated with both changes in resting and recruitable EF, as well as in several arterial parameters, it remains unknown and/or controversial. *Objectives.* To simultaneously and noninvasively assess in healthy pregnant (HP) and nonpregnant (NP) women central parameters in conjunction with "basal and recruitable" EF, employing new complementary approaches. *Methods.* HP ($n = 11$, 34.2 ± 3.3 weeks of gestation) and age- and cardiovascular risk factors-matched NP ($n = 22$) were included. Aortic blood pressure (BP), AIx@75, PWVcf, common carotid stiffness, and intima-media thickness, as well as FMD, L-FMC, and ΔPWVcr %, were measured. *Results.* Aortic BP, stiffness, and AIx@75 were reduced in HP. ΔPWVcr% and FMD were enhanced in HP in comparison to NP. No differences were found in L-FMC between groups. *Conclusion.* HP is associated with reduced aortic stiffness, central BP, wave reflections, and enhanced recruitable, but not resting, EF.

1. Introduction

Arterial structure and function can now be simple and noninvasively assessed by different accurate methods, which have been extensively used in patients with cardiovascular risk factors. In this context, Celermajer et al.'s technique, commonly known as *flow-mediated dilation* (FMD), which utilizes the vasoreactivity test (VRT), has stood the test of time and remains the most popular method to assess endothelial function [1, 2]. The VRT consists in positioning a pneumatic cuff around the forearm and provoking an arterial occlusion for five minutes (i.e., transient ischemia). This maneuver elicits an increase in blood flow in the brachial artery once the cuff is deflated (i.e., reactive hyperemia, *RH*),

which subsequently stimulates endothelium to release several vasoactive biochemical factors (i.e., nitric oxide). Finally, locally produced factors result in a dilation of the brachial artery (measured by B-Mode ultrasound) [2] and a reduction in arterial stiffness (changes in pulse wave velocity [PWV] assessed by mechanotransducers [3]). The VRT has also been also applied in healthy pregnancy and in pregnancy-related diseases [4, 5]. Independently of the setting, the magnitude of the arterial dilation is used as an indicator of endothelial function and healthy pregnant women show an enhanced vascular response evaluated by this method compared with healthy nonpregnant women [6, 7]. However, whereas FMD provides information about the "recruitability" of endothelial function (i.e., its responsiveness to a specific stimulus), it does not provide information concerning basal/tonic endothelial function (i.e., release of endothelial autacoids before FMD measures are initiated) [8]. In this context, Gori et al. described a novel index for assessing the response of the artery to low flow, which utilizes data obtained from the cuff occlusion period of an FMD scan [9]. Synonymous to FMD, the vasoconstriction observed under conditions of reduced blood flow has been named low-flow-mediated vasoconstriction (L-FMC) [9]. Inclusion of L-FMC data to traditional measurement of FMD could provide additional and/or complementary information, which, they propose, may improve the detection of patients with cardiovascular disease and profile the vascular response to exercise among healthy volunteers [10]. Whether healthy pregnancy is associated with changes in L-FMC remains to be established. In this context, it is also unknown if the integration of L-FMC into traditional FMD studies will be able to provide additional/complementary information among pregnant women.

In addition, changes in carotid-to-radial PWV (PWVcr) due to the same maneuver have been proposed as an alternative tool for the evaluation of recruitable endothelial function [3, 11]. PWV is recognized as the "gold standard" parameter for the evaluation of regional arterial stiffness and has had a wide biomedical application [12, 13]. A reduction in PWVcr values has been reported in response to VRT in healthy young adults [3] whereas a blunted reduction has been reported in pathophysiological circumstances, such as hypertension [14] and congestive heart failure [11]. A preliminary report suggested that changes in PWVcr due to VRT offer additional information of endothelial dynamics and thus could have a potential role in the assessment of endothelial function during pregnancy with a potential clinical application in predicting pregnancy-induced hypertension and preeclampsia [15].

Finally, there is still a lack of knowledge about the expected changes for several structural and functional parameters widely used in noninvasive arterial studies. In this regard, if pregnancy is associated with changes in central aortic pressure, wave reflections levels and/or elastic and muscular arteries stiffness remains to be determined. Changes in arterial structure and function of both maternal muscular and elastic arteries could be of value in accommodating pregnancy-induced increasing cardiac output and blood volume for a correct maternal-fetal hemodynamic interaction [16, 17]. Therefore, we here hypothesize that normal pregnancy, in contraposition to the nonpregnant status and particularly during the third trimester stage in which profound cardiovascular changes are expected, will evidence notable vascular adaptations (i.e., reduction in wave reflections levels and arterial stiffness), features capable of being assessed and quantified by using promising and complementary noninvasive arterial parameters.

In this context, the work aims were firstly to determine and analyze "basal and recruitable" endothelial function through the measurement of brachial artery FMD and L-FMC and PWVcr RH-related changes in a group of healthy nonpregnant and pregnant women and, secondly, to determine noninvasively central and peripheral arterial parameters, by using validated and gold standard techniques.

2. Methods

2.1. Subjects, Demographic Characteristics, and Laboratory Samples.
This was an analytic observational case-control study involving 11 healthy pregnant (HP) and 22 healthy nonpregnant women (NP). The HP women were recruited from the routine antenatal clinic where they were asked and agreed to participate in the study (convenience sampling). NP group was obtained from our database (CUiiDARTE Project and Centre, Republic University) once HP women were matched based on age, height, and cardiovascular risk factors [18–20]. Baseline demographic and anthropometric data were obtained by an obstetrician/physician during a clinical interview and exam, and laboratory samples were extracted prior to the examination. They were all healthy (with the exception of dyslipidemia in some of them) and without family history of premature cardiovascular disease. All HP women had uncomplicated pregnancies before and during the study. None of them received any vasoactive drugs.

Exclusion criteria for HP and NP included previous history of pregnancy-induced hypertension (including preeclampsia), gestational diabetes, or current chronic hypertension and/or diabetes mellitus. Significant unexplained proteinuria (>300 mg total protein in a 24 h urine collection) developing in obstetric controls was also an exclusion criterion for HP. The definitions for pathologies used for exclusion criteria took into account the one recommended by the National Institute for Health and Clinical Excellence guidelines [21, 22].

Participants were asked to abstain from physical activity, tobacco products, and vitamin supplementation for at least 4 hours prior to the examination. The study protocol was approved by the Ethics Research Committee of the Republic University (Uruguay) and all participants gave written informed consent.

2.2. Baseline Noninvasive Arterial Evaluation.
Subjects were instructed to lie in a left lateral position (particularly for HP, to avoid vena cava compression by the uterus) in a temperature-controlled (21°–23°C) room, for at least 15 minutes, in order to establish stable hemodynamic conditions. Heart rate (HR) and right brachial (peripheral) systolic and diastolic blood pressure (pSBP and pDBP, resp.) were measured using an oscillometric device (Omron HEM-433INT Oscillometric System; Omron Healthcare Inc., Illinois, USA) at 5–8-minute intervals during the whole procedure. Mean blood pressure (MBP) was determined using classic empirical formula currently used at the peripheral level as pDBP plus one-third times of peripheral pulse pressure (pPP = pSBP − pDBP).

2.2.1. Carotid-to-Femoral Pulse Wave Velocity and Pulse Wave Analysis.
The carotid-femoral pulse-wave velocity (PWVcf) was measured to analyze aortic regional stiffness. To this end, carotid and femoral artery waveforms were consecutively obtained with a high-fidelity applanation tonometer from the carotid and femoral regions simultaneously with continuous ECG monitoring (SphygmoCor 7.01, AtCor Medical, Sydney, Australia) (Figure 1). Then, carotid-femoral propagation time

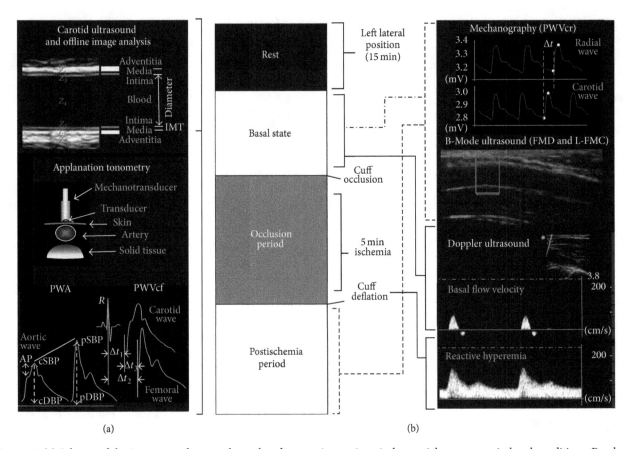

(a)   (b)

FIGURE 1: (a) Schema of the instrumental approach employed to acquire noninvasively arterial parameters in basal conditions. Employed techniques: carotid-to-femoral PWV and PWA (applanation tonometry) and carotid arterial diameter and CIMT (B-Mode ultrasound). (b) Representative diagram of the study protocol of Vasoreactivity Test (VRT) applied to evaluate changes in carotid-to-radial PWV and brachial arterial diameter. Z: acoustic impedance; CIMT: carotid intima-media thickness; PWA: pulse wave analysis; PWVcf: carotid-to-femoral pulse wave velocity; Δt_1, Δt_2: time delay between R wave from ECG and central (carotid) foot wave and peripheral (femoral or radial) foot wave, respectively; Δt_3: time delay between carotid foot wave and radial foot wave; AP: augmentation pressure; cSBP and pSBP: central and peripheral systolic blood pressure, respectively; cDBP and pDBP: central and peripheral diastolic blood pressure, respectively; PWVcr: carotid-to-radial pulse wave velocity; FMD: flow-mediated dilation; L-FMC: low flow-mediated constriction.

(Δt_3) was determined by subtracting the time delay between the peak of R wave of the ECG recording to femoral foot of the pressure waveform (Δt_2) of the corresponding cardiac cycle and the time delay between the peak of R wave to carotid foot of the pressure waveform (Δt_1). The algorithm utilized to detect the so-called "foot of the wave" was the *intersecting tangents*, explained elsewhere [23]. Straight distance between the recording sites (carotid-to-femoral distance [C-F Δx]) was then carefully measured using tape on the body surface to reduce the influence of altered body contour in pregnancy. Finally, PWVcf was automatically calculated as the quotient between C-F Δx and Δt_3 (Figure 1). The reported value of PWVcf for a subject was always the average of at least eight consecutive beats.

Pulse wave analysis (PWA) was used to assess central hemodynamics as well as systemic arterial stiffness and wave reflections. For this porpoise, mean radial artery waveform was obtained (through the acquisition of many cycles) with the applanation tonometer from the wrist, and a corresponding mean ascending aortic pressure waveform was generated with a validated generalized transfer function using the same

mentioned customized software (SphygmoCor 7.01, AtCor Medical, Sydney, Australia) [24]. The radial pulse waveform was then calibrated using the diastolic and mean arterial pressure obtained at the brachial artery [12]. Central systolic, diastolic, and pulse pressure (cSBP, cDBP, and cPP, resp.), heart rate corrected central augmentation index (AIx@75, adjusted to a rate of 75 beats/minute), and amplification ratio (pPP/cPP) were determined with the integrated software.

2.2.2. Carotid Artery Studies. Ultrasound assessment of carotid arteries was based on the techniques and recommendations described in international consensus [25]. High-resolution B-Mode ultrasound images of both (right and left) common carotid arteries (CCA) were obtained using a linear-array transducer connected to a portable Ultrasound System (Probe L38e, 5–10 MHz, SonoSite, MicroMaxx, SonoSite Inc., 21919 30th Drive SE, Bothell, WA 98021, USA). Measurements (still images and video clips/cine loops) were digitally stored for offline analysis (Figure 1). Near and far walls were analyzed and images were obtained from anterior, lateral, and posterior angles. At first, a carotid plaque screening was performed, for which the definition used was a focal wall thickening at least 50% greater than that of the surrounding vessel, a thickening that protrudes into the lumen 0.5 mm or as a region with carotid intima-media thickness (CIMT) greater than 1.5 mm [25]. Then, longitudinal views of the CCAs were acquired and a video (cine loop) of at least 30 seconds was recorded and stored. The CIMT and beat-to-beat diameter waveforms were obtained and analyzed offline using a step-by-step border detection algorithm (based in changes in acoustic impedance [Z]), applied to each digitized image (Hemodyn-4M software, Buenos Aires, Argentina). A region 1.0 cm proximal to the carotid bulb was identified, and the far wall CIMT was determined as the distance between the lumen-intima and the media-adventitia interfaces (Figure 1). The software performs multiple automated or semiautomated measurements along the centimeter and averages them, increasing the accuracy of the measures.

The instantaneous mean diameter (from the leading edge of the near wall intima-media interface to the intima-media interface of the far wall) waveform was obtained during pulsation in order to obtain diastolic and systolic diameter. Then, the pressure strain or Peterson's elastic modulus (E_p) was calculated relating these measures with central blood pressure as follows [12]:

$$E_P = \frac{(cSBP - cDBP)}{(SD - DD)/DD},\qquad(1)$$

where cSBP, cDBP, SD, and DD are central systolic and diastolic blood pressure and carotid systolic and diastolic diameter, respectively (Figure 1). E_p measures the ability of the arteries to change its dimensions in response to the pulse pressure caused by cardiac pulsatile ejection (pressure change required for (theoretic) 100% increase in diameter) [12, 26, 27].

2.3. Vascular Reactivity: Resting and Recruitable Endothelial Function.

Once baseline noninvasive arterial evaluation was carried out, we utilized the theoretical basis, general protocol, and methodological aspects of the VRT recommended by the guidelines for the ultrasound assessment of endothelial-dependent flow-mediated vasodilation of the brachial artery [2, 28]. For this purpose, participants were submitted to five minutes of ischemia by occluding left radial and cubital arteries using a pneumatic cuff placed around the left forearm (just below the elbow to at least 50 mm Hg above pSBP) and several parameters of vascular reactivity were measured before, during, and after ischemia (Figure 1). The parameters used for the evaluation of endothelial function are listed below.

2.3.1. L-FMC, FMD, and Shear Rate.

Taking into account "gold standard" accepted methodology for the evaluation of endothelial function "recruitability" and simultaneously PWVcr measurement (see later), left brachial artery was visualized longitudinally above the antecubital crease using the same high resolution B-Mode ultrasound device mentioned earlier (Sonosite; MicroMaxx; USA) (Figure 1). Similarly, video sequences were recorded at rest (1 minute), during forearm occlusion (5 minutes), and after cuff deflation

(4 minutes). Subsequently and similarly to the processing of carotid images, recordings were analyzed offline using same automated step-by-step algorithm applied to each digitalized image that allows for the brachial diameter waveform obtainment and L-FMC and FMD calculation [29].

L-FMC was quantified as the percentage of change in brachial artery diastolic diameter (DD), considering the basal levels and the DD before cuff deflation:

$$L\text{-FMC}\% = \frac{DD_{before\ cuff\ deflation} - DD_{baseline}}{DD_{baseline}} \times 100.\qquad(2)$$

FMD was quantified as the percentage of change in brachial DD, considering the basal levels and the maximal diastolic diameter after cuff deflation:

$$FMD\% = \frac{DD_{after\ cuff\ deflation} - DD_{baseline}}{DD_{baseline}} \times 100.\qquad(3)$$

In addition, Doppler signals were performed to acquire blood flow velocity in baseline conditions and at specific moments during the RH period. Doppler signals were used to obtain the brachial *shear rate* (SR) and its percentage of change, relating mean blood flow velocity (V_m [cm/s]) to brachial mean diameter (D_m) according to the following equations:

$$SR = \frac{V_m}{D_m},$$
$$SR\% = \frac{SR_{after\ cuff\ deflation} - SR_{baseline}}{SR_{baseline}} \times 100.\qquad(4)$$

SR is an estimate of *shear stress* without accounting for blood viscosity [30] and was obtained for the characterization of the endothelial stimulus. All measurements were done by the same trained operator. The study protocol is represented in Figure 1.

2.3.2. Carotid-to-Radial Pulse Wave Velocity.

Noninvasively, carotid and radial pressure waveforms were simultaneously obtained using strain gauge mechanotransducers (Motorola MPX 2050, Motorola Inc., Corporate 1303 E. Algonquin Road, Schaumburg, Illinois 60196, USA) by placing them on the skin over the carotid and radial sites (left hemibody). PWVcr was determined taking into account the given distance between these arterial sites (C-R Δx) and the time delay (Δt) between the carotid and radial waveforms onset (Figure 1). The algorithm used for the detection of the foot waves was described and explained in previous work [31]. Although a four-minute recording postcuff release was obtained, one-minute postischemia was the specific moment where the analysis was especially taken, according to previous reports [14, 31, 32]. The PWVcr accepted variation coefficient was less than 7%.

PWVcr levels corresponding to baseline and to post-ischemia period were determined by averaging eight consecutive beats. After that, percent of change of PWVcr (with respect to basal levels) was quantified as follows:

$$\Delta PWVcr\% = \frac{PWVcr_{after\ cuff\ deflation} - PWVcr_{baseline}}{PWVcr_{baseline}} \quad (5)$$

$$\times\ 100.$$

2.4. Statistics. The statistical analyses were performed using the Statistical Package for Social Sciences (version 19.0). All data were expressed as mean value (MV) ± standard deviation (SD) and a $P < 0.05$ indicates significant statistical differences. Comparisons between pregnant and nonpregnant women were performed using two-tailed unpaired Student t-test. Differences in prevalence were analyzed using χ^2 Test with or without Yates's correction if appropriate. Differences in percentage of change of variables determined before and after the VRT (arterial diameter, PWV and shear rate) were evaluated using two-tailed paired Student t-test. Linear regression analyses were used to assess relationships between variables.

3. Results

Recordings were successfully obtained from all women and all studies were included in the analysis. The mean duration of the studies was one hour approximately and they were all well tolerated (without symptoms and/or complications). The mean gestational age at examination in HP women was 34.2 ± 3.3 weeks. Demographic, anthropometric, and clinical data are shown in Table 1. As was mentioned above, age, height, and cardiovascular risk factors were taken into account in order to match groups. Body mass index was significantly higher in HP compared with NP ($P < 0.05$).

Baseline cardiovascular characteristics are given and compared in Table 2. The mean heart rate was higher in pregnancy compared to the nonpregnant controls. In addition, baseline pDBP and MBP levels were significantly higher in NP in comparison with HP ($P < 0.05$). No pSBP differences were found between the groups. However, in addition to differences in cDBP, significantly higher values in cSBP were evidenced in NP women.

Mean AIx@75 was higher in NP with respect to HP ($18.8 \pm 10.1\%$ versus $8.9 \pm 8.6\%$; resp.; $P = 0.019$), whereas amplification ratio was significantly reduced (Table 2).

When analyzing geometrical and biomechanical characteristics of muscular peripheral arteries important differences were found between groups. In concrete, basal brachial SD and DD were significantly increased in HP versus NP ($P < 0.001$) and PWVcr values were higher in NP compared with HP ($P = 0.003$). Elastic arteries such as aorta and CCAs were also analyzed by both regional and local arterial stiffness parameters (Table 2). Meaningfully differences in stiffness were only evidenced in regional stiffness (PWVcf), which was significantly reduced in HP. Values of local stiffness (E_P) of both right and left CCA did not reach statistical differences

TABLE 1: Demographic, anthropometric, and clinical characteristics.

Variable	NP	HP	P value[*]
N	22	11	
Age (years)	27.9 ± 6.2	29.1 ± 4.7	0.475
Gestational age (weeks)	N/A	34.2 ± 3.3	N/A
Weight (kg)	61.8 ± 7.1	66.9 ± 7.4	0.065
Height (cm)	158.6 ± 8.2	157.9 ± 7.1	0.755
BMI (kg/m^2)	24.7 ± 2.9	$27.0 \pm 3.7^*$	0.048
Carotid-to-radial distance (cm)	60.2 ± 9.1	61.6 ± 4.2	0.550
Carotid-to-femoral distance (cm)	59.0 ± 2.6	58.5 ± 3.2	0.665
SSN-to-carotid distance (cm)	8.0 ± 1.1	7.6 ± 0.8	0.262
Hypertension (%)	0.0	0.0	N/A
Dyslipidemia (%)	20.0	18.1	0.700
Diabetes (%)	0.0	0.0	N/A
Cardiovascular disease (%)	0.0	0.0	N/A

Values are expressed as means ± SD or as prevalence in %. ∗ indicates $P < 0.05$. All comparisons were determined using two-tailed unpaired student t-test and χ^2 Test with or without Yates's correction if appropriate. n: number of patients per group; N/A: not applicable; NP: nonpregnant women; HP: healthy pregnant women; BMI: body mass index; SSN: suprasternal notch.

among groups, despite the lower mean values that were found in HP.

None of the groups presented atherosclerotic plaques. Structural differences were only noticed on the right CCA, where CIMT was significantly reduced in HP with respect to NP women ($P = 0.044$).

Taking into account the VRT, all groups evoked endothelial stimulus (reactive hyperemia) evaluated by changes in SR before and after cuff deflation ($P < 0.001$) (Table 3). Pregnancy was associated with increased baseline SR values in comparison with NP controls ($66.2 \pm 24.4\,s^{-1}$ versus $110.8 \pm 40.1\,s^{-1}$; $P < 0.001$). Nevertheless, after cuff deflation, peak SR and $\Delta SR\%$ were not different between groups ($P = 0.079$ and $P = 0.525$, resp.), ensuring a similar hyperemic stimulus (Table 3). As was expected, no significant changes were found in heart rate or blood pressure intra- and intergroup before and after the cuff deflation (data not shown).

Regarding the FMD, both groups showed dilatation of the brachial artery with respect to basal state, but as was expected, HP women showed quantitatively the highest FMD response ($9.6 \pm 3.4\%$ versus $7.1 \pm 2.3\%$; $P < 0.05$) (Table 3), despite the higher basal brachial artery diameter existing in HP (Table 2). One minute after cuff deflation, PWVcr significantly decreased in both HP (6.8 ± 1.4 to 5.8 ± 0.9 m/s; $P = 0.005$) and NP (8.4 ± 1.1 to 7.4 ± 0.9 m/s; $P < 0.001$). The mean absolute change of the study groups was similar; however PWVcr response in % differed comparing HP women with NP women (-14.0% versus -8.5%; $P < 0.05$) (Table 3). L-FMC of the brachial artery occurred in both groups independently of the physiological status ($P < 0.001$). However, even though maximal vasoconstriction of the brachial artery (negative values) was observed in HP women ($-7.0 \pm 4.7\%$; $P < 0.001$) in comparison to NP ($-5.7 \pm 2.4\%$; $P < 0.001$), the magnitude of the reduction of

TABLE 2: Central (aortic) and peripheral arterial structural and functional parameters.

Variable	NP	HP	P value[*]
Heart rate (beats/minute)	73.8 ± 10.8	$85.0 \pm 10.0^{*}$	0.007
Peripheral SBP (mmHg)	113.0 ± 11.2	112.0 ± 9.2	0.740
Peripheral DBP (mmHg)	72.4 ± 8.2	$62.5 \pm 8.9^{*}$	0.004
MBP (mmHg)	89.0 ± 8.5	$78.6 \pm 5.7^{*}$	0.002
Peripheral PP (mmHg)	45.9 ± 9.3	49.8 ± 17.8	0.235
Central SBP (mmHg)	104.2 ± 9.9	$95.8 \pm 6.8^{*}$	0.043
Central DBP (mmHg)	72.2 ± 8.2	$63.4 \pm 9.4^{*}$	0.016
Central PP (mmHg)	32.0 ± 4.3	32.4 ± 11.0	0.683
Amplification ratio (pPP/cPP)	1.31 ± 0.21	$1.51 \pm 0.16^{*}$	0.006
AIx@75 (%)	18.8 ± 10.1	$8.9 \pm 8.6^{*}$	0.019
Carotid-to-radial PWV (m/s)	8.4 ± 1.1	$6.8 \pm 1.4^{*}$	0.003
Brachial SD (mm)	3.1 ± 0.3	$3.9 \pm 0.3^{*}$	<0.001
Brachial DD (mm)	2.9 ± 0.3	$3.7 \pm 0.3^{*}$	<0.001
Carotid-to-femoral PWV (m/s)	8.1 ± 1.3	$6.8 \pm 0.9^{*}$	0.022
Right CCA SD (mm)	6.8 ± 0.6	7.0 ± 0.5	0.311
Right CCA DD (mm)	6.7 ± 0.5	6.9 ± 0.7	0.388
Right CCA E_P (mmHg)	416.9 ± 157.6	350.6 ± 110.0	0.301
Right CIMT (mm)	0.550 ± 0.077	$0.462 \pm 0.089^{*}$	0.044
Left CCA SD (mm)	6.6 ± 0.6	$7.2 \pm 0.4^{*}$	0.040
Left CCA DD (mm)	6.0 ± 0.5	6.5 ± 0.3	0.062
Left CCA E_P (mmHg)	401.8 ± 155.7	352.7 ± 179.0	0.702
Left CIMT (mm)	0.572 ± 0.090	0.519 ± 0.080	0.146

Values are expressed as means $\pm$ SD. $*$ indicates $P < 0.05$. All comparisons were determined using two-tailed unpaired Student t-test. NP: nonpregnant women; HP: healthy pregnant women; SBP, DBP, MBP, and PP: systolic, diastolic, mean, and pulse pressure, respectively. pPP and cPP: peripheral and central pulse pressure, respectively. AIx@75: augmentation index adjusted to a heart rate of 75 beats/minute; PWV: pulse wave velocity; SD and DD: systolic and diastolic diameter, respectively; E_P: Peterson's or pressure-strain elastic modulus; CCA: common carotid artery; CIMT: carotid intima-media thickness.

TABLE 3: Vascular reactivity parameters: endothelial function.

Variable	NP	HP	P value[*]
Basal SR (s^{-1})	66.2 ± 24.4	$110.8 \pm 40.1^{*}$	<0.001
Peak SR (s^{-1})	180.0 ± 73.7	227.0 ± 67.8	0.079
ΔSR (%)	132.5 ± 59.9	110.9 ± 88.5	0.525
FMD (%)	7.1 ± 2.3	$9.6 \pm 3.4^{*}$	0.039
ΔPWVcr (%)	-8.5 ± 6.4	$-14.0 \pm 7.8^{*}$	0.035
L-FMC (%)	-5.7 ± 2.4	-7.0 ± 4.7	0.208

Values are expressed as means $\pm$ SD. $*$ indicates $P < 0.05$. All comparisons were determined using two-tailed unpaired Student t-test. NP: nonpregnant women; HP: healthy pregnant women; FMD: flow-mediated dilation; L-FMC: low-flow-mediated constriction; PWVcr: carotid-to-radial pulse wave velocity; SR: shear rate.

arterial diameters was not statistically different between the groups (Table 3).

Finally, there were no significant correlations between endothelial function parameters (FMD, L-FMC, or ΔPWVcr%) and AIx@75, PWVcf, or central blood pressure (data not shown). However, FMD correlated with L-FMC ($R = 0.54$, $P = 0.038$) and ΔPWVcr% ($R = 0.419$, $P = 0.037$), whereas no significant correlation was evidenced between ΔPWVcr% and L-FMC ($R = 0.30$, $P = 0.198$). A positive correlation between L-FMC (negative number) and basal SR (positive number) was found across the whole studied population ($R = 0.587$, $P = 0.017$).

4. Discussion

The present study is, to our knowledge, the first one to determine and assess simultaneously, in a group of healthy pregnant women, the endothelial function by using three different but complementary methods in conjunction with the determination of central and peripheral structural and functional arterial validated parameters. These approaches allow us to conclude that, with respect to nonpregnant women matched by age, anthropometric features and cardiovascular risk factors, pregnant women showed (1) reduced aortic and "upper limb" arterial stiffness levels, in coherence with the higher basal brachial artery diameters that were found in this group; (2) reduced central (aortic), but not peripheral, systolic blood pressure, determined by a reduced contribution of reflected waves to central aortic pressure waveform (lower AIx@75); (3) an enhanced recruitable (FMD), but not resting (L-FMC), endothelial function, despite higher basal brachial diameters.

4.1. Physiological Considerations. Regarding the hemodynamic parameters, we found that HP women showed, in comparison to controls, increased HR and reduced pDBP and MBP in basal state. These findings are in consonance with an expected pregnancy-induced decrease in peripheral vascular resistance and increased cardiac output at rest. However, pregnancy-related changes were also notable when central hemodynamics is analyzed. Central (aortic) systolic blood pressure and PWVcf (aortic stiffness) were lower in HP comparing to controls, independently of brachial systolic blood pressure levels. In addition, AIx@75, a composite parameter of systemic arterial stiffness and wave reflection amplitude, was different between HP and NP. This suggests that healthy pregnancy is associated with reduced wave reflection contribution to the central aortic pressure waveform and central arterial (aortic) stiffness. However, changes in CCA stiffness (E_p) related with pregnancy were not statistically significant, despite lower mean levels in HP. This finding supports Kärkkäinen et al. report, since these authors evidenced that carotid arterial distensibility (inverse of E_P) decreased towards the end of the pregnancy reaching the lowest values in the third trimester [27]. Nevertheless, taking our results together, we evidenced that healthy pregnancy is associated with reduced aortic stiffness, central systolic pressure, and wave reflections.

Among the methods that allow for measurement of endothelial function in the clinical setting, FMD has rapidly gained popularity because of its simplicity, reproducibility, and noninvasiveness [2, 28]. However, as was mentioned earlier, one important limitation of FMD is that it only provides information about the "recruitability" of endothelial function (i.e., its responsiveness to a specific stimulus) and not about "resting" endothelial function (i.e., release of endothelial autacoids before FMD measures are initiated) [8]. We here analyze, in healthy pregnant women, both types of functional aspects of endothelial function, "endothelial recruitability" through FMD and PWVcr changes and "resting endothelial tone" through L-FMC. As it was expected, the magnitude of FMD observed in HP in response to VRT surpassed that observed in NP. This finding, which is similar to that described in previous reports, is in coherence with an enhanced endothelial function assessed by this method [6, 7]. On another side, when analyzing changes in arterial stiffness due to VRT, even though both groups showed a reduction in PWVcr values, HP showed the major decrease ($P < 0.05$). It is noteworthy that both groups showed a similar "endothelial stimulus," since peak SR and ΔSR% were similar between them. In addition, even though starting (basal) levels of brachial diameter and PWVcr (basal state) in HP were higher and lower, respectively, these values were not correlated with the vascular response (i.e., FMD and ΔPWVcr%). When examining the relationship between FMD and PWVcr the analysis should take into account the Moens and Korteweg equation. In that sense, PWV is determined by both arterial diameter and the elastic modulus, among other factors [12]. In a previous study, we evidenced in healthy subjects that changes in PWVcr due to the VRT may be also provoked by a smooth muscle relaxation. If there were a right shift in the brachial pressure-volume loop, post-cuff deflation, in addition to a slope decrease due to smooth muscle relaxation, the global response might suit our results (as PWVcr changes were even higher than those only expected by changes in VMF) [3]. In light of our results, we hypothesize that besides an enhanced vasodilatory response, smooth muscle relaxation could be pronounced in healthy pregnancy.

Taking into account "resting" endothelial tone, our results show that, during the cuff inflation, L-FMC occurred in the brachial artery independently of the physiological status. However, mean L-FMC was not different between the groups. Although L-FMC was firstly described at the radial artery as a specific phenomenon [9], in the 90's it had been already reported in the brachial artery in response to the cuff occlusion in subjects with hypercholesterolemia [33]. Later, Spiro et al. evidenced that this specific phenomenon also occurs in healthy subjects at the brachial artery and it can be measured reliably [34]. Studies agree that vasoconstriction of the radial artery occurs during the cuff inflation in nonpregnant women, although the mechanisms involved remain not completely understood [9, 35, 36]. L-FMC of the brachial artery has been controversial and several studies demonstrated conflicting results [33–35, 37, 38]. Indeed, Weissgerber et al. did not evidence L-FMC in the brachial artery in pregnant women [35], in contraposition with our results. Differences in cardiovascular profile, technical aspects, methodological issues, and/or interobserver variability could explain the widely variable results, as it occurs with FMD measurements [39–41]. For example, we here measure L-FMC of the brachial artery in a regimen of low but not zero blood flow (as it occurs in the radial artery) in a level that is upstream of the occlusion site. Therefore, the magnitude of reduced blood flow in the brachial artery and its relationship with the basal levels (endothelial "negative" stimulus for vasoconstriction) should surely yield different brachial responses. Nevertheless, our results indicate that the more the basal blood flow (or SR), the more the vasoconstriction of the brachial artery provoked by the occlusion of the pneumatic cuff. Even though we did not measure "the residual" brachial blood flow during the cuff occlusion, it is expected that the absolute change in brachial blood flow may be of greater amount with the same occlusion protocol, if the starting point of blood flow in basal conditions is increased (i.e., increased "negative" stimulus for vasoconstriction).

We found a significant correlation between FMD and L-FMC, FMD and ΔPWVcr%, but not between L-FMC and ΔPWVcr%. Our results indicate that brachial artery responses to inflation and deflation of the cuff related with endothelial dynamics could share some vascular mechanism. However, there are confusing results around the FMD and L-FMC correlation, with variable results depending on the analyzed artery (brachial versus radial) and type of physiological or pathophysiological circumstance [8–10, 34]. This emphasizes again the complexity of studying "endothelial functions." Although both L-FMC and FMD are an expression of the vascular reactivity in response to changes in blood flow, their relationship is neither conceptually simple nor mathematically linear [10]. Nevertheless, it is reasonable to think that the same vasodilatatory mechanisms (i.e., nitric oxide) involved in response to increased blood flow (shear stress) will diminish (with the consequent vasoconstriction) when the stimulus for its production is reduced/abolish.

4.2. Interpretation of Findings. The important additional information brought by the introduction of changes in PWVcr and L-FMC, together with the information of central and peripheral hemodynamics, is that these variables provide information concerning different aspects of vascular reactivity and endothelial function, therefore complementing (and not overlapping) the information provided by FMD. An enhanced response and/or increased vasodilator reserve to changes in blood flow in a concrete vascular ledge (i.e., brachial artery) implicates an elevated capability of the arterial system to accomplish an appropriate vascular adjustment against hemodynamic changes in the long term (fetal growth) and even in the short term (exercise, change of position, etc.). In addition, these could be associated with cardiovascular benefits reported by other authors like reduced left ventricle afterload and improve diastolic function and reduced myocardial oxygen demand in the maternal circulation [42–44]. Previous results of our group suggested that pregnancy-induced hypertension (i.e., preeclampsia-eclampsia syndrome) could be associated with increased central aortic pressure, elastic arteries stiffness, and wave reflections, in conjunction with both resting and recruitable endothelial dysfunctions [45]. These arterial disturbances would not only blunt the mentioned hemodynamic benefits of the pregnancy physiological condition but also add extra load to the maternal circulation in the context of increased cardiac output and fetal requirements. However, although this comprehensive arterial assessment would improve our understanding of the haemodynamics of both healthy pregnancy and pregnancy-related diseases, the inclusion of this information together with the recognized validated clinical, obstetric, and laboratory variables remains to be addressed during the first trimester of pregnancy, since at this time they could have an additional/complementary value in the prediction of preeclampsia [46, 47]. In this small study, that addresses the feasibility of measuring these parameters simultaneously, simply, and noninvasively, we found encouraging results that, we believe, warrant further investigation.

4.3. Limitations and Perspectives. The sample size of our study was relatively small. However, our findings were statistically significant and, by definition, this indicates that the study was adequately statistically powered. Our technical approaches including the use of both multiple types of automated and semiautomated edge-detection/point software in ultrasound image and pressure wave assessment are largely operator independent and also empower our findings [28]. Given the means of the different variables and SDs observed in previous works and in the present sample, twenty-eight subjects ($n = 28$) of the total sample size (the sum of the sizes of comparison groups) would be required to detect a statistically significant effect of the pregnancy status with at least 80% of power [45]. Secondly, even groups were properly matched, women with dyslipidemia were included in the analysis, and this could have an impact in our results, being a limitation of the "healthy groups."

This vascular approach may provide a more comprehensive assessment of vascular state and endothelial function in normal pregnancy. Future studies will have to determine if accounting of this information, particularly during the early stages of pregnancy (i.e., first trimester), in conjunction with recognized important clinical, obstetric, laboratory variables, will be able to improve early detection of pathophysiological circumstances like pregnancy-induced hypertension.

5. Conclusion

With respect to nonpregnant women matched by age, anthropometric features and cardiovascular risk factors, pregnant women showed (1) reduced aortic and "upper limb" arterial stiffness levels, in coherence with the higher basal brachial artery diameters that were found in this group; (2) reduced central (aortic), but not peripheral, systolic blood pressure, determined by a reduced contribution of reflected waves to central aortic pressure waveform; and (3) an enhanced recruitable, but not resting, endothelial function, despite higher basal brachial diameters.

Conflict of Interests

The authors declare that there is no conflict of interests regarding the publication of this paper.

Acknowledgments

The authors wish to acknowledge the technical assistance given by Manuela Pereira. This work was supported by the CUiiDARTE Centre and Project, Agencia Nacional de Investigación e Innovación (ANII-Uruguay), Comisión Sectorial de Investigación Científica and Espacio Interdisciplinario (Universidad de la República).

References

[1] D. S. Celermajer, K. E. Sorensen, V. M. Gooch et al., "Noninvasive detection of endothelial dysfunction in children and adults at risk of atherosclerosis," *The Lancet*, vol. 340, no. 8828, pp. 1111–1115, 1992.

[2] M. C. Corretti, T. J. Anderson, E. J. Benjamin et al., "Guidelines for the ultrasound assessment of endothelial-dependent flow-mediated vasodilation of the brachial artery: a report of the International Brachial Artery Reactivity Task Force," *Journal of the American College of Cardiology*, vol. 39, no. 2, pp. 257–265, 2002, Erratum in: *Journal of the American College of Cardiology*, vol. 39, no. 6, p. 1082, 2002.

[3] J. Torrado, D. Bia, Y. Zocalo et al., "Reactive hyperemia-related changes in carotid-radial pulse wave velocity as a potential tool to characterize the endothelial dynamics," in *Proceedings of the Annual International Conference of the IEEE Engineering in Medicine and Biology Society (EMBC '09)*, pp. 1800–1803, IEEE, Minneapolis, Minn, USA, September 2009.

[4] B. Takase, T. Goto, A. Hamabe et al., "Flow-mediated dilation in brachial artery in the second half of pregnancy and prediction of pre-eclampsia," *Journal of Human Hypertension*, vol. 17, no. 10, pp. 697–704, 2003.

[5] E. V. D. C. Filho, C. Mohr, B. J. A. Filho et al., "Flow-mediated dilatation in the differential diagnosis of preeclampsia syndrome," *Arquivos Brasileiros de Cardiologia*, vol. 94, no. 2, pp. 182–186, 2010.

[6] I. Dørup, K. Skajaa, and K. E. Sørensen, "Normal pregnancy is associated with enhanced endothelium-dependent flow-mediated vasodilation," *The American Journal of Physiology—Heart and Circulatory Physiology*, vol. 276, no. 3, part 2, pp. H821–H825, 1999.

[7] M. D. Savvidou, N. A. Kametas, A. E. Donald, and K. H. Nicolaides, "Non-invasive assessment of endothelial function in normal pregnancy," *Ultrasound in Obstetrics and Gynecology*, vol. 15, no. 6, pp. 502–507, 2000.

[8] T. Gori, J. D. Parker, and T. Münzel, "Flow-mediated constriction: further insight into a new measure of vascular function," *European Heart Journal*, vol. 32, no. 7, pp. 784–787, 2011.

[9] T. Gori, S. Dragoni, M. Lisi et al., "Conduit artery constriction mediated by low flow. A novel noninvasive method for the assessment of vascular function," *Journal of the American College of Cardiology*, vol. 51, no. 20, pp. 1953–1958, 2008.

[10] T. Gori, S. Grotti, S. Dragoni et al., "Assessment of vascular function: flow-mediated constriction complements the information of flow-mediated dilatation," *Heart*, vol. 96, no. 2, pp. 141–147, 2010.

[11] K. K. Naka, A. C. Tweddel, S. N. Doshi, J. Goodfellow, and A. H. Henderson, "Flow-mediated changes in pulse wave velocity: a new clinical measure of endothelial function," *European Heart Journal*, vol. 27, no. 3, pp. 302–309, 2006.

[12] S. Laurent, J. Cockcroft, L. Van Bortel et al., "Expert consensus document on arterial stiffness: methodological issues and clinical applications," *European Heart Journal*, vol. 27, no. 21, pp. 2588–2605, 2006.

[13] L. M. Van Bortel, S. Laurent, P. Boutouyrie et al., "Expert consensus document on the measurement of aortic stiffness in daily practice using carotid-femoral pulse wave velocity," *Journal of Hypertension*, vol. 30, no. 3, pp. 445–448, 2012.

[14] H. Kamran, L. Salciccioli, Eun Hee Ko et al., "Effect of reactive hyperemia on carotid-radial pulse wave velocity in hypertensive participants and direct comparison with flow-mediated dilation: a pilot study," *Angiology*, vol. 61, no. 1, pp. 100–106, 2010.

[15] J. Torrado, I. Farro, F. Farro et al., "Carotid-radial pulse wave velocity as an alternative tool for the evaluation of endothelial function during pregnancy: potential role in identifying hypertensive disorders of pregnancy," in *Proceedings of the Annual International Conference of the IEEE Engineering in Medicine and Biology Society (EMBC '12)*, pp. 5603–5606, IEEE, San Diego, Calif, USA, August-September 2012.

[16] J. P. van den Wijngaard, B. E. Westerhof, D. J. Faber, M. M. Ramsay, N. Westerhof, and M. J. van Gemert, "Abnormal arterial flows by a distributed model of the fetal circulation," *American Journal of Physiology—Regulatory, Integrative and Comparative Physiology*, vol. 291, no. 5, pp. R1222–R1233, 2006, Erratum in: *American Journal of Physiology—Regulatory, Integrative and Comparative Physiology*, vol. 292, no. 1, p. R663, 2007.

[17] J. S. Morton and S. T. Davidge, "Arterial endothelium-derived hyperpolarization: potential role in pregnancy adaptations and complications," *Journal of Cardiovascular Pharmacology*, vol. 61, no. 3, pp. 197–203, 2013.

[18] D. B. Santana, Y. A. Zócalo, and R. L. Armentano, "Integrated e-health approach based on vascular ultrasound and pulse wave analysis for asymptomatic atherosclerosis detection and cardiovascular risk stratification in the community," *IEEE Transactions on Information Technology in Biomedicine*, vol. 16, no. 2, pp. 287–294, 2012.

[19] D. Bia, Y. Zócalo, I. Farro et al., "Integrated evaluation of age-related changes in structural and functional vascular parameters used to assess arterial aging, subclinical atherosclerosis, and cardiovascular risk in uruguayan adults: CUiiDARTE project," *International Journal of Hypertension*, vol. 2011, Article ID 587303, 112 pages, 2011.

[20] D. B. Santana, Y. A. Zócalo, I. F. Ventura et al., "Health informatics design for assisted diagnosis of subclinical atherosclerosis, structural, and functional arterial age calculus and patient-specific cardiovascular risk evaluation," *IEEE Transactions on Information Technology in Biomedicine*, vol. 16, no. 5, pp. 943–951, 2012.

[21] National Collaborating Centre for Women's and Children's Health, *Hypertension in Pregnancy. The Management of Hypertensive Disorders During Pregnancy*, Clinical Guideline; no. 107, National Institute for Health and Clinical Excellence (NICE), London, UK, 2010.

[22] National Collaborating Centre for Women's and Children's Health, *Diabetes in Pregnancy: Management of Diabetes and Its Complications from Preconception to the Postnatal Period*, (Clinical Guideline), National Collaborating CentreNational Institute for Health and Clinical Excellence (NICE), London, UK, 2015.

[23] Y. C. Chiu, P. W. Arand, S. G. Shroff, T. Feldman, and J. D. Carroll, "Determination of pulse wave velocities with computerized algorithms," *American Heart Journal*, vol. 121, no. 5, pp. 1460–1470, 1991.

[24] A. L. Pauca, M. F. O'Rourke, and N. D. Kon, "Prospective evaluation of a method for estimating ascending aortic pressure from the radial artery pressure waveform," *Hypertension*, vol. 38, no. 4, pp. 932–937, 2001.

[25] J. H. Stein, C. E. Korcarz, R. T. Hurst et al., "Use of carotid ultrasound to identify subclinical vascular disease and evaluate cardiovascular disease risk: a consensus statement from the American society of echocardiography carotid intima-media thickness task force endorsed by the society for vascular medicine," *Journal of the American Society of Echocardiography*, vol. 21, no. 2, pp. 93–111, 2008.

[26] M. F. O'Rourke, J. A. Staessen, C. Vlachopoulos, D. Duprez, and G. E. Plante, "Clinical applications of arterial stiffness; definitions and reference values," *American Journal of Hypertension*, vol. 15, no. 5, pp. 426–444, 2002.

[27] H. Kärkkäinen, H. Saarelainen, P. Valtonen et al., "Carotid artery elasticity decreases during pregnancy—the Cardiovascular Risk in Young Finns study," *BMC Pregnancy and Childbirth*, vol. 14, article 98, 2014.

[28] D. H. J. Thijssen, M. A. Black, K. E. Pyke et al., "Assessment of flow-mediated dilation in humans: a methodological and physiological guideline," *The American Journal of Physiology—Heart and Circulatory Physiology*, vol. 300, no. 1, pp. H2–H12, 2011.

[29] D. Craiem, G. Chironi, A. Simon, and J. Levenson, "New assessment of endothelium-dependent flow-mediated vasodilation to characterize endothelium dysfunction," *American Journal of Therapeutics*, vol. 15, no. 4, pp. 340–344, 2008.

[30] K. E. Pyke, E. M. Dwyer, and M. E. Tschakovsky, "Impact of controlling shear rate on flow-mediated dilation responses in the brachial artery of humans," *Journal of Applied Physiology*, vol. 97, no. 2, pp. 499–508, 2004.

[31] J. Torrado, D. Bia, Y. Zócalo et al., "Carotid-radial pulse wave velocity as a discriminator of intrinsic wall alterations during evaluation of endothelial function by flow-mediated dilatation," in *Proceedings of the Annual International Conference of the IEEE Engineering in Medicine and Biology Society (EMBC '11)*, pp. 6458–6461, IEEE, Boston, Mass, USA, August-September 2011.

[32] J. Torrado, D. Bia, Y. Zócalo, I. Farro, F. Farro, and R. L. Armentano, "Hyperemia-related changes in arterial stiffness: comparison between pulse wave velocity and stiffness index in the vascular reactivity assessment," *International Journal of Vascular Medicine*, vol. 2012, Article ID 490742, 7 pages, 2012.

[33] V. Filitti, P. Giral, A. Simon, I. Merli, M. Del Pino, and J. Levenson, "Enhanced constriction of the peripheral large artery in response to acute induction of a low-flow state in human hypercholesterolemia," *Arteriosclerosis and Thrombosis*, vol. 11, no. 1, pp. 161–166, 1991.

[34] J. R. Spiro, J. E. Digby, G. Ghimire et al., "Brachial artery low-flow-mediated constriction is increased early after coronary intervention and reduces during recovery after acute coronary syndrome: characterization of a recently described index of vascular function," *European Heart Journal*, vol. 32, no. 7, pp. 856–866, 2011.

[35] T. L. Weissgerber, G. A. L. Davies, and M. E. Tschakovsky, "Low flow-mediated constriction occurs in the radial but not the

brachial artery in healthy pregnant and nonpregnant women," *Journal of Applied Physiology*, vol. 108, no. 5, pp. 1097–1105, 2010.

[36] E. A. Dawson, A. Alkarmi, D. H. J. Thijssen et al., "Low-flow mediated constriction is endothelium-dependent: effects of exercise training after radial artery catheterization," *Circulation: Cardiovascular Interventions*, vol. 5, no. 5, pp. 713–719, 2012.

[37] B. A. Parker, S. J. Ridout, and D. N. Proctor, "Age and flow-mediated dilation: a comparison of dilatory responsiveness in the brachial and popliteal arteries," *American Journal of Physiology—Heart and Circulatory Physiology*, vol. 291, no. 6, pp. H3043–H3049, 2006.

[38] K. E. Pyke and M. E. Tschakovsky, "Peak vs. total reactive hyperemia: which determines the magnitude of flow-mediated dilation?" *Journal of Applied Physiology*, vol. 102, no. 4, pp. 1510–1519, 2007.

[39] D. H. J. Thijssen, M. M. van Bemmel, L. M. Bullens et al., "The impact of baseline diameter on flow-mediated dilation differs in young and older humans," *The American Journal of Physiology—Heart and Circulatory Physiology*, vol. 295, no. 4, pp. H1594–H1598, 2008.

[40] M. L. Bots, J. Westerink, T. J. Rabelink, and E. J. P. De Koning, "Assessment of flow-mediated vasodilatation (FMD) of the brachial artery: effects of technical aspects of the FMD measurement on the FMD response," *European Heart Journal*, vol. 26, no. 4, pp. 363–368, 2005.

[41] K. E. Pyke and M. E. Tschakovsky, "The relationship between shear stress and flow-mediated dilatation: implications for the assessment of endothelial function," *The Journal of Physiology*, vol. 568, no. 2, pp. 357–369, 2005.

[42] S. H. Kubo, T. S. Rector, A. J. Bank, R. E. Williams, and S. M. Heifetz, "Endothelium-dependent vasodilation is attenuated in patients with heart failure," *Circulation*, vol. 84, no. 4, pp. 1589–1596, 1991.

[43] M. Spasojevic, S. A. Smith, J. M. Morris, and E. D. M. Gallery, "Peripheral arterial pulse wave analysis in women with pre-eclampsia and gestational hypertension," *BJOG*, vol. 112, no. 11, pp. 1475–1478, 2005.

[44] E. V. Tyldum, B. Backe, A. Støylen, and S. A. Slørdahl, "Maternal left ventricular and endothelial functions in preeclampsia," *Acta Obstetricia et Gynecologica Scandinavica*, vol. 91, no. 5, pp. 566–573, 2012.

[45] J. Torrado, I. Farro, Y. Zócalo et al., "Preeclampsia is associated with increased central aortic pressure, elastic arteries stiffness and wave reflections, and resting and recruitable endothelial dysfunction," *International Journal of Hypertension*, vol. 2015, Article ID 720683, 12 pages, 2015.

[46] K. H. Nicolaides, R. Bindra, O. M. Turan et al., "A novel approach to first-trimester screening for early pre-eclampsia combining serum PP-13 and Doppler ultrasound," *Ultrasound in Obstetrics and Gynecology*, vol. 27, no. 1, pp. 13–17, 2006.

[47] E. Scazzocchio and F. Figueras, "Contemporary prediction of preeclampsia," *Current Opinion in Obstetrics & Gynecology*, vol. 23, no. 2, pp. 65–71, 2011.

18

The Desire for Multiple Pregnancy among Patients with Infertility and Their Partners

Ida Lilywaty Md Latar and Nuguelis Razali

Department of Obstetrics & Gynaecology, Universiti Malaya, 59100 Kuala Lumpur, Malaysia

Correspondence should be addressed to Nuguelis Razali; nuguelis@ummc.edu.my

Academic Editor: Hind A. Beydoun

Objective. To study the predictors for desire for multiple pregnancies and the influence of providing information regarding the maternal and fetal complications associated with multiple pregnancies on their preference for multiple pregnancies. *Methods.* Couples attending an infertility clinic were offered to fill up a questionnaire separately. Following this, they were handed a pamphlet with information regarding the risks associated with multiple pregnancies. The patients will then be required to answer the question on the number of pregnancies desired again. *Results.* Two hundred fifty three out of 300 respondents completed the questionnaires adequately. A higher proportion of respondents, 60.3% of females and 57.9% of males, prefer singleton pregnancy. Patients who are younger than 35 years, with preexisting knowledge of risks associated with multiple pregnancies and previous treatment for infertility, have decreased desire for multiple pregnancies. However, for patients who are older than 35, with longer duration of infertility, and those patients who have preexisting knowledge of the increased risk, providing further information regarding the risks did not change their initial preferences. *Conclusion.* Providing and reinforcing knowledge on the risks to mother and fetus associated with multiple pregnancies did not decrease the preference for multiple pregnancies in patients.

1. Introduction

Assisted reproductive techniques (ART) have enabled many childless couples to achieve their dream of having a child of their own. The number of women undergoing ART treatment has increased tremendously over the past three decades, leading to more than 5 million children conceived by this treatment [1]. However, as ART traditionally involved ovarian stimulation and replacement of more than one embryo, it had contributed to a significantly higher number of multiple births.

The multiple birth rate from 376,971 European IVF treatment cycles in 2007 was reported as 22.3% (21.3% twins and 1% triplets), similar to rates in 2005 and 2006 (21.8 and 20.8%, resp.) [2]. The data from the Society for Assisted Reproduction Technology (SART) registry in the USA, based on 108,130 ART cycles, revealed a multiple birth rate of 35.4, of which 31.8% were twins, 3.5% were triplets, and 0.1% were higher order multiple [3].

As compared to singleton, twin and higher order pregnancies have contributed significantly to preterm deliveries. Prematurity, which is a main cause of neonatal morbidity and mortality, occurs in nearly one-half of all multiple pregnancies. It was reported that 42% of twins are born before 37 completed weeks, compared to 8% of singletons [4, 5]. The risk of mortality is increased six-fold in twins and 10–20-fold in triplets compared to singletons [6]. Multiple pregnancies are also associated with higher rate of spontaneous abortion and intrauterine fetal demise. It is also more likely to result in neonatal and infant death, cerebral palsy, and congenital birth defects [7].

Maternal complications that may be associated with multiple pregnancies are hypertensive disorders, abruptio placentae, caesarean delivery, and postpartum haemorrhage [8]. Women who had multiple births are at increased risk for depression and experiencing higher parenting stress [9].

Furthermore, the economic effect on society and the economic and emotional stresses on families that are associated with raising twins, triplets, and more children are becoming increasingly apparent [8, 10]. Following these concerns, multiple pregnancies are considered as a serious complication of assisted reproductive techniques (ART) and the American Society for Reproductive Medicine has actually designated reduction in the incidence of multifetal pregnancy resulting from ART "an essential goal for ART programs and their patients" [11].

Single embryo transfer (SET) is increasingly practiced worldwide in an effort to reduce rates of multiple births associated with ART. The rate of single embryo transfer was about 20% in Europe in 2005, but much higher rates are reported in some countries (69% in Sweden in 2005 and 57% in Australia and New Zealand in 2006) [12]. Although SET prevents multiple pregnancies, there are concerns that it might reduce pregnancy rates. The data from the Cochrane database 2014 showed that a live births rate (LBR) following a single cycle of double embryo transfer was 45% while the LBR following a single cycle of single embryo transfer was between 24% and 33%. The LBR following repeated single embryo transfer would be between 31% and 44%. However, the risk of twins was about seven times higher after double embryo transfer [13]. In Sweden, SET represented 67% of all transfers in 2004, with an almost unchanged delivery rate of 27% per transfer, whereas the IVF multiple birth rate was reduced to 5.6% [14]. The Turkish government implemented a new legislation starting March 2010 in an attempt to promote single-embryo transfer. According to the new regulation, only one embryo transfer is permitted in the first and second treatment cycles of patients under 35, a maximum of two embryos can be transferred in the third or further cycles, and a maximum of two embryos can be transferred to patients aged above 35 years [15].

A study by Kutlu et al. following the implementation of the new legislation showed that the overall clinical pregnancy rates were decreased from 39.9% to 34.5% and multiple pregnancy rates were decreased from 23.1% to 5.3%. The difference in pregnancy rates was not statistically significant while the difference in multiple pregnancy rates was statistically highly significant [16].

Regardless of the concerns above, a large proportion of infertility patients still appear to favour multiple pregnancies as an ideal treatment outcome [17]. For infertile patients who want more than one child, twin deliveries represent a favourable and cost effective treatment outcome that should be encouraged, in contrast to the current medical consensus [18, 19]. These preferences have been strongly associated with the patients' lack of knowledge about fertility treatment and multiple pregnancy as well as the associated risks [17, 20]. Previous data has shown that simple educational materials can improve knowledge of twin pregnancy risks and affect decision making [21]. In developing practices and policies of ARTs, it is important to take into account the interest of all parties involved. At a minimum, providers and patients need to be educated about the risks of multiple gestations so that steps can be taken to prevent adverse outcomes [14].

In Malaysia, very few data has been published to evaluate these matters. As ART in Malaysia is considered costly and not financially supported by the government, it would be beneficial to assess the patients' knowledge and preferences on this particular ground to further assist the clinician in fertility treatment and management of the patients.

The aim of this study is to determine the preferences on the number of pregnancies among infertility patients and their partners and to assess the effect of providing or reinforcing the information regarding the risks associated with multiple births. These include their demographic picture, their desire towards multiple pregnancies, and their knowledge about its risks as well as other factors that may affect their preferences such as age, sex, financial level, and prior knowledge on the risks of multiple pregnancies.

2. Materials and Methods

All the women and their spouses attending the infertility clinic in University Malaya Medical Centre (UMMC), Kuala Lumpur, during the period of six months from December 2009 until June 2010 were offered to fill in a pre-prepared questionnaire comprising 3 sections (Appendix A). The questionnaire was prepared in 2 languages (Bahasa Malaysia and English) as preferred by the subjects recruited. The patients and their partners were required to self-complete the questionnaire separately without consulting each other. The subjects include those first time attendees as well as patients coming for follow-up visits. The patients were required to respond to the questionnaire only once throughout their course of treatment in the infertility unit. The research was reviewed and approved by the UMMC Research Ethical Board (IRB reference number: 782.3).

The first section of the questionnaire includes subjects' demographic data such as age, sex, ethnicity, level of education, occupation, and estimated total family income. The next section of the questionnaire includes data on their fertility as well as any prior treatment received. At the end of the second section, subjects will be asked in order of preferences regarding the number of pregnancies they desire. This was prepared in a 4-point scale fashion with 1 indicating the most desirable number of pregnancies and 4 indicating the least. Following this, subjects will be given a pre-prepared multiple languages pamphlet that will provide information on the association of multiple pregnancies with fertility treatment as well as its risks (Appendix B). Subjects will then be required to answer the question on the number of pregnancy desired that was previously asked again.

Our analysis focused on the patients and their partners' desire for multiple pregnancies, their knowledge of the risks associated with it, and the association between demographic, infertility and treatment history, and knowledge and its effects on their desire for multiple pregnancies. Data was analysed using multiple logistic regression analysis (SPSS version 17). We identified independent variable associated with positive response as desire for multiple pregnancies. Continuous variables were analysed by means of 2-sample t-test and categorical responses were analysed by Fisher exact or chi-square test.

3. Results

A total of 300 questionnaires were distributed throughout the study. Out of these, 253 respondents completed the questionnaire while the remaining questionnaires were not included in the analysis as they were not fully completed with omitted answers. The 253 respondents included 107 men and 146 women.

Demographic data with the baseline characteristics of the respondents are shown in Table 1. The mean age of the female and male respondents was 31.7 years and 33.5 years, respectively. The mean duration of infertility for both groups was 51 months for female and 42.5 months for male respondents. Both groups have the mean total monthly income of around RM3500. Most of our respondents were well educated with almost 50% of the female and male respondents having at least a diploma or a degree in their respective fields. A smaller proportion of the female respondents already had children prior to this treatment as compared to their male partners (9.3% versus 14.4%). As expected, more women had received previous treatment as compared to their male counterparts (52.1% versus 33.6%).

More female and male respondents desired singleton pregnancy rather than multiple pregnancies but the difference between the two genders was not significant ($P = 0.71$) (Table 1). The possible associated factors were cross-tabulated according to desired number of foetuses in Table 2. A significant number of younger patients (<35 years old taken as the baseline) actually preferred singleton pregnancy compared to the older age group. Similarly, preexisting knowledge of risks of multiple pregnancies also significantly influenced the desire for singleton pregnancy. Total income and previous fertility treatment did not affect desire for multiple or singleton pregnancy.

Among those who desired twins and higher orders pregnancies, 46.7% of male and 44.8% of female respondents gave advancing age as the reason for preferences. 11.1% of male and 15.5% of female respondents, respectively, stated long duration of trying to conceive as the reason of preferring twins or higher orders pregnancies. Other reasons given were high cost of fertility treatment (2.2% versus 5.1%), wanting to complete family faster, worry of inability, or difficulties to get pregnant again or health factor.

Univariate and multivariate analysis was carried out to look for predictors of preference of multiple pregnancies (Table 3). Age more than 35 years is associated with increased preference while previous fertility treatment and preexisting knowledge on the risks of multiple pregnancies was associated with reduced preference.

Out of those who desired multiple pregnancies prior to exposure to knowledge of its risks, only 24.1% of female respondents and 37.8% of male respondents changed their preference from multiple pregnancies to singleton after being exposed to the information about multiple pregnancies. Univariate and multivariate analysis was performed to identify factors that are associated with continuous desire for multiple pregnancy even after given information regarding the risks of multiple pregnancies (Table 4). Respondents who are more than 35 years old and those with preexisting recognition regarding the risks of multiple pregnancy were significantly more likely to continue with their preference even after given additional information.

4. Discussion

Contrary to the previous data, more patients in our setting considered singleton pregnancy as an ideal treatment outcome even before being exposed to the knowledge of multiple pregnancies itself [19, 22]. Initially, we hypothesized that more patients would desire multiple pregnancies as ART is not funded in our country; therefore, multiple pregnancy is deemed as more cost effective for them. This positive finding might be because of the background of our patients who are mostly well educated with more exposure to the information itself even before being informed to them and perhaps cost really is not an issue. This finding is similar to other studies [23].

Our study has found that there is no significant difference in the desire of multiple pregnancies among our male and female respondents. This is in accordance with the previous data available which has shown that patient's sex did not affect desire for multiple births [22, 24].

Another interesting finding is that those patients who are younger have been found to have a significant desire for singleton as compared to multiple pregnancies as the ideal treatment outcome. This is in contrast to the study by Ryan et al. which showed that younger women preferred multiple pregnancies [17]. A possible explanation for this may be that younger patients are not pressured to complete their family earlier as compared to the older patients. However, on the other hand, there was no clear evidence to show significant preferences towards multiple pregnancies among older age groups.

Patients who are aware of the increased fetal risks associated with multiple pregnancies were significantly less likely to desire this outcome. This suggests that patients' prior information and knowledge regarding the risks will reduce their desire of having multiple pregnancies as the treatment outcome.

After the patients have been given the information regarding the risks of multiple pregnancies following fertility treatment, only a small proportion of those who had first chosen multiple pregnancies changed their decision to singleton pregnancy and this finding was not statistically significant. This may be due to the fact that those who opted for multiple pregnancies were already aware of the risks but still prefer multiple pregnancies due to reasons such as increasing age or desire to complete family faster. Other reasons such as desire for siblings, a positive attitude towards twins, and a wish to minimize physical and psychological stress through having as few IVF treatments as possible were given in a Danish study [25].

Various methods have been employed in order to provide patients with information regarding the risks associated with multiple pregnancies. This includes provision of information leaflets, additional discussion sessions, risk perception survey, and communication strategies utilizing the framing effect and fear appeal [21, 26, 27]. An empowerment programme which consisted of a decision aid kit, support of a nurse, and reimbursement of an additional treatment cycle was developed by van Perperstraten et al. in an attempt to persuade patients to choose elective SET. Their study reported

TABLE 1: Demographic data and baseline characteristics of respondents.

	Female (*n* = 146)	Male (*n* = 107)	*P* value
Age (years), mean (SD)	31.7 (4.4)	33.5 (5.5)	*P* 0.004
Duration of infertility (months), mean (SD)	51.0 (34.8)	42.5 (26.4)	*P* 0.29
Total income (RM), mean (SD)	3574.7 (1479.1)	3532.7 (1401.7)	*P* 0.82
Level of education, *n* (%)			
Primary school	2 (1.4%)	4 (3.7%)	
Secondary school	76 (52.1%)	57 (53.3%)	
Diploma/degree	63 (43.2%)	43 (40.2%)	
Postgraduate	5 (3.4%)	3 (2.8%)	
History of previous children, *n* (%)	10 (9.3%)	21 (14.4%)	
Previous treatment received, *n* (%)	76 (52.1%)	36 (33.6%)	
Desired number of babies with next fertility treatment, *n* (%)			
Singleton	88 (60.3%)	62 (57.9%)	*P* 0.71
Multiple pregnancies	58 (39.7%)	45 (42.1%)	
Decision changed following information regarding multiple pregnancies, *n* (%)	14 (24.1%)	17 (37.8%)	*P* 0.13

TABLE 2: Desire in order of pregnancy of 253 infertility patients and their partners with associated information.

	Desired singleton (*n* = 150)	Desired multiple pregnancies (*n* = 103)	*P* value
Total income > RM 3500	78 (52.0%)	54 (52.4%)	*P* 0.95
Age < 35 years old	121 (80.7%)	65 (63.1%)	*P* 0.02
Age > 35 years old	29 (19.3%)	38 (26.9%)	
Previous treatment received	63 (42.0%)	49 (47.6%)	*P* 0.38
Preexisting recognition of risks of multiple pregnancies	121 (80.7%)	66 (64.1%)	*P* 0.002

that patients who were administered the empowerment strategy were more likely to choose elective SET, but the differences between the empowerment and control group was much lower than the estimated goal of 25% based upon power calculations [28]. The results for these studies have been conflicting. Thus, the value of providing information regarding risks associated with multiple births to infertile patients and empowerment program with reimbursement has been shown to be limited [28].

Although more of our patients preferred singleton pregnancy compared to multiple pregnancies during the survey, we do acknowledge the fact that this might not translate to increase preference of single embryo transfer (SET) over double embryo transfer (DET). Højgaard et al. noted that the majority of their infertile couples currently in treatment preferred twins (58.7%) to one child at a time (37.9%) but a larger majority (78.5%) planned to have two embryos transferred in the next treatment. There was no association between opting for twins and having received information and feeling well informed [25]. The preference for DET is not only explained by a wish to have a high success rate and, thus, avoiding more treatments but also reflects a deliberate wish to have twins in the majority of couples [25]. In a review of twenty papers by Leese and Denton, patients in most studies would rather choose double-embryo transfer than single, mainly to maximize their chances of achieving a pregnancy

and did not necessarily reflect a preference for twins [29]. Similarly, Newton et al. also noted both women and men in their study tended to view 2ET as the most desirable option. However, attitudes toward SET changed markedly after providing patients with information about the risks of twin pregnancy [23].

The patients' preference for a singleton pregnancy as the preferred treatment outcome may indirectly assist the decision making process for the clinician in treating them. Based on our finding, with adequate counselling, younger patients might be more accepting of SET. Apart from providing risk information, patients also should be informed regarding the success rate of SET. To further improve the acceptability of SET, the outcome with cryopreserved embryos and protocols for frozen embryo transfer also need to be improved. It is worthwhile to note that even though most of our patients preferred singleton pregnancy, there is still a sizeable proportion of patients who preferred multiple pregnancy and are willing to take the risks associated with it. Thus, clinicians may need to take this preference into account after appropriate counselling and the absence of any medical conditions.

5. Conclusion

A higher proportion of patients with infertility actually prefer singleton pregnancy compared to multiple pregnancy.

TABLE 3: Univariate and multivariate analysis of predictors for multiple pregnancies outcome.

	Number of patients	Univariate analysis Hazard ratio (95% CI)	P	Multivariate analysis Hazard ratio (95% CI)	P
Total	253				
Age < 35 years	186	1.00		1.00	
Age ≥ 35 years	67	2.44 (138–4.31)	0.002	2.29 (1.26–4.16)	0.014
Treatment IUI					
No	230	1.00			
Yes	23	0.41 (0.17–0.98)	0.044		
Preexisting recognition of risks of multiple pregnancy					
No	54	1.00		1.00	
Yes	187	0.30 (0.16–0.56)	<0.001	0.30 (0.16–0.57)	<0.001

TABLE 4: Univariate and multivariate analysis of predictors for a continuous desire of multiple pregnancies outcome.

	Number of patients	Univariate analysis Hazard ratio (95% CI)	P	Multivariate analysis Hazard ratio (95% CI)	P
Total	103				
Age < 35 years	65	1.00		1.00	
Age ≥ 35 years	38	3.33 (1.22–9.11)	0.019	3.57 (1.24–10.43)	0.019
Duration of infertility					
<5 year	70	1.00			
≥5 years	33	3.31 (1.14–9.63)	0.028		
Preexisting recognition of risks of multiple pregnancy					
No	35	1.00	0.001	1.00	
Yes	66	4.32 (1.76–10.60)		4.59 (1.79–11.72)	0.001

The desire on multiple pregnancies among patients with infertility is not affected by sex or financial factors. Younger patients significantly prefer singleton as compared to multiple pregnancies. Patients with prior knowledge on the risks of multiple pregnancies were significantly less likely to desire this outcome. However, for those patients who prefer multiple pregnancies, reinforcing the knowledge on risks of multiple pregnancies did not reduce their desire.

Limitations

The limitation of this study was the pamphlet of information given to the patients. Different respondents may interpret the magnitude of the risks implied by the pamphlets differently.

Appendices

A. The Desire for Multiple Pregnancies among Patients with Infertility and Their Partners

A.1. Questionnaire

(1) Age: ....years old

(2) Sex: ....Male/Female

(3) Race: ....Malay/Chinese/Indian/Others

(4) Level of education: Primary school/Secondary school/Degree/Postgraduate

(5) Occupation (please state): ....

(6) Clinic attendance: First visit/Follow up

(7) How long have you and your partner have been trying to conceive? .... years and ....months

(8) Number of children you had before (including with previous partners, if any?) ....

(9) Which of the following fertility treatments have you had before? (Please tick correct answer)

.... Fertility pills

.... Surgery to open /repair blocked tubes

.... IUI (Stimulation of ovaries & insemination of sperm into uterus)

.... IVF (In Vitro Fertilization/test tube baby treatment)

.... others.

(10) Have you ever been counseled before regarding the risk of multiple pregnancies following fertility treatment? YES/NO.

(11) If the current fertility treatment is successful, what would be the preferred number of babies that you would like to have (please put in order of numbers, 1 for most desirable, followed by 2, 3 and 4).

……… Singleton pregnancy (1 baby)

……… Twins (2 babies)

……… Triplets (3 babies)

……… Quadruplets (4 babies)

Please state your reasons for making the choices above:
……………………………………

(12) Do you think that there are more dangers for the babies in a multiple pregnancy (2 or more babies) compared to singleton (1 baby)? YES/NO.

A.2. Please Answer This Question Again after You Have Read the Information Leaflet Provided (Your Answer May Be Different from the Previous Answer that You Have Given).

(11) If the current fertility treatment is successful, what would be the preferred number of babies that you would like to have (please put in order of numbers, 1 for most desirable, followed by 2, 3 and 4)

………… Singleton pregnancy (1 baby)

………… Twins (2 babies)

………… Triplets (3 babies)

………… Quadruplets (4 babies)

B. Information Leaflet

Dear participants,

Please read through this information leaflet before answering the last question:

Fertility treatments are associated with increased number of multiple pregnancies

Multiple pregnancies have generally higher risks as compared to single (one baby) pregnancy. The risks involve the mother as well as the fetus/baby.

The mother is at increased risk of several pregnancy complications, including:

(1) Miscarriage

(2) Hyperemesis (Severe vomiting in early pregnancy)

(3) Premature labour and delivery

(4) Anaemia (reduced red blood cells)

(5) Pre-eclampsia (complicated hypertension in pregnancy)

(6) Antepartum hemorrhage (vaginal bleeding during pregnancy)

(7) Postpartum hemorrhage (excessive vaginal bleeding after delivery)

(8) Polyhydramnios (Excessive amniotic fluid) which may lead to abdominal discomfort and breathlessness

(9) Operative delivery (caesarean section)

(10) Prolonged stay in hospital

The babies are at increased risk of:

(1) Preterm labour: Twins are 5 times more likely to be born preterm compared to singleton. Almost 15% of triplets (pregnancies with 3 babies) deliver before 30 weeks of gestation. Preterm babies have higher risks of:

  (i) Neurological problems like encephalopathy, cerebral palsy and intraventricular hemorrhage

  (ii) (Bleeding in brain)

  (iii) Retinopathy (poor development of the retina of the eye)

  (iv) Developmental disability

  (v) Heart problems

  (vi) Respiratory problems: Respiratory distress syndrome, chronic lung disease

  (vii) Gastrointestinal and metabolic issues can arise from low sugar level, feeding difficulties, low calcium, inguinal hernia and necrotizing enterocolitis (immature gut)

  (viii) Hematologic complications include anemia, low platelet and jaundice.

  (ix) Severe infection including sepsis, pneumonia and urinary tract infection.

(1) Intrauterine growth restriction (babies born below the normal weight range): 25-33% risks

(2) Single fetal death

(3) Cerebral Palsy

(4) Abnormal babies

(5) Twin to twin transfusion syndrome (TTTS): Complication of unequal blood supply when two or more fetuses share a single sac and placenta. Severe TTTS has a 60-100% fetal death rate.

Conflict of Interests

The authors declare that there is no conflict of interests regarding the publication of this paper.

References

[1] S. D. McDonald, K. Murphy, J. Beyene, and A. Ohlsson, "Perinatel outcomes of singleton pregnancies achieved by in vitro fertilization: a systematic review and meta-analysis," *Journal of Obstetrics and Gynaecology Canada*, vol. 27, no. 5, pp. 449–459, 2005.

[2] J. de Mouzon, V. Goossens, S. Bhattacharya et al., "Assisted reproductive technology in Europe, 2007: results generated from European registers by ESHRE," *Human Reproduction*, vol. 27, no. 4, pp. 954–966, 2012.

[3] Society for Assisted Reproductive Technology and American Society for Reproductive Medicine, "Assisted reproductive technology in the United States: 2001 results generated from

the American Society for Reproductive Medicine/Society for Assisted Reproductive Technology registry," *Fertility and Sterility*, vol. 87, pp. 1253–1266, 2001.

[4] J. Moise, A. Laor, Y. Armon, I. Gur, and R. Gale, "The outcome of twin pregnancies after IVF," *Human Reproduction*, vol. 13, no. 6, pp. 1702–1705, 1998.

[5] W. N. Spellacy, A. Handler, and C. D. Ferre, "A case-control study of 1253 twin pregnancies from a 1982–1987 perinatal data base," *Obstetrics and Gynecology*, vol. 75, no. 2, pp. 168–171, 1990.

[6] O. Ozturk and A. Templeton, "Multiple pregnancy in assisted reproduction techniques," in *Current Practices and Controversies in Assisted Reproduction*, E. Vayena, P. J. Rowe, and P. D. Griffin, Eds., pp. 220–234, WHO, Geneva, Switzerland, 2002.

[7] M. Dhont, P. De Sutter, G. Ruyssinck, G. Martens, and A. Bekaert, "Perinatal outcome of pregnancies after assisted reproduction: A case-control study," *American Journal of Obstetrics and Gynecology*, vol. 181, no. 3, pp. 688–695, 1999.

[8] FIGO Committee for the Ethical Aspects of Human Reproduction and Women's Health, "Ethical guidelines in the prevention of iatrogenic multiple pregnancy," *European Journal of Obstetrics & Gynecology and Reproductive Biology*, vol. 96, pp. 209–210, 2001.

[9] K. Thorpe, J. Golding, I. MacGillivray, and R. Greenwood, "Comparison of prevalence of depression in mothers of twins and mothers of singletons," *British Medical Journal*, vol. 302, no. 6781, pp. 875–878, 1991.

[10] W. L. Kinzler, C. V. Ananth, and A. M. Vintzileos, "Medical and economic effects of twin gestations," *Journal of the Society for Gynecologic Investigation*, vol. 7, no. 6, pp. 321–327, 2000.

[11] "ASRM Guidelines on number of embryos transferred. A Practice Committee Report," pp. 1-2, November 1999.

[12] American Society for Reproductive Medicine, "Elective single embryo transfer," *Fertility and Sterility*, vol. 97, pp. 835–842, 2012.

[13] Z. Pandian, S. Bhattacharya, O. Ozturk, G. I. Serour, and A. Templeton, "Number of embryos for transfer following in-vitro fertilisation or intra-cytoplasmic sperm injection," *Cochrane Database of Systematic Reviews*, vol. 15, no. 2, 2004.

[14] C. Bergh, A. T. Kjellberg, and P. O. Karlstrom, "Single-embryo fertilization in vitro. Maintained birth rate in spite of dramatically reduced multiple birth frequency," *Läkartidningen*, vol. 102, pp. 3444–3447, 2005.

[15] B. Urman and K. Yakin, "New Turkish legislation on assisted reproductive techniques and centres: a step in the right direction?" *Reproductive BioMedicine Online*, vol. 21, no. 6, pp. 729–731, 2010.

[16] P. Kutlu, O. Atvar, O. F. Vanlioglu et al., "Effect of the new legislation and single embryo transfer policy in Turkey on assisted reproduction outcomes: preliminary results," *Reproductive BioMedicine Online*, vol. 22, no. 2, pp. 208–214, 2011.

[17] G. L. Ryan, S. H. Zhang, A. Dokras, C. H. Syrop, and B. J. Van Voorhis, "The desire of infertile patients for multiple births," *Fertility and Sterility*, vol. 81, no. 3, pp. 500–504, 2004.

[18] N. Gleicher and D. Barad, "Twin pregnancy, contrary to consensus, is a desirable outcome in infertility," *Fertility and Sterility*, vol. 91, no. 6, pp. 2426–2431, 2009.

[19] N. Gleicher, D. P. Campbell, C. L. Chan et al., "The desire for multiple births in couples with infertility problems contradicts present practice patterns," *Human Reproduction*, vol. 10, no. 5, pp. 1079–1084, 1995.

[20] M. D'Alton, "Infertility and the desire for multiple births," *Fertility and Sterility*, vol. 81, no. 3, pp. 523–525, 2004.

[21] G. L. Ryan, A. E. T. Sparks, C. S. Sipe, C. H. Syrop, A. Dokras, and B. J. van Voorhis, "A mandatory single blastocyst transfer policy with educational campaign in a United States IVF program reduces multiple gestation rates without sacrificing pregnancy rates," *Fertility and Sterility*, vol. 88, no. 2, pp. 354–360, 2007.

[22] T. J. Child, A. M. Henderson, and S. L. Tan, "The desire for mulitple pregnancy in male and female infertility patients," *Human Reproduction*, vol. 19, no. 3, pp. 558–561, 2004.

[23] C. R. Newton, J. McBride, V. Feyles, F. Tekpetey, and S. Power, "Factors affecting patients' attitudes toward single- and multiple-embryo transfer," *Fertility and Sterility*, vol. 87, no. 2, pp. 269–278, 2007.

[24] S. K. Kalra, M. P. Milad, S. C. Klock, and W. A. Grobman, "Infertility patients and their partners: differences in the desire for twin gestations," *Obstetrics and Gynecology*, vol. 102, no. 1, pp. 152–155, 2003.

[25] A. Højgaard, L. D. M. Ottosen, U. Kesmodel, and H. J. Ingerslev, "Patient attitudes towards twin pregnancies and single embryo transfer—a questionnaire study," *Human Reproduction*, vol. 22, no. 10, pp. 2673–2678, 2007.

[26] S. Murray, A. Shetty, A. Rattray, V. Taylor, and S. Bhattacharya, "A randomized comparison of alternative methods of information provision on the acceptability of elective single embryo transfer," *Human Reproduction*, vol. 19, no. 4, pp. 911–916, 2004.

[27] O. B. A. Van Den Akker and S. Purewal, "Elective single-embryo transfer: Persuasive communication strategies can affect choice in a young British population," *Reproductive BioMedicine Online*, vol. 23, no. 7, pp. 838–850, 2011.

[28] A. van Peperstraten, W. Nelen, R. Grol et al., "The effect of a multifaceted empowerment strategy on decision making about the number of embryos transferred in in vitro fertilisation: randomised controlled trial," *British Medical Journal*, vol. 341, article c2501, 2010.

[29] B. Leese and J. Denton, "Attitudes towards single embryo transfer, twin and higher order pregnancies in patients undergoing infertility treatment: A review," *Human Fertility*, vol. 13, no. 1, pp. 28–34, 2010.

19

Total Laparoscopic Hysterectomy with Prior Uterine Artery Ligation at Its Origin

Vidyashree Ganesh Poojari,[1] Vidya Vishwanath Bhat,[1] and Ravishankar Bhat[2]

[1] Department of OBG, Radhakrishna Multispeciality Hospital, Bangalore, Karnataka, India
[2] Department of General Surgery, Radhakrishna Multispeciality Hospital, Bangalore, Karnataka, India

Correspondence should be addressed to Vidyashree Ganesh Poojari; drvidyaganesh@gmail.com

Academic Editor: Lauren A. Wise

We compared the duration of surgery, blood loss, and complications between patients in whom both uterine arteries were ligated at the beginning of total laparoscopic hysterectomy (TLH) and patients in whom ligation was done after cornual pedicle. Using a prospective study in a gynecologic laparoscopic center, a total of 52 women who underwent TLH from June 2013 to January 2014 were assigned into two groups. In group A, uterine arteries were ligated after the cornual pedicles as done conventionally. In group B, TLH was done by ligating both uterine arteries at the beginning of the procedure. All the other pedicles were desiccated using harmonic scalpel or bipolar diathermy. Uterus with cervix was removed vaginally or by morcellation. The indication for TLH was predominantly dysfunctional uterine bleeding and myomas in both groups. In group A, the average duration of surgery was 71 minutes, when compared to 60 minutes in group B ($P < 0.001$). In group A, the total blood loss was 70 mL, when compared to 43 mL in group B (P value < 0.001). There were no major complications in both groups. To conclude, prior uterine artery ligation at its origin during TLH reduces the blood loss and surgical duration as well as the complications during surgery.

1. Introduction

Hysterectomy is a common gynecological procedure worldwide for benign uterine disease. Traditionally, this has been via the abdominal or vaginal routes [1]. In the present era, hysterectomies are undertaken using minimal access techniques. Total laparoscopic hysterectomy (TLH) is performed entirely by the laparoscopic route, including closure of the vaginal vault, with the uterus being removed vaginally or by morcellation [2].

Today, lap hysterectomy is a safe and feasible technique to manage benign uterine pathology as it offers minimal postoperative discomfort, shorter hospital stay, rapid convalescence, and early return to the activities of daily living [3]. Considerable technical advances in this procedure have occurred during the last few years.

In our study, we have modified the steps and started with the ligation of the uterine artery at its origin from the internal iliac artery on both sides causing transient uterine ischemia as most blood enters the uterus through these vessels especially its ascending branch [4]. The hypothesis of this study proposes that, soon after occlusion, blood within the myometrium clots and the myometrium becomes hypoxic.

The aim of this study was to compare conventional TLH to prior uterine artery ligation at its origin.

2. Materials and Methods

It was a prospective randomized controlled study conducted from June 2013 to January 2014. Total of 52 cases were included in the study of which 26 underwent conventional total laparoscopic hysterectomy and another 26, underwent uterine artery ligation at its origin prior to total laparoscopic hysterectomy. Ethical clearance and informed consent were obtained for the study.

All patients underwent preoperative evaluation. Patients were kept nil by mouth 12 hours before the procedure and no bowel preparation was done prior to surgery. Catheterization of the urinary bladder was done preoperatively. Antibiotic prophylaxis was given to all patients included in the study. Compression devices were given to all patients for prophylaxis against possible thromboembolic episodes. Subcutaneous low molecular weight heparin was given postoperatively in obese patients.

3. Surgical Technique

Under general anesthesia, the patient was placed in modified lithotomy position. A Veress needle is inserted at the umbilicus or supraumbilical site depending on the size of the uterus and abdomen is insufflated with carbon dioxide at initial pressure of 20 mm Hg and maintenance at 15 mm Hg. A 10 mm trocar is inserted blindly and 10 mm telescope is introduced through this port. Uterus and the adnexa were visualized. Three additional 5mm ports are introduced: one along the left spinoumbilical line at the junction of medial 2/3rd and lateral 1/3rd, second port at right angles to the previous port two ports, and a third 5 mm port placed around 2 cm below and to the right of umbilicus. The entire abdomen is surveyed before starting the procedure. The size of the uterus, presence of myomas, and adnexa and course of ureters are visualized. Manipulation of the uterus was done with a 5 mm myoma spiral laparoscopically. No vaginal manipulators were used. Uterine artery was dissected by a lateral approach. A window was created in the broad ligament, close to the uterine vessels. The ascending branch of the uterine artery is identified close to the isthmus (Figure 1). The uterine vessels are ligated at this level close to the uterus using 1-0 delayed absorbable suture material or coagulated using bipolar diathermy (Figure 2). The uterine artery is not sutured away from the uterus as the ureters cross beneath them at that level. Dissecting the uterovesical fold and pushing the bladder down move the ureters laterally and decrease the risk of including them in the suture. The vasculature of the uterus is thus secured and this is evidenced by the color change in the fundus, which becomes pale. The cornual pedicles on one side are then desiccated and cut either using bipolar diathermy or the harmonic ultracision. The ligated uterine pedicles are cut. The uterosacral and cardinal ligaments are desiccated and cut. The position of the myoma spiral is then changed so that the opposite side pedicles can be taken care of.

If both ovaries need to be removed, the infundibulopelvic ligaments are desiccated and cut. Now a vaginal cuff is introduced through the vagina to identify the vault and the anterior lip of cervix held with a tenaculum. Vault cut laparoscopically using monopolar hook and the specimen is detached completely. The uterus with cervix is delivered vaginally if small. In case of large uteri, the specimen can be retrieved by morcellation through abdominal port. We prefer to use the contralateral ports for suturing. The right midquadrant port and the left lower quadrant port are ergonomically apt for suturing. The vaginal vault is sutured with number 1 delayed absorbable suture (vicryl). Ports

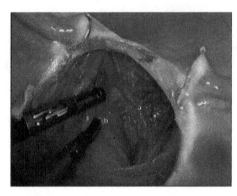

FIGURE 1: Identifying (a) uterine artery and (b) ureter by lateral dissection.

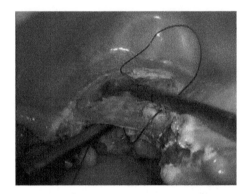

FIGURE 2: Prior ligation of uterine vessels.

closed using staples. The total blood loss is calculated from the suction apparatus. The blood in the suction tube is also measured to give the accurate value. No irrigation is used throughout the procedure until the calculation of the total blood loss. Peritoneal lavage is given with normal saline solution and 500 mL of normal saline is left in the peritoneal cavity. The catheter is removed after 6 hours and liquid diet started after peristalsis is established. The patient is discharged the following day and called for follow-up after 7 days.

4. Results

52 cases were included in the study, of which 26 underwent conventional TLH (Group A) and another 26 underwent TLH with prior uterine artery ligation at its origin (Group B). Sociodemographic data were similar in both groups. The main symptoms of patients were similar in both groups, with the predominant being menorrhagia (74.9% in group A and 74.1% in group B). Indication for surgery also revealed similar results in both groups as shown in Table 1. In group A, 72.9% of women had previous normal delivery and 27.1% had previous cesarean section and in group B 68% had previous normal delivery and 22% had previous cesarean section. In patients with previous cesarean section, because of dense bladder adhesions in some cases, there were difficulties in dissection.

TABLE 1: Indications for surgery in both groups.

Diagnosis	Group A		Group B	
	No.	%	No.	%
Abnormal uterine bleeding (AUB)*	13	50.0	14	53.8
Endometriosis	3	11.5	3	11.5
Fibroid	10	38.4	10	38.4
Total	26	100.0	26	100.0

* AUB are those cases where medical management failed.

TABLE 2: Comparison of blood loss and duration of surgery between groups A and B.

Parameters	Group A	Group B	P value
Duration of surgery (min)	71.35 ± 5.21	60.77 ± 5.04	<0.001
Blood loss (mL)	70.96 ± 18.33	43.08 ± 5.67	<0.001

Clinical size of the uterus ranged from 10 weeks to 22 weeks in both groups. The hemoglobin levels in all patients of both groups were above 9 g/dL. None of them required preoperative blood transfusion. In group A, 64.6% of specimens were retrieved vaginally and 35.4% of specimens were morcellated and retrieved. In group B, 68.4% of specimens were removed vaginally and 31.6% were retrieved by morcellation.

Total duration of surgery and blood loss in both groups were compared (Table 2). In group A, the average duration of surgery was 71 minutes. In group B, the average duration of surgery was 60 minutes. The comparison between the 2 groups revealed a statistically significant difference ($P < 0.001$) in duration of surgery between the 2 groups. The time taken was less in patients where the uterine artery was prior ligated.

In group A, the total blood loss was 70 mL. In group B, the total blood loss was 43 mL. The comparison between the 2 groups revealed a statistically significant difference (P value < 0.001). The data reveal that a significant decrease in blood loss and need for blood transfusion existed in group B where the uterine arteries were ligated before dividing the cornual structures.

There were no major complications in both of the groups. One patient in Group B with multiple fibroids and previous 2 lower segment cesarean section (LSCS) had bladder injury, detected postoperatively, and was treated conservatively with catheterization for 2 weeks.

5. Discussion

Total laparoscopic hysterectomy is currently accepted as an alternative to standard abdominal hysterectomy.

The vascular supply of the uterus is mainly derived from the uterine and ovarian arteries. Because most blood enters the uterus through the uterine arteries, transient uterine ischemia occurs after uterine artery ligation [5]. Bilateral uterine vessel ligation is an efficient method to obliterate the blood flow to the uterus [6].

Like most studies, we believe that the main step in hysterectomy is securing the uterine vascular pedicle [7]. Enlarged uteri allow limited access to uterine vascular pedicles depending on the size and location of myomas and may be associated with high risk of complications such as hemorrhage, ureteric injury. Prior dissection of uterine artery at its origin and ligating helps in reducing the blood supply and also lowering the risk of ureteral injury [7, 8].

To reduce the total blood loss and the duration of surgery, in this study we ligated the uterine arteries as the first step before tackling the other pedicles. In case of very large uterus, it may sometimes be difficult to dissect the ureter away from the uterine arteries properly. In such situations, coagulation of uterine vessels poses the risk of thermal damage to the ureters if they were not fully mobilized. Therefore, it is best to perform intracorporeal suturing of uterine vessels.

Our study showed that the average blood loss during the procedure is considerably reduced if the uterine vessels are primarily handled at its origin as compared to the study done by Sinha et al. [7]. The fear of ureteric injury is mostly caused by lack of familiarity with the pelvic anatomy. Once the bladder is dissected down, the ureters fall laterally and move away with the peritoneum. Hence, the risk of including the ureters in the suture is practically negligible. The risk of ureteric injuries is lower using suture compared with bipolar desiccation or staples [9].

No major complications occurred in our study. Only one patient in Group B with multiple fibroids and previous 2 LSCS had bladder injury, detected postoperatively, and was treated conservatively with catheterization for 2 weeks comparable to Sinha et al. [7].

6. Conclusion

Prior uterine artery ligation at its origin during TLH reduces the blood loss and surgical duration as well as the complications during surgery. As the expertise of the surgeon increases in retroperitoneal dissection, the duration of the procedure also reduces considerably.

Conflict of Interests

The authors declare that there is no conflict of interests regarding the publication of this paper.

References

[1] R. D. Clayton, "Hysterectomy," *Best Practice & Research Clinical Obstetrics & Gynaecology*, vol. 20, no. 1, pp. 73–87, 2006.

[2] H. Reich and L. Roberts, "Laparoscopic hysterectomy in current gynecological practice," *Reviews in Gynaecological Practice*, vol. 3, no. 1, pp. 32–40, 2003.

[3] H. Reich, F. McGlynn, and L. Sekel, "Total laparoscopic hysterectomy," *Gynaecological Endoscopy*, vol. 2, no. 2, pp. 59–63, 1993.

[4] M. Lichtinger, F. Burbank, L. Hallson, S. Herbert, J. Uyeno, and M. Jones, "The time course of myometrial ischemia

and reperfusion after laparoscopic uterine artery occlusion—theoretical implications," *Journal of the American Association of Gynecologic Laparoscopists*, vol. 10, no. 4, pp. 553–565, 2003.

[5] R. Sinha, A. Hegde, N. Warty, and N. Patil, "Laparoscopic excision of very large myomas," *Journal of the American Association of Gynecologic Laparoscopists*, vol. 10, no. 4, pp. 461–468, 2003.

[6] F. Nezhat, C. Nezhat, S. Gordon, and E. Wilkins, "Laparoscopic versus abdominal hysterectomy," *Journal of Reproductive Medicine for the Obstetrician and Gynecologist*, vol. 37, no. 3, pp. 247–250, 1992.

[7] R. Sinha, M. Sundaram, Y. A. Nikam, A. Hegde, and C. Mahajan, "Total laparoscopic hysterectomy with earlier uterine artery ligation," *Journal of Minimally Invasive Gynecology*, vol. 15, no. 3, pp. 355–359, 2008.

[8] W. Bateman, "Treatment of intractable menorrhagia by bilateral uterine vessel interruption," *American Journal of Obstetrics & Gynecology*, vol. 89, no. 6, pp. 825–827, 1964.

[9] M. K. Whiteman, S. D. Hillis, D. J. Jamieson et al., "Inpatient hysterectomy surveillance in the United States, 2000–2004," *American Journal of Obstetrics and Gynecology*, vol. 198, no. 1, pp. 34–e7, 2008.

20

Body Mass Index and Pregnancy Outcome after Assisted Reproduction Treatment

Khaled Kasim[1] and Ahmed Roshdy[2]

[1] Department of Public Health and Community Medicine, Faculty of Medicine, Al-Azhar University, Nasr City, Cairo, Egypt
[2] Assisted Reproductive Technology (ART) Unit, International Islamic Centre for Population Studies and Research (IICPSR), Al-Azhar University, Cairo, Egypt

Correspondence should be addressed to Khaled Kasim; kasimyhr@yahoo.com

Academic Editor: Hind A. Beydoun

The present study aimed to evaluate the impact of body mass index (BMI) on pregnancy outcome after intracytoplasmic sperm injection (ICSI). The study analyzed pregnancy outcome of 349 women who underwent ICSI by their BMI: <25, 25–<30, and ≥30 kg/m^2. The associations were generated by applying logistic regression models. A significant reduction in positive pregnancy outcome was observed among overweight and obese women (odds ratio (OR) = 0.50; 95% confidence interval (CI) = 0.25–0.99 for overweight women and OR = 0.45; 95% CI = 0.20–0.89 for obese women). These estimates show that the pregnancy rates are reduced with increasing BMI. The effect of obesity on pregnancy outcome was absent when three and more embryos were transferred. Our study contributes to the reports linking overweight and obesity with decreased positive pregnancy outcome after ICSI and suggests women's age, infertility type, and number of embryos transferred to modify this reducing effect.

1. Introduction

Body mass index (BMI) has an adverse effect on reproduction [1]. Overweight women have a higher incidence of menstrual dysfunction and anovulation, possibly because of altered secretion of gonadotropin releasing hormone, sex hormone binding globulin, ovarian and adrenal androgen, and luteinising hormone and also because of altered insulin resistance [2]. A body mass index that was either high or low was associated with reduced probability of achieving pregnancy in women receiving assisted reproduction treatment. Mechanisms through which body mass affects reproduction that have been cited include menstrual disturbance and anovulation [3] but these problems can be overcome through assisted reproduction treatment. There is no evidence that body mass affects the quality of the embryo and therefore the pregnancy rate. Other mechanisms may be proposed such as altered receptivity of the uterus after transfer of embryos, possibly because of disturbed endometrial function [2].

The prevalence of obesity in infertile women is high, and there is growing evidence that BMI is associated with pregnancy outcome after ART. Several recent and previous studies have linked overweight and obesity to low pregnancy rate [4–8] and spontaneous abortion [9] in ART programs. Obesity is also potentially modifiable, possibly amenable to low cost, noninvasive self-management by patients. These studies, however, did not examine the interaction (effect modification) between BMI and other related factors on the probability of pregnancy outcome in these women. According to published studies [10, 11], patient's age, infertility type, and number of transferred embryos appeared to be the most important factors affecting pregnancy outcome after ICSI. The current study aimed to examine the association of pregnancy outcome with BMI and to assess the possible effect modification of women's age, infertility type, and number of transferred embryos on the probability of positive pregnancy outcome associated with body mass index in infertile women receiving assisted reproduction treatment.

2. Methods

A retrospective study was designed to examine the association of pregnancy outcome with BMI and to examine the

TABLE 1: Distribution of the studied women by body mass index in relation to their characteristics.

Characteristics	Body mass index (kg/m^2)			P value
	<25 (n = 51)	25–<30 (n = 184)	≥30 (n = 114)	
Age (years)	27.3 ± 4.5	29.8 ± 5.4	32.8 ± 5.7	0.001*
Infertility duration (years)	5.4 ± 3.9	7.5 ± 4.7	8.5 ± 5.3	0.001*
Cycle length (days)	27.6 ± 3.4	28.9 ± 8.1	31.5 ± 13.2	0.03*
FSH (MIU/mL)	6.5 ± 2.5	6.2 ± 2.9	6.4 ± 2.6	0.78
LH†	6.7 ± 3.4	5.3 ± 2.7	5.1 ± 2.4	0.004*
PRL**	18.1 ± 16.6	15.5 ± 10.1	15.4 ± 10.9	0.45
E2 (pg/mL)	76.7 ± 59.9	74.2 ± 55.8	70.1 ± 51.6	0.82
Endometrial thickness	10.5 ± 2.2	10.5 ± 2.2	10.7 ± 2.1	0.68
HCG days	13.2 ± 2.4	13.7 ± 2.6	13.2 ± 2.2	0.10
Number of embryo transfer	2.8 ± 1.0	2.8 ± 0.9	2.8 ± 0.9	0.99
Infertility type				
Primary	46 (15%)	158 (53%)	94 (32%)	0.41
Secondary	5 (10%)	26 (50%)	20 (40%)	

*Significant.
†Luteinizing hormone.
**Prolactin hormone.

possible effect modification of women's age, infertility type, and number of transferred embryos on the observed association. The study extracted data from the files of 349 infertile women who underwent assisted fertilization at the ART Unit, the International Islamic Center for Population Researches and Studies (IICPRS), Al-Azhar University, during 2011. Three hundred forty-nine files were selected randomly from the ART medical data archives according to the estimated sample size. Because of missing outcome data, only one file was excluded from study analyses. The sample size is calculated according to the estimated average pregnancy rate in the studied center during the previous years (25%) and to an assumed precision of 0.04 with confidence interval of 95% and probability value of 0.05. According to pregnancy outcome, a nested case-control approach is designed where women with positive pregnancy outcome were considered as cases and those with negative pregnancy outcome as controls. The study design was approved by medical ethical committee at ART Unit. The collected data were managed and analyzed confidentially and anonymously.

The main outcome variable was the pregnancy outcome. Urine and/or serum Human Chorionic Gonadotrophin (HCG) measurement was routinely obtained on days 14–17 after embryo transfer, and positive pregnancy is confirmed following HCG rise. The main studied variables were categorized for the clarity of data analysis and presentation of results as follows: age is classified into three categories according to tertile distribution of the studied women: <27 years, 27–33 years, and >33 years; and three BMI subgroups were formed: <25 kg/m^2 (normal), 25–>30 kg/m^2 (overweight), and ≥30 kg/m^2(obese) [12]. The number of transferred embryos was classified into three categories (one embryo transfer, two embryos transfer, and three and more embryos transfer).

The collected data were analysed by using the statistical analysis system (SAS) software package [13]. Chi-square and t-tests were used as appropriate to compare the studied women by BMI in relation to their characteristics. Logistic regression models were used to estimate odds ratios and their 95% confidence intervals for the association of positive pregnancy outcome and BMI. To explore the possible effect modification of patient's age, type of infertility, and number of embryo transfer on the probability of positive pregnancy outcome associated with BMI, we incorporated the main effect variables and their cross-product terms into logistic regression models for testing of interaction based on a multiplicative model. P values of Wald test <0.05 were considered as evidence of statistical interaction.

3. Results

Of the studied 349 women, 52% were overweight and 32% were obese. The positive pregnancy rate among the whole studied women was 21% (75 of 349). The positive pregnancy rate is varied by BMI where it was 33%, 22%, and 18% in normal, overweight, and obese women, respectively. Table 1 presents the women characteristics by BMI strata. There were significant differences among BMI strata regarding age, infertility duration, cycle length, and luteinising hormone (LH) level, where the highest mean age, infertility duration, cycle length, and the lowest mean LH level were among obese women. On the other hand, no significant differences among the three BMI strata were observed regarding other studied factors.

Table 2 shows odds ratios (ORs) and their 95% confidence intervals for the association of positive pregnancy outcome with BMI in the unadjusted and adjusted logistic model. The results of both models were nearly the same with no

TABLE 2: Odds ratios (OR) and their 95% confidence intervals (CI) for the association of BMI with positive pregnancy outcome.

Studied factor	Positive pregnancy women	Negative pregnancy women	OR	95% CI	P-trend
Body mass index (kg/m^2)[*]					
<25	17	34	1.00	Ref.	
25–<30	37	147	0.50	0.25–0.99	
≥30	21	93	0.45	0.21–0.95	0.04
Body mass index (kg/m^2)[†]					
<25	17	34	1.00	Ref.	
25–<30	37	147	0.50	0.25–0.99	
≥30	21	93	0.45	0.20–0.99	

[*]Unadjusted model.
[†]Model adjusted by age groups, type of infertility, number of embryo transfer, HCG days endometrial thickness, and hormonal profiles.

TABLE 3: Positive pregnancy outcome associated with body mass index (kg/m^2) by age groups, infertility type, and number of embryo transfer (ET).

Studied factor	Body mass index (BMI) kg/m^2						P-interaction
	<25		25–<30		≥30		
	OR	95% CI	OR	95% CI	OR	95% CI	
Age groups							
<27 years	1.00	—	0.30	0.10–0.85	0.23	0.05–1.00	
27–33 years	1.00	—	1.02	0.50–1.95	0.95	0.30–2.45	0.46
>33 years	1.00	—	0.20	0.10–0.98	0.30	0.15–1.30	
Type of infertility							
Primary	1.00	—	0.27	0.15–0.98	0.35	0.12–0.99	0.76
Secondary	1.00	—	0.45	0.05–2.85	0.50	0.10–3.65	
Number of ET[*]							
One ET	1.00	—	0.20	0.05–1.90	—	—	
Two ET	1.00	—	0.50	0.12–2.56	0.45	0.10–2.89	0.33
Three and more ET	1.00	—	1.60	0.74–4.68	0.98	0.20–3.89	

[*]Number of embryo transfer.

confounding effects of the controlled confounders being observed. The odds ratio of positive pregnancy is found to be negatively and significantly associated with overweight and obesity. Among overweight and obese women, the probability of positive pregnancy is reduced by 50% and 55%, respectively, in overweight and obese women (OR = 0.50; 95% CI = 0.25–0.99 among overweight women; OR = 0.45; 95% CI = 0.20–0.99 among obese women).

Table 3 shows the adjusted ORs of positive pregnancy outcome and their 95% CIs for the two-way interactions between BMI and patient's age, infertility type, and ET. Although no relation was detected between BMI and pregnancy outcome among women aged 27–33 years, a varying degree of reduction was observed for other age groups. The highest reduction was among overweight women aged >33 years (80%) and obese women aged <27 years (77%). Also, there has been a reduction in pregnancy outcome among overweight and obese women with primary and secondary infertility with the highest and significant reductions being for primary infertile women (OR = 0.27; 95% CI = 0.15–0.98

for overweight, and OR = 0.35; 95% CI = 0.12–0.99 for obese women). The reduction in pregnancy rate among overweight and obese women who had one or two ET was not seen among women who had more than two embryos transferred. In this group, the probability of positive pregnancy outcome was increased by 1.6-fold (OR = 1.60; 95% CI = 0.74–4.68).

4. Discussion

This study contributes to the previous reports of decreased probability of positive pregnancy outcome in overweight and obese women after infertility treatment [4, 6–8]. The endocrinological and/or biochemical milieu associated with obesity, operating through a functional state such as insulin resistance, can create a hostile intraovarian or intrauterine environment for the oocytes or embryos. Also, plausibility for a causal link between obesity and reproductive hormones can be found in studies that link modest weight loss and a reduction of central fat to improved insulin sensitivity, resulting in ovulation and pregnancy in overweight infertile women [14]. Moreover, obesity is associated with alterations in carbohydrate and fat metabolism central to the development of insulin resistance. A diet with a high-glycemic index has been associated with infertility, fetal loss, congenital anomalies, and prematurity, as well as macrosomia. Greater carbohydrate intake and dietary glycemic load have been associated with an increased risk of infertility due to anovulation [15].

The striking negative association of positive pregnancy outcome with overweight and obesity, observed in our study as in previous ones [3, 5, 16, 17], directed us to examine if the probability of positive pregnancy varies according to other known risk factors. The results suggest the reducing effect of overweight and obesity on the probability of positive pregnancy outcome to increase more in primary infertile women and among those aged <27 years and more than 33 years. However, this reducing effect disappeared among women aged 27–33 years and those have had two ET. The practice of multiple embryos transfer in ART has also been suggested to decrease early pregnancy loss among normal and overweight women [18, 19]. The mechanism by which age, infertility type, and number of ET can modify the probability of positive pregnancy associated with overweight and obesity is unclear. But these results may open a number of avenues for subsequent research to shed more light on such mechanisms. However, there is a still controversy about the dangerous effect of transferring multiple embryos. Multiple birth is related to the number of transferred embryos and is associated with adverse fetal and infant outcomes, and they also pose increased risks of maternal morbidity and mortality [20, 21]. Accordingly, weight reduction among obese women undergoing ART may be of value in reducing the number of transferred embryos and hence reducing the associated complications. However, a recent study [22] reported that short-term weight loss was unrelated to positive β-hCG, clinical pregnancy, or live birth rates, particularly among obese and overweight women.

To our knowledge, this study is the first to search for the possible effect modification of some women's characteristics as well as the number of embryo transfer on the reported negative association between BMI and positive pregnancy outcome. A potential concern in this study is the lack of data, due to the retrospective nature of the study. Accordingly, other factors were not available about women lifestyle factors (such as smoking, physical exercise, and dietary habit) to investigate their modification effect on the probability of pregnancy outcome associated with BMI.

In summary, this study confirms the reported reducing effect of overweight and obesity on positive pregnancy outcome in infertile women after assisted reproduction treatment. Our study also suggests a possible effect modification of patient's age, infertility type, and number of ET on such association. The latter observation deserves further investigation.

Conflict of Interests

The authors declare that there is no conflict of interests regarding the publication of this paper.

Acknowledgment

The authors would like to thank all health team of ART Unit, Al-Azhar University, for their help during performance of this study.

References

[1] R. E. Frisch, "Body weight and reproduction," *Science*, vol. 246, no. 4929, p. 432, 1989.

[2] J. X. Wang, M. Davies, and R. J. Norman, "Body mass and probability of pregnancy during assisted reproduction treatment: retrospective study," *British Medical Journal*, vol. 321, no. 7272, pp. 1320–1321, 2000.

[3] L. Lake, C. Power, and T. J. Cole, "Women's reproductive health: the role of body mass index in early and adult life," *Internal Journal of Obstetric Related Metabolic Disorders*, vol. 21, no. 6, pp. 432–438, 1997.

[4] B. Luke, M. B. Brown, J. E. Stern, S. A. Missmer, V. Y. Fujimoto, and R. Leach, "Female obesity adversely affects assisted reproductive technology (ART) pregnancy and live birth rates," *Human Reproduction*, vol. 26, no. 1, pp. 245–252, 2011.

[5] J. Bellver, Y. Ayllón, M. Ferrando et al., "Female obesity impairs in vitro fertilization outcome without affecting embryo quality," *Fertility and Sterility*, vol. 93, no. 2, pp. 447–454, 2010.

[6] E. C. A. M. van Swieten, L. van der Leeuw-Harmsen, E. A. Badings, and P. J. Q. van der Linden, "Obesity and clomiphene challenge test as predictors of outcome of in vitro fertilization and intracytoplasmic sperm injection," *Gynecologic and Obstetric Investigation*, vol. 59, no. 4, pp. 220–224, 2005.

[7] B. Vural, K. Sofuoglu, E. Caliskan et al., "Predictors of intracytoplasmic sperm injection (ICSI) outcome in couples with and without male factor infertility," *Clinical and Experimental Obstetrics and Gynecology*, vol. 32, no. 3, pp. 158–162, 2005.

[8] S. Shen, A. Khabani, N. Klein, and D. Battaglia, "Statistical analysis of factors affecting fertilization rates and clinical outcome associated with intracytoplasmic sperm injection," *Fertility and Sterility*, vol. 79, no. 2, pp. 355–360, 2003.

[9] D. Hamilton-Fairley, D. Kiddy, H. Watson, C. Paterson, and S. Franks, "Association of moderate obesity with a poor pregnancy outcome in women with polycystic ovary syndrome treated with low dose gonadotrophin," *British Journal of Obstetrics and Gynaecology*, vol. 99, no. 2, pp. 128–131, 1992.

[10] F. J. Broekmans, J. Kwee, D. J. Hendriks, B. W. Mol, and C. B. Lambalk, "A systematic review of tests predicting ovarian reserve and IVF outcome," *Human Reproduction Update*, vol. 12, no. 6, pp. 685–718, 2006.

[11] B. Luke, M. B. Brown, J. E. Stern, D. A. Grainger, N. Klein, and M. Cedars, "Effect of embryo transfer number on singleton and twin implantation pregnancy outcomes after assisted reproductive technology," *Journal of Reproductive Medicine*, vol. 55, no. 10, pp. 387–394, 2010.

[12] World Health Organization (WHO), "Obesity: preventing and managing the global epidemic," World Health Organization Technical Report Series 894, WHO Consultation, 2000.

[13] SAS Institute, *Proprietary Software Release 8. 2*, SAS Institute, Cary, NC, USA, 1999.

[14] M.-M. Huber-Buchholz, D. G. P. Carey, and R. J. Norman, "Restoration of reproductive potential by lifestyle modification in obese polycystic ovary syndrome: role of insulin sensitivity and luteinizing hormone," *Journal of Clinical Endocrinology and Metabolism*, vol. 84, no. 4, pp. 1470–1474, 1999.

[15] J. E. Chavarro, J. W. Rich-Edwards, B. A. Rosner, and W. C. Willett, "A prospective study of dietary carbohydrate quantity and quality in relation to risk of ovulatory infertility," *European Journal of Clinical Nutrition*, vol. 63, no. 1, pp. 78–86, 2009.

[16] J. Bellver, Y. Ayllón, M. Ferrando et al., "Female obesity impairs in vitro fertilization outcome without affecting embryo quality," *Fertility and Sterility*, vol. 93, no. 2, pp. 447–454, 2010.

[17] V. Rittenberg, S. Seshadri, S. K. Sunkara, S. Sobaleva, E. Oteng-Ntim, and T. El-Toukhy, "Effect of body mass index on IVF treatment outcome: an updated systematic review and meta-analysis," *Reproductive BioMedicine*, vol. 23, no. 4, pp. 421–439, 2011.

[18] C. Simón, J. Landeras, J. L. Zuzuarregui, J. C. Martín, J. Remohí, and A. Pellicer, "Early pregnancy losses in in vitro fertilization and oocyte donation," *Fertility and Sterility*, vol. 72, no. 6, pp. 1061–1065, 1999.

[19] P. Fedorcsák, R. Storeng, P. O. Dale, T. Tanbo, and T. Åbyholm, "Obesity is a risk factor for early pregnancy loss after IVF or ICSI," *Acta Obstetricia et Gynecologica Scandinavica*, vol. 79, no. 1, pp. 43–48, 2000.

[20] M. A. Reynolds, L. A. Schieve, G. Jeng, H. B. Peterson, and L. S. Wilcox, "Risk of multiple birth associated with in vitro fertilization using donor eggs," *American Journal of Epidemiology*, vol. 154, no. 11, pp. 1043–1050, 2001.

[21] L. A. Schieve, B. Cohen, A. Nannini et al., "A population-based study of maternal and perinatal outcomes associated with assisted reproductive technology in Massachusetts," *Maternal and Child Health Journal*, vol. 11, no. 6, pp. 517–525, 2007.

[22] J. E. Chavarro, S. Ehrlich, D. S. Colaci et al., "Body mass index and short-term weight change in relation to treatment outcomes in women undergoing assisted reproduction," *Fertility and Sterility*, vol. 98, no. 1, pp. 109–116, 2012.

21

Correlation between Abortion and Infertility among Nonsmoking Women with a History of Passive Smoking in Childhood and Adolescence

Jila Amirkhani,[1] Soheila Yadollah-Damavandi,[2] Seyed Mohammad-Javad Mirlohi,[3] Seyede Mahnaz Nasiri,[3] Yekta Parsa,[2] and Mohammad Gharehbeglou[4]

[1] *Medical Science Research Center, Medical Department, Islamic Azad University, Tehran Medical Sciences Branch, Tehran, Iran*
[2] *Young Researchers Club, Islamic Azad University, Tehran Medical Sciences Branch, Tehran, Iran*
[3] *Student Research Committee, Islamic Azad University, Tehran Medical Sciences Branch, Tehran, Iran*
[4] *Department of Medicine, Islamic Azad University, Qom Branch, Qom, Iran*

Correspondence should be addressed to Yekta Parsa; yekta.parsa@gmail.com

Academic Editor: Stefania A. Nottola

The aim of this study is to evaluate the correlation of exposing to the cigarette smoke in childhood and adolescence with infertility and abortion in women. This case-control study evaluated 178 women who had been attended to at the Amir-al-Momenin Hospital in Tehran in 2012-2013. Seventy-eight women with chief complaint of abortion, infertility, and missed abortion and 100 healthy women were considered as case and control groups, respectively. The tool was a questionnaire with two parts. In the first part demographic information was gathered and in the second part the information regarding the history of passive smoking in childhood and adolescence period, abortion, and infertility was gathered. The mean age in case and control groups was 26.24 $\pm$ 3.1 and 27.3 $\pm$ 4.2 years, respectively. The mean body mass index (BMI) was 25.74 $\pm$ 1.38 Kg/m^2. Abortion rates among passive smoker and nonpassive smoker patients were statistically significant ($P = 0.036$). Based on findings of this study, the experience of being a passive smoker in childhood and adolescence in women will increase the risk of abortion and infertility in the future, which could be the reason to encourage the society to step back from smoking cigarettes.

1. Introduction

Currently, smoking is one of the most important causative factors in human death. World annual death among smokers is more than 4 million, which is predicted to reach 10 million in 2020 without interfering [1–3]. There are more than 10 million smokers in Iran, of those, 2.5% are women. Even though the cigarette consumption is higher among males, it is predicted to be equal in the near future, regarding the habitual change in society [4]. Cigarette has more than 4000 antigenic and carcinogenic factors such as cyclic aromatic benzene, cadmium, ethylbenzene, cotinine, and nicotine [5]. In some studies, it was shown that the risk of exposure to cancerous substances in passive smokers is 2.5 times more than the risk in direct smokers [6, 7]. Pregnant women are more susceptible to the injuries and smokes. There are studies

in benefit of preterm birth and low birth weight, related to passive smoking [8]. The immature and low-birth-weight neonates need special care and budget, and these babies are susceptible to have anatomical and mental damage in the future [8]. Cigarette is one of the agents that have potential risk to cause abortion and infertility. Abortion means the termination of pregnancy before the fetus reaches viability. Infertility is a condition in which a woman has not become pregnant after one year of regular sexual intercourse, without contraception [9, 10]. Studies showed that cigarette smoking in 2 last months of pregnancy increases the risk of preterm birth and stillbirth [11]. Direct exposure to the cigarette smoke in women caused unsuccessful pregnancy, delay in fertilization, ectopic pregnancy, and placental defects. The nicotine in cigarette might affect the follicular growth negatively, by inducing apoptosis. On the other hand, the chemical agents in cigarette might affect function of the fallopian tubes. Menstrual disorders and premature menopause are also the other side effects of smoking, which might cause infertility [12–20]. Some studies in the United States demonstrated the effects of cigarette smoke on granulosa cells and aromatase enzyme that decreases the production of estrogen. In addition, the alkaloids in cigarette inhibit the production of progesterone [15]. In another study, hyperplasia of syncytial cells and cytotrophoblasts beside the false nodes in the umbilical cord and thickening of the basal membrane of placenta induced by cigarette smoke might cause the necrosis and abruption placentae have been reported [11]. Other effects of cigarette smoke during pregnancy include missed abortion, placenta previa, premature rupture of the amniotic membrane, increasing risk of fetal death after 12 weeks of pregnancy, and bleeding [21]. Regardless of physical and mental problems, abortion is responsible for 15–20% of maternal death; it places a huge economic burden on healthcare system, especially in developing countries [8]. Knowing the factors like cigarette which leads to infertility and abortion is very important for the healthcare system. It is also essential to consider those factors in their planning to decrease the abortion and infertility rates. Therefore, the aim of this study is to evaluate the correlation of exposing to the cigarette smoke in childhood and adolescence with infertility and abortion in women.

2. Methods and Materials

This case-control study was performed on 178 nonsmoker women who had been attended to at Amir Hospital, Tehran, Iran, during 2012-2013. Seventy-eight women with chief complaint of abortion, infertility, and missed abortion and 100 healthy women were considered as case and control groups, respectively. Patients over 40 years with the history of genital infectious diseases, systemic diseases, metabolic disorders, recurrent miscarriage (the loss of three or more consecutive pregnancies), drug addiction, using antidepressants, and an anatomic disorder of uterus and ovaries were excluded from the study. A questionnaire consisting of two parts was prepared; the first part was dedicated to the demographic information and, in the second part, information about experience of cigarette smoking, being a passive smoker, and having experience of missed abortion and infertility was gathered.

Data were analyzed by statistical SPSS15 software, using chi-square test. The significant level was considered $P < 0.05$.

3. Results

The mean age in case and control groups was 26.24 ± 3.1 and 27.3 ± 4.2 years, respectively. The mean body mass index (BMI) was 25.74 ± 1.38 kg/m^2. Among the participants, 85.4% were housewives. In the case group, 71.7% ($n = 56$) and, in the control group, 44% ($n = 44$) were passive smokers.

According to Table 1, abortion rates among passive smoker and nonpassive smoker patients were statistically significant ($P = 0.036$); also, the difference between infertility rate in the two groups was statistically significant (12.5%

TABLE 1: The frequency of abortion and infertility in the case group with positive or negative history of passive smoking in childhood and adolescent.

	History of passive smoking	
	Positive ($n = 56$) N (%)	Negative ($n = 22$) N (%)
Abortion	36 (64.2)	8 (36.3)
Infertility	7 (12.5)	1 (4.5)
Miss abortion	7 (12.5)	3 (13.6)
Family history of abortion	1 (1.7)	0 (0)
Family history of infertility	2 (3.5)	1 (4.5)
Family history of miss abortion	0 (0)	0 (0)

versus 4.5%, resp., $P = 0.02$), while there was not a significant correlation between family histories of abortion and missed abortion in patients ($P = 0.84$). There was no significant correlation between family history of abortion and infertility ($P = 0.65$) and family history of infertility with abortion in patients ($P = 0.71$). In addition, the correlation between family history of infertility and infertility in patients was not seen ($P = 0.93$).

4. Discussion

Cigarette smoking causes unsatisfactory changes in female's genital system, which is due to substances like nicotine that produce oxidative stress. Therefore, oxidative stress not only causes infertility, but also increases the risk of missed abortion as well. In animal studies, higher rate of abortion among passive smokers has been reported. The lowest rate of fertility compared to nonsmoker mice also has been reported [6].

In this study, 71.7% of participants were passive smokers. 64.2% of passive smokers and 36.3% of those with no experience of cigarette contact had an abortion, and the difference was statistically significant ($P = 0.002$). It was also a report of infertility among 12.5% of passive smokers and 4.5% of those without cigarette contact, in which the difference was statistically significant ($P = 0.02$). In a study by Meeker et al. in 2007 in the United States, the risk for the abortion among women who were passive smokers in comparison to others was 4.35 times higher, and the fertility rate was lower [22], which is similar to the current study. In another study by Neal et al., the same lower rate of fertility among active and passive smoker women was shown [23].

In a study by Depa-Martynów et al., the success rates of in vitro fertilization (IVF) among smoker women in comparison to control group were lower [24]. On the other hand, in the study by Sterzik et al., the success rates of IVF among infertile smoker women and passive smoker women were the same as the control group [25], which is different from the current study.

In a study by George et al., 19% of women without experience of abortion and 24% of women with experience of abortion were passive smokers, which was statistically significant [26].

Cigarette smoking is a high-risk behavior which can lead to many social problems [27], as Patrick et al. [28] state that it causes premature morbidity and mortality. As a result, gathering data about this behavior seems to be necessary. Self-reports of smoking are usually conducted to see tendencies in cigarette smoking [29] and whether or not interventions towards this habitual desire are effective [28]. The validity of self-reported smoking is usually compromised by many reasons. For example, Patrick et al. [28] mention that smokers often deny or underestimate their smoking and its quantity. Another point of view is established by Pokorski et al. [30], which indicates that smoking is often an occasional habit among adolescents; therefore estimating the exact amount and pattern of smoking is not easy, as well. People may also be embarrassed by finding themselves as someone who commits an action which is not well accepted and desirable in the society; this can prevent them from reporting their information accurately and creating bias in smoking self-reports [27–30].

5. Conclusion

In conclusion, according to results of this study and compared to other studies, it seems that the experience of being passive smoker in childhood and adolescence will increase the risk of abortion and infertility in the future, and informing the society about the disadvantages of cigarette is recommended.

Conflict of Interests

The authors declare that there is no conflict of interests regarding the publication of this paper.

References

[1] M. M. Haenle, S. O. Brockmann, M. Kron et al., "Overweight, physical activity, tobacco and alcohol consumption in a cross-sectional random sample of German adults," *BMC Public Health*, vol. 6, article 233, 2006.

[2] World Health Organization, *Process for a Global Strategy on Diet Physical Activity and Health Geneva*, World Health Organization, Geneva, Switzerland, 2003.

[3] J. I. Herrero, F. Pardo, D. D'Avola et al., "Risk factors of lung, head and neck, esophageal, and kidney and urinary tract carcinomas after liver transplantation: the effect of smoking withdrawal," *Liver Transplantation*, vol. 17, no. 4, pp. 402–408, 2011.

[4] K. Schilling, B. Toth, S. Rösner, T. Strowitzki, and T. Wischmann, "Prevalence of behaviour-related fertility disorders in a clinical sample: results of a pilot study," *Archives of Gynecology and Obstetrics*, vol. 286, no. 5, pp. 1307–1314, 2012.

[5] J. D. Meeker and M. D. Benedict, "Infertility, pregnancy loss and adverse birth outcomes in relation to maternal secondhand tobacco smoke exposure," *Current Women's Health Reviews*, vol. 9, no. 1, pp. 41–49, 2013.

[6] L. N. Anderson, M. Cotterchio, L. Mirea, H. Ozcelik, and N. Kreiger, "Passive cigarette smoke exposure during various periods of life, genetic variants, and breast cancer risk among never smokers," *The American Journal of Epidemiology*, vol. 175, no. 4, pp. 289–301, 2012.

[7] K. S. Louie, X. Castellsague, S. De Sanjos et al., "Smoking and passive smoking in cervical cancer risk: pooled analysis of couples from the IARC multicentric case-control studies," *Cancer Epidemiology Biomarkers and Prevention*, vol. 20, no. 7, pp. 1379–1390, 2011.

[8] C. Iñiguez, F. Ballester, R. Amorós, M. Murcia, A. Plana, and M. Rebagliato, "Active and passive smoking during pregnancy and ultrasound measures of fetal growth in a cohort of pregnant women," *Journal of Epidemiology & Community Health*, vol. 66, no. 6, pp. 563–570, 2012.

[9] S. Gurunath, Z. Pandian, R. A. Anderson, and S. Bhattacharya, "Defining infertility-a systematic review of prevalence studies," *Human Reproduction Update*, vol. 17, no. 5, Article ID dmr015, pp. 575–588, 2011.

[10] C. Gnoth, E. Godehardt, P. Frank-Herrmann, K. Friol, J. Tigges, and G. Freundl, "Definition and prevalence of subfertility and infertility," *Human Reproduction*, vol. 20, no. 5, pp. 1144–1147, 2005.

[11] L. B. Strand, A. G. Barnett, and S. Tong, "Maternal exposure to ambient temperature and the risks of preterm birth and stillbirth in Brisbane, Australia," *The American Journal of Epidemiology*, vol. 175, no. 2, pp. 99–107, 2012.

[12] R. Bordel, M. W. Laschke, M. D. Menger, and B. Vollmar, "Nicotine does not affect vascularization but inhibits growth of freely transplanted ovarian follicles by inducing granulosa cell apoptosis," *Human Reproduction*, vol. 21, no. 3, pp. 610–617, 2006.

[13] S. R. Soares and M. A. Melo, "Cigarette smoking and reproductive function," *Current Opinion in Obstetrics and Gynecology*, vol. 20, no. 3, pp. 281–291, 2008.

[14] R. Shao, S. Zou, X. Wang et al., "Revealing the hidden mechanisms of smoke-induced fallopian tubal implantation," *Biology of Reproduction*, vol. 86, no. 4, article 131, 2012.

[15] A. Kokcu, "Premature ovarian failure from current perspective," *Gynecological Endocrinology*, vol. 26, no. 8, pp. 555–562, 2010.

[16] L. D. Dorn, S. Negriff, B. Huang et al., "Menstrual symptoms in adolescent girls: association with smoking, depressive symptoms, and anxiety," *Journal of Adolescent Health*, vol. 44, no. 3, pp. 237–243, 2009.

[17] W. C. Strohsnitter, E. E. Hatch, M. Hyer et al., "The association between in utero cigarette smoke exposure and age at menopause," *American Journal of Epidemiology*, vol. 167, no. 6, pp. 727–733, 2008.

[18] K. D. Henderson, L. Bernstein, B. Henderson, L. Kolonel, and M. C. Pike, "Predictors of the timing of natural menopause in the multiethnic cohort study," *The American Journal of Epidemiology*, vol. 167, no. 11, pp. 1287–1294, 2008.

[19] J. L. V. Shaw, E. Oliver, K. Lee et al., "Cotinine exposure increases fallopian tube PROKR1 expression via nicotinic AChRα-7: a potential mechanism explaining the link between smoking and tubal ectopic pregnancy," *American Journal of Pathology*, vol. 177, no. 5, pp. 2509–2515, 2010.

[20] J. Leonardi-Bee, A. Smyth, J. Britton, and T. Coleman, "Environmental tobacco smoke and fetal health: systematic review and meta-analysis," *Archives of Disease in Childhood: Fetal and Neonatal Edition*, vol. 93, no. 5, pp. F351–F361, 2008.

[21] M. H. Aliyu, O. Lynch, R. E. Wilson et al., "Association between tobacco use in pregnancy and placenta-associated syndromes: a population-based study," *Archives of Gynecology and Obstetrics*, vol. 283, no. 4, pp. 729–734, 2011.

[22] J. D. Meeker, S. A. Missmer, D. W. Cramer, and R. Hauser, "Maternal exposure to second-hand tobacco smoke and pregnancy outcome among couples undergoing assisted reproduction," *Human Reproduction*, vol. 22, no. 2, pp. 337–345, 2007.

[23] M. S. Neal, E. G. Hughes, A. C. Holloway, and W. G. Foster, "Sidestream smoking is equally as damaging as mainstream smoking on IVF outcomes," *Human Reproduction*, vol. 20, no. 9, pp. 2531–2535, 2005.

[24] M. Depa-Martynów, L. Pawelczyk, G. Taszarek-Hauke, M. Jósiak, K. Derwich, and P. Jedrzejczak, "The effect of smoking on infertility treatment in women undergoing assisted reproduction cycles," *Przegląd Lekarski*, vol. 62, no. 10, pp. 973–975, 2005.

[25] K. Sterzik, E. Strehler, M. De Santo et al., "Influence of smoking on fertility in women attending an in vitro fertilization program," *Fertility and Sterility*, vol. 65, no. 4, pp. 810–814, 1996.

[26] L. George, F. Granath, A. L. V. Johansson, G. Annerén, and S. Cnattingius, "Environmental tobacco smoke and risk of spontaneous abortion," *Epidemiology*, vol. 17, no. 5, pp. 500–505, 2006.

[27] N. D. Brener, J. O. G. Billy, and W. R. Grady, "Assessment of factors affecting the validity of self-reported health-risk behavior among adolescents: evidence from the scientific literature," *Journal of Adolescent Health*, vol. 33, no. 6, pp. 436–457, 2003.

[28] D. L. Patrick, A. Cheadle, D. C. Thompson, P. Diehr, T. Koepsell, and S. Kinne, "The validity of self-reported smoking: a review and meta-analysis," *The American Journal of Public Health*, vol. 84, no. 7, pp. 1086–1093, 1994.

[29] S. L. Wong, M. Shields, S. Leatherdale, E. Malaison, and D. Hammond, "Assessment of validity of self-reported smoking status," *Health Reports*, vol. 23, no. 1, pp. 47–53, 2012.

[30] T. L. Pokorski, W. W. Chen, and R. L. Bertholf, "Use of urine cotinine to validate smoking self-reports in U.S. Navy recruits," *Addictive Behaviors*, vol. 19, no. 4, pp. 451–454, 1994.

22

Comparative Evaluation of the Impact of Subacute Exposure of Smokeless Tobacco and Tobacco Smoke on Rat Testis

Jonah Sydney Aprioku and Theresa Chioma Ugwu

Department of Pharmacology, Faculty of Basic Medical Sciences, University of Port Harcourt, PMB 5323, Port Harcourt, Nigeria

Correspondence should be addressed to Jonah Sydney Aprioku; sydaprio@yahoo.com

Academic Editor: Robert Gaspar

This study investigated the effects of 30-day exposure to tobacco smoke (TS), smokeless tobacco (ST), and nicotine on reproductive parameters and oxidative biomarkers in prepubertal and adult male rats. Sperm motility was reduced by 77.5 and 89.0% in TS and ST exposed prepubertal rats and 71.1 and 86.4% in adult rats, respectively. Sperm count was also reduced by 64.7 and 89.9% in prepubertal rats and 64.9 and 47.0% in adult rats, respectively. Nicotine decreased sperm motility (82.2%) and count (62.6%) in prepubertal rats but caused no effect in adult rats. There were no changes in sperm morphology; testosterone was decreased, while LH and FSH were increased in exposed rats, when compared with control. Malondialdehyde levels in testes of exposed rats were increased, and GSH, SOD, and catalase were altered. Results indicate that subacute exposure of tobacco products alters sperm characteristics in a rank order of ST > TS > nicotine, which may be linked to increase in oxidative stress in the testis.

1. Introduction

Tobacco is known to cause several negative health consequences in both animals and humans [1, 2], and cigarette smoking (tobacco inhalation) and ingestion of smokeless tobacco (e.g., nasal snuff, snus, and moist snuff) are among the major sources of human exposure to tobacco. Aside from the principal biologically active component (nicotine), tobacco products also contain several potentially toxic compounds, including polycyclic aromatic hydrocarbons, cyanide, carbon-monoxide, heavy metals, nitrosamines, and insecticides [3, 4].

Cigarette smoking has been shown not only to cause cancers but also to be associated with increased incidences of chronic obstructive pulmonary diseases, COPDs [5–7], and coronary heart disease [8]. Increasing public awareness of the negative health implications of cigarette smoking, coupled with its restriction in public places by different regulatory bodies, may have controlled the level of smoking in some way. However, this may have at the same time increased the use of smokeless tobacco products as alternatives [9, 10]. In Nigeria, nasal snuff is the most popular form of smokeless tobacco product, and it is consumed in both rural and urban areas not only as alternative to tobacco smoke but also for various other reasons which include medicinal and sociocultural purposes [11]. Furthermore, it has been reported that the use of smokeless tobacco products is becoming more common among young males, and there has been an increase in their production and consumption [12]. This has been partly attributed to the promotion of novel smokeless tobacco products as safer alternatives to smoked tobacco products [10], with the consequence of increasing the potential risk of nicotine poisoning [9]. Unfortunately, there is limited data on the effects of smokeless tobacco, especially on reproductive function because most previous studies have been focused on cigarette smoking [11, 13, 14].

Reproductive dysfunction is a major cause of infertility among couples and tobacco smoke has been shown to cause different forms of reproductive dysfunction in both male and female: low birth weight [14, 15], prenatal and neonatal mortality [16], reduction in uterine blood flow [17, 18], and reduced penile erection [19, 20]. However, the effects of tobacco products on reproductive function continue to be investigated as existing data are not conclusive. Earlier works of Vine et al. [21] and Trummer et al. [22] have reported opposing results on the influence of cigarette smoking on male reproductive hormones. In addition, in spite of the growing knowledge of adverse reproductive effects of smoking on reproduction, it is not certain whether or not nicotine has similar effects and mechanism of action as cigarette smoking on the reproductive system. There are also concerns of the impact of tobacco exposure, particularly smokeless tobacco, on reproductive activity in the young or juvenile male, with the increasing rate of smokeless tobacco consumption in the young.

Earlier studies have shown that cigarette smoke induces apoptosis and degenerative effects on testicular tissues which was associated with increase in oxidative stress [23]. Abdul-Ghani et al. [24] have also shown that cigarette smoke exposure causes impairment of spermatogenesis in rats, which was partly attributed to induction of DNA damage and oxidative stress. In other studies, exposure to cigarette smoke has been reported to induce lipid peroxidation and changes in the oxidative enzyme levels in rat testis [25, 26]. In this study, it is logical to hypothesize that tobacco smoke and smokeless tobacco will produce more deleterious effects than nicotine, attributable to their additional components. In addition, tobacco smoke and smokeless tobacco would alter male reproductive function, mediated through increased oxidative stress, which would be more pronounced in the juvenile animals than the adult [27, 28]. The present study intends to investigate the response of reproductive tissues to subacute exposures of tobacco smoke, smokeless tobacco, and nicotine in prepubertal and adult male rats.

2. Materials and Methods

2.1. Materials. Benson and Hedges cigarettes (1.0 mg nicotine/stick), locally prepared nasal snuff (16 mg nicotine/g), and nicotine hydrogen tartrate, 98% (BDH Chemicals Ltd., Poole, England), were used.

2.2. Animals. Forty-two (42) prepubertal male Wistar albino rats of 5 weeks of age, weighing 80 to 130 g, and 42 adult male Wistar albino rats of 12 weeks of age, weighing 250 to 280 g, were obtained from the Animal House of the University of Port Harcourt. The animals were housed four per cage and fed with standard rat chow and allowed access to tap water *ad libitum*. They were maintained in a well-ventilated room with a 12 h light/dark cycle at room temperature and handled in accordance with the international, national, and institutional guidelines for care and use of laboratory animals as promulgated by the Canadian Council of Animal Care [29].

2.3. Experimental Design. The prepubertal and adult rats were each divided into 7 groups containing 6 rats per group and exposed to cigarette smoke, smokeless tobacco, and nicotine. A pilot experiment was done to determine the tolerability of rats to different amounts of cigarette smoke equivalent to 0.25, 0.5, and 1 mg of nicotine using the whole body exposure method as described by Dorman et al. [30] and Wong [31]. Using cigarette containing 1 mg nicotine per stick, the equivalent tobacco smoke doses were 1/4, 1/2, and 1 stick, respectively. None of the doses caused death of animals, so tobacco smoke exposure levels equivalent to 0.5 and 1 mg

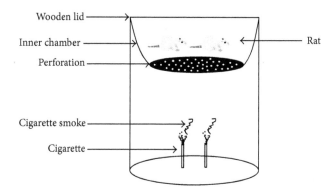

FIGURE 1: Inhalational chamber showing perforated inner chamber with wooden lid.

nicotine were used in the study. Groups I and II of prepubertal or adult rats were exposed to tobacco smoke at target nicotine concentrations of 0.5 or 1 mg daily. To standardize animal exposure, all the exposures were carried out with the same brand of cigarette. Groups III and IV were given smokeless tobacco, nasal snuff ($\approx$0.5 or 1 mg nicotine/kg) daily. Groups V and VI were given nicotine (0.5 or 1 mg/kg) daily. Group VII (control group) animals were allowed to inhale tobacco-free air.

The doses of nicotine used are standard doses in most toxicological investigations [30–32]. Nicotine was serially diluted with normal saline to obtain suitable working concentrations and animals were injected subcutaneously. Nasal snuff (smokeless tobacco) powder was dissolved in distilled water and given by oral gavage. All solutions of nicotine and nasal snuff were stored in foil-wrapped glass bottles at 4°C for no longer than seven days.

2.4. Tobacco Smoke Exposure. Whole body exposure is the commonly used method for long-duration exposure studies and for large numbers of test subjects [31]. The model used in this study consists of acrylic plastic cylindrical inhalation chambers (diameter: 30 cm; height: 38 cm; breath: 91 cm). Each chamber has an inner chamber, about 24 cm from the bottom, where the test animals are placed. There is also a wooden lid at the top of the main chambers which ensures minimal leakage of air from the cage and also to restrain the animals.

The cigarette was lit (1/2 or 1 stick) at the base of the main chamber and the animals (two at a time) were quickly introduced into the inner chamber and the wooden lid was closed and kept for 5–7.5 min or 10–15 min, respectively (each cigarette produces nearly 10–15 min of smoke). The inner chamber has a perforated base, which permits smoke into the inner chamber from the cigarette that is lit at the base of the main chamber (Figure 1). After that, the procedure was repeated with 10-minute interval of rest, and so all the animals received 1/2 or 1 cigarette smoke per day. Each cigarette used contained 1.0 mg nicotine, 10 mg tar, and 10 mg CO. The control group was left free in the interior of chambers and only received compressed air. Tobacco smoke exposures were done under static conditions, and temperatures of the chamber before and during tobacco smoke exposure were monitored (31.5–32°C and 34-35°C, resp.).

At the end of 30 days of treatment, the rats were anesthetized with diethyl ether and sacrificed. Blood samples were collected by cardiac puncture into plain and lithium heparinized tubes. The blood samples were centrifuged at 3000 rpm for 10 minutes and serum was separated and assayed for hormonal levels of testosterone, luteinizing hormone (LH), and follicle stimulating hormone (FSH), using tube-based enzyme linked immunoassay (EIA) technique. Also, the testis was removed along with the epididymis. The caudal epididymis was separated from the testis and lacerated to collect sperm for measurement of sperm indices. Thereafter, the testis was carefully excised, cleared of adhering tissues, and washed in an ice cold 1.15% KCl solution and blotted. Tissues were then homogenized with 0.1 M phosphate buffer (pH 7.2), using a homogenizer. The homogenate was centrifuged at 2500 rmp speed for 15 minutes, and the supernatant was stored at −20°C for estimation of antioxidant enzymes: superoxide dismutase (SOD), reduced glutathione (GSH), and catalase activities and malondialdehyde (MDA) level.

2.5. Sperm Analysis. Sperm was placed on a clean dry glass slide and emulsified with equal volume of 1% NaHCO$_3$ buffered Tyrodes Lactate solution. Slide was examined under the microscope to measure sperm motility, count, and morphology as described by Baker [33] and Ochei and Kolhatker [34]. Briefly, sperm motility was determined by counting motile and nonmotile spermatozoa in 10 randomly selected fields under the microscope, using 40x objective. Sperm count was done using the improved Neubauer hemocytometer. The Neubauer counting chamber was prepared and charged with diluted seminal fluid and allowed to stand in a moist chamber for 15 minutes. Complete morphologically mature sperm cells were then counted using 40x magnification. Sperm morphology was evaluated by staining sperm smears on microscope slides with a nigrosin-eosin stain after they were air-dried. The slides were examined under the microscope with 100x objective and with oil immersion. The number and percentage of abnormal sperm cells were noted.

2.6. Analysis of Oxidative Biomarkers

2.6.1. Superoxide Dismutase (SOD) Enzyme Assay. Superoxide dismutase activity was determined according to the method described by Sun and Zigman [35]. The principle is based on the ability of SOD to inhibit autooxidation of epinephrine determined by the increase in absorbance at 480 nm. To initiate the reaction, testis homogenate (0.02 mL) was allowed to react with 2.95 mL of sodium carbonate buffer (0.05 M, pH 10.2) and 0.03 mL of epinephrine in 0.005 N HCl. The reference cuvette contained 2.95 mL buffer, 0.03 mL of substrate (epinephrine), and 0.02 mL of water. Enzyme activity was calculated by measuring the change in absorbance at 480 nm for 5 min, $\sum = 4020\,M^{-1}\,cm^{-1}$.

2.6.2. Catalase Enzyme Assay. Catalase activity was assayed colorimetrically at 620 nm and expressed as μmoles of H$_2$O$_2$

consumed/min/mg protein at 25°C, according to the method described by Aebi [36]. The reaction mixture (1.5 mL) contained 1.0 mL of 0.01 M phosphate buffer (pH 7.0), 0.1 mL of testis homogenate, and 0.4 mL of 2 M H$_2$O$_2$. The reaction was stopped by the addition of 2.0 mL of dichromate-acetic acid reagent (5% potassium dichromate and glacial acetic acid were mixed in 1 : 3 ratio), $\sum = 40\,M^{-1}\,cm^{-1}$.

2.6.3. Reduced Glutathione (GSH) Enzyme Assay. Reduced glutathione content of the testis as nonprotein sulfhydryls was estimated according to the method described by Sedlak and Lindsay [37]. To the homogenate, 10% tricarboxylic acid (TCA) was added and centrifuged. The supernatant (1.0 mL) was then treated with 0.5 mL of Ellman's reagent (19.8 mg of 5,5-dithiobisnitrobenzoic acid, DTNB, in 100 mL of 0.1% sodium nitrate) and 3.0 mL of phosphate buffer (0.2 M, pH 8.0). The absorbance was read at 412 nm, $\sum = 1.34 \times 10^4\,M^{-1}\,cm^{-1}$.

2.6.4. Malondialdehyde (MDA) Assay. Malondialdehyde was determined using the method of Buege and Aust [38]. Testis homogenate (1.0 mL) was added to 2 mL mixture of 15% TCA (tricarboxylic acid), 0.37% TBA (thiobarbituric acid), and 0.24 N HCl (hydrochloric acid) reagents (0.37% TBA, 15% TCA, and 0.24 N HCl) in a 1 : 1 : 1 ratio and boiled at 100°C for 15 minutes and allowed to cool. Flocculent materials were removed by centrifuging at 3000 rpm for 10 min. The supernatant was then removed and the absorbance read at 532 nm against a blank. MDA was calculated using the molar extinction coefficient for MDA-TBA complex of $1.56 \times 10^5\,M^{-1}\,cm^{-1}$.

2.6.5. Statistical Analysis. The results are presented as mean ± SEM for each group ($n = 6$). Differences among groups were analyzed using one-way analysis of variance (ANOVA) followed by Dunnett's multiple range post hoc test for pairwise comparisons. Data were analyzed using GraphPad Prism Version 5.

3. Results

3.1. Sperm Parameters. Sperm morphology was not altered in all exposed rats (Figures 2(c) and 2(f)), while sperm motility and counts obtained in tobacco smoke (TS) and smokeless tobacco (ST) exposed prepubertal rats were dose-dependently decreased, compared to non-tobacco exposed control rats (Figures 2(a) and 2(b)). Sperm motility and counts in TS and ST exposed adult rats were also decreased dose-dependently. However, only the results obtained in the rats that were exposed to the higher doses were significantly ($p < 0.05$) different from the controls in both prepubertal and adult rats (Figures 2(a), 2(b), 2(d), and 2(e)). In nicotine treated adult rats, sperm motility, counts, and morphology were not altered, but sperm motility was decreased in all nicotine treated prepubertal rats, while sperm count decreased only in prepubertal rats that received 1 mg/kg, when compared to the control rats (Figures 2(a), 2(b), 2(d), and 2(e)). The levels of reduction of motility produced by the tobacco

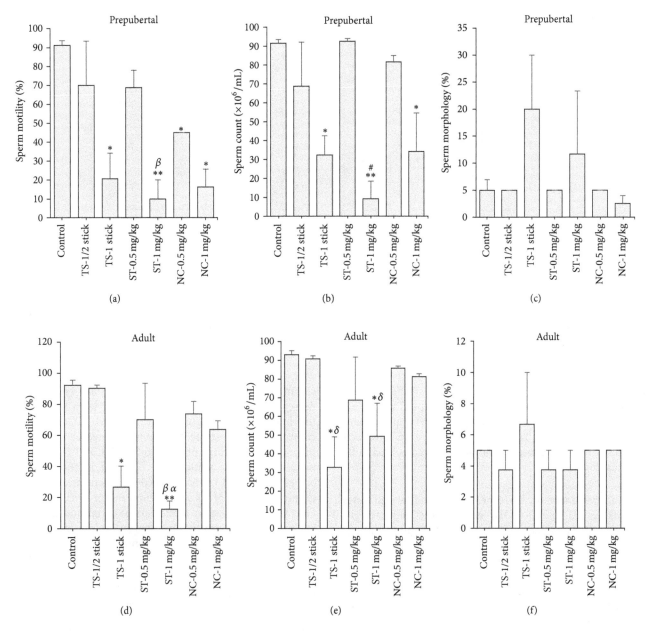

FIGURE 2: Effects of 30-day daily exposure to cigarette smoke (tobacco smoke, TS), smokeless tobacco (ST), and nicotine on sperm motility, count, and morphology in prepubertal ((a), (b), and (c)) and adult rats ((d), (e), and (f)). Data are expressed as mean $\pm$ SEM ($n = 6$). $^*p < 0.05$ compared to control; $^{**}p < 0.01$ compared to control; $^{\beta}p < 0.05$ compared to TS-1 stick; $^{\alpha}p < 0.01$ compared to NC-1 mg/kg; $^{\#}p < 0.05$ compared to TS-1 stick and NC-1 mg/kg; $^{\delta}p < 0.05$ compared to NC-1 mg/kg.

smoke, smokeless tobacco, and nicotine treatments were 77.5, 89, and 82.2%, respectively, in prepubertal rats and 71.1, 86.4, and 0%, respectively, in adult rats. The corresponding levels of reductions of sperm counts were 64.7, 89.9, and 62.6%, respectively, in prepubertal rats and 64.9, 47, and 0%, respectively, in adult rats. When compared, the motility and sperm counts in prepubertal and adult groups that were exposed to the higher doses of tobacco smoke, smokeless tobacco, and nicotine were also statistically different from each other (Figures 2(a), 2(b), 2(d), and 2(e)).

3.2. Oxidative Biomarkers

3.2.1. Lipid Peroxidation (LPO).
In tobacco smoke (TS) exposed prepubertal rat testes, the LPO product, malondialdehyde (MDA) level, was increased (596.4%), compared to non-tobacco exposed control rats (Figure 3(a)). MDA level was also increased in smokeless tobacco (ST) and nicotine exposed prepubertal rats (432.7 and 585.5%, resp.), when compared with non-tobacco exposed control rats (Figure 3(a)). Intragroup comparison showed that the MDA

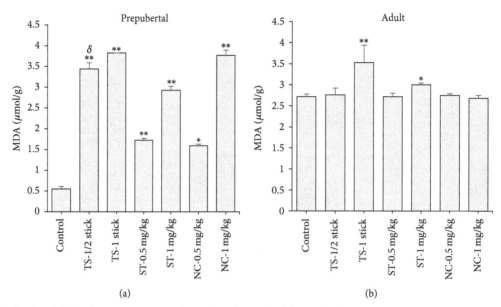

FIGURE 3: Levels of malondialdehyde (MDA) in testis of prepubertal (a) and adult rats (b) following daily exposure to cigarette smoke (tobacco smoke, TS), smokeless tobacco (ST), and nicotine for 30 days. Data are expressed as mean ± SEM ($n = 6$). $^*p < 0.05$ compared to control; $^{**}p < 0.01$ compared to control; $^\delta p < 0.05$ compared to ST-0.5 mg/kg and NC-0.5 mg/kg.

level in TS (1/2 stick) exposed group was different from ST and nicotine (0.5 mg/kg) exposed groups (Figure 3(a)). Furthermore, MDA was elevated in TS and ST exposed adult rats (29.8 and 102.9%, resp.), but there were no significant changes in nicotine treated adult rats, when compared to the controls (Figure 3(b)).

3.2.2. Antioxidants. In TS exposed prepubertal rat testes, superoxide dismutase (SOD) activity and reduced glutathione (GSH) content were not altered (Figures 4(a) and 4(b)), but catalase was reduced (19.7%), compared to nontobacco exposed control rats (Figure 4(c)). There were no changes in SOD and catalase activities in ST and nicotine exposed prepubertal rats. GSH was decreased at the higher dose of ST (42.0%), whereas it was increased dose-dependently in nicotine exposed rats, 77.7 and 155.4%, respectively (Figures 4(a), 4(b), and 4(c)). Intragroup comparison showed that the GSH levels in nicotine exposed groups were statistically different from ST and TS exposed groups (Figure 4(c)). Furthermore, SOD was unaffected in TS exposed adult rats (Figure 4(d)), but catalase and GSH were increased, though nonsignificantly (Figures 4(e) and 4(f)). In the ST exposed adult rats, SOD and catalase activities were not altered (Figures 4(d) and 4(e)), but GSH level was elevated, 115.1% (Figure 4(f)). In the nicotine treated adult rats, SOD activity was reduced, 14.6%, but there were no changes in catalase and GSH, when compared to control rats (Figures 4(d), 4(e), and 4(f)). Intragroup comparison showed that the GSH level in ST (1 mg/kg) exposed group was statistically different from nicotine (1 mg/kg) exposed group (Figure 4(f)).

3.3. Reproductive Hormones. In tobacco smoke, smokeless tobacco, and nicotine exposed prepubertal and adult rats,

serum testosterone levels were significantly ($p < 0.05$) decreased but mostly in the groups that were treated with the higher doses (Figures 5(a) and 5(d)). Compared to control rats, the testosterone levels obtained in the exposed prepubertal rats corresponded to 73, 75.9, and 71.6% reductions, respectively, while those obtained in the adult rats corresponded to 63.8, 53.8, and 0% reductions, respectively (Figures 5(a) and 5(d)). In addition, serum levels of LH and FSH were increased in treated prepubertal and adult rats, but this was also mostly observed in the groups that were treated with the higher doses (Figures 5(b), 5(c), 5(e), and 5(f)). The respective serum levels of LH that were obtained in tobacco smoke, smokeless tobacco, and nicotine exposed prepubertal rats were equivalent to 116.0, 93.3, and 19.2% increases (Figure 5(b)), while the serum levels of FSH were equivalent to 114.2, 91.7, and 40.8% increases, respectively (Figure 5(c)). Similarly, the respective serum levels of LH in exposed adult rats were equivalent to 89, 0, and 0% increases, (Figure 5(e)), while those of FSH were equivalent to 120.5, 100.0, and 0% increases, (Figure 5(f)). When compared among the treatment groups, the testosterone level in tobacco smoke (1 stick) exposed adult group was statistically different from nicotine (1 mg/kg) exposed group (Figure 5(d)).

4. Discussion

Reproductive organs are highly sensitive to xenobiotics and, in view of the high prevalence of infertility among couples [39, 40], evaluation of xenobiotic exposure to reproductive (male or female) tissues remains pertinent.

Cigarette smoking has been shown to cause several adverse effects on animal and human health, including reproductive toxicity. Previous studies have reported infertility and poor pregnancy outcomes among female smokers [13, 18, 41],

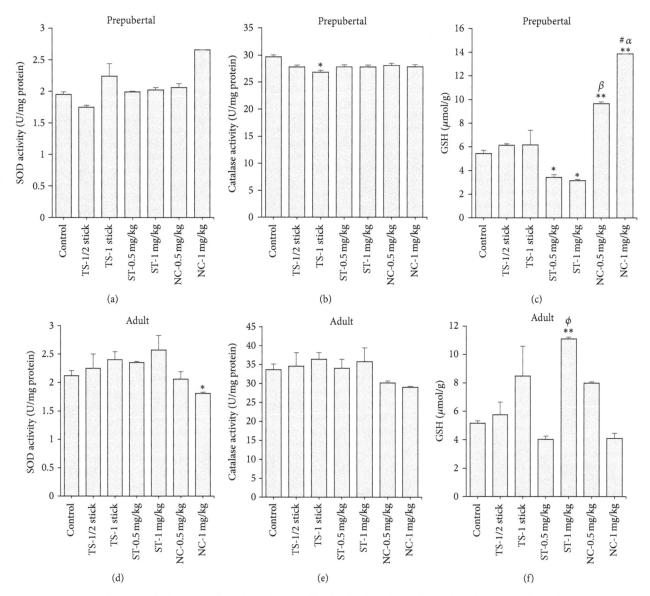

FIGURE 4: Activities of superoxide dismutase (SOD), catalase, and levels of reduced glutathione (GSH) in testis of prepubertal ((a), (b), and (c)) and adult rats ((c), (d), and (e)) following daily exposure to cigarette smoke (tobacco smoke, TS), smokeless tobacco (ST), and nicotine for 30 days. Data are expressed as mean ± SEM ($n = 6$). $^{*}p < 0.05$ compared to control; $^{**}p < 0.01$ compared to control; $^{\beta}p < 0.05$ compared to ST-0.5 mg/kg.; $^{\#}p < 0.05$ compared to TS-1 stick; $^{\alpha}p < 0.01$ compared to ST-0.5 mg/kg; $^{\delta}p < 0.05$ compared to ST-0.5 mg/kg and NC-0.5 mg/kg; $^{\phi}p < 0.05$ compared to NC-1 mg/kg.

as well as alteration of semen parameters in cigarette smoke exposed males [21, 42, 43]. However, similar studies on other tobacco products are limited. Also, the relative impact of tobacco products in juvenile animals has not been well studied.

In this study, tobacco smoke (TS), smokeless tobacco (ST), and nicotine were exposed to prepubertal and adult rats daily at different doses for 30 days and sperm parameters were measured to evaluate the effects of subacute exposure to tobacco products on reproductive function in the male. TS and ST had no significant effect on sperm morphology but reduced sperm motility and also sperm count in both prepubertal and adult rats in a dose-dependent fashion.

Sperm production (spermatogenesis) takes place primarily in the seminiferous tubules in the testis and spermatogenic activity is conventionally assessed by measurement of sperm parameters. Reduction in sperm count and motility observed in exposed rats reflects a reduction in the number and quality of sperm produced in the rats. Further, the observation of these reductions occurring mostly in the rats that were exposed to the higher doses of TS and ST indicates that low levels of TS and ST exposures may not affect testicular activity in the rat. The levels of reduction of the semen indices were observed to be higher in the prepubertal rats in comparison with the adult rats, which also indicates an inverse relationship of toxicity of tobacco products and

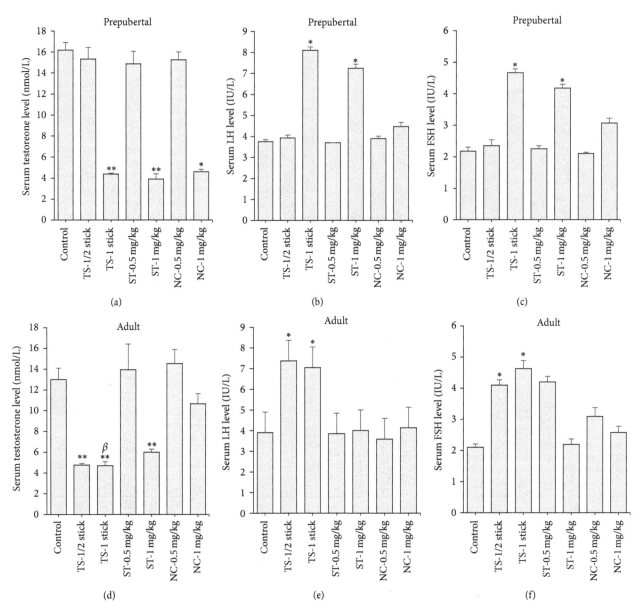

FIGURE 5: Serum levels of testosterone, luteinizing hormone (LH), and follicle stimulating hormone (FSH) in prepubertal ((a), (b), and (c)) and adult rats ((d), (e), and (f)) following daily exposure to cigarette smoke (tobacco smoke, TS), smokeless tobacco (ST), and nicotine for 30 days. Data are expressed as mean ± SEM ($n = 6$). $^*p < 0.05$ compared to control; $^{**}p < 0.01$ compared to control; $^\beta p < 0.05$ compared to NC-1 mg/kg.

testicular age. Additionally, ST may produce greater level of testicular toxicity, as the ST induced alterations of sperm motility and count were higher, compared to those of TS. This surprising finding evidences that ST products are not safer alternatives to TS.

Previous reports from several studies have provided contrasting reports on the effect of cigarette smoke on semen parameters. Trummer et al. [22] and de Jong et al. [44] have reported that smoking does not affect semen parameters in humans. On the contrary, Vine et al. [21] and Künzle et al. [43] showed negative effects of cigarette smoking on semen parameters in humans, which is consistent with our results. Unfortunately, the reasons for these different results

are not yet fully understood. Some previous studies had attributed the effects of tobacco products mostly to nicotine. Interestingly, our results showed that nicotine treatment had no significant effect on the sperm parameters measured in the adult rats but caused 82.2 and 62.6% reductions in sperm motility and count, respectively, in the prepubertal rats. This provides evidence that the components of tobacco smoke and smokeless tobacco contribute significantly to their testicular effects. Tobacco smoke and smokeless tobacco contain known mutagenic compounds in addition to other compounds that have been shown to be potentially toxic to normal testicular function, including cadmium, lead, and benzo(a)pyrene diol epoxide [4, 45, 46]. The different types and proportions of these components in tobacco smoke and smokeless tobacco products may account for their different degrees of toxicities. Even though there are many publications on the effects of cigarette smoking on semen parameters, limited data exist on the effects of smokeless tobacco, particularly in prepubertal animals. Further, comparative effects of tobacco products and nicotine on semen parameters had been sparsely studied prior to this study, which makes the findings of this study relevant.

Spermatogenesis is regulated by the androgen, testosterone, which is produced and secreted by the Leydig cells of the testis. The secretion of testosterone is in turn regulated by anterior pituitary and hypothalamic factors. Reduction in testosterone levels by tobacco smoke, smokeless tobacco, and nicotine exposures correlates positively with the reduction in sperm count and motility caused by the agents. This was accompanied by elevations of luteinizing hormone (LH) and follicle stimulating hormone (FSH) levels. Earlier, opposing results have also been reported on the hormonal influences of cigarette smoking in males. Ramlau-Hansen et al. [47] reported a positive dose-response relationship between smoking and reproductive hormones (testosterone and LH) in male humans; Trummer et al. [22] reported elevation of serum testosterone in smokers, while Pasqualotto et al. [48] reported absence of any significant difference between cigarette smokers and nonsmokers in levels of FSH, LH, or testosterone. These varying observations may partly be related to differences in the dose and duration of cigarette smoke exposure, animal species, or experimental procedure. The elevations of LH and FSH observed in this study suggest that the negative feedback control of testosterone secretion by the anterior pituitary gonadotropic hormones may be preserved. It thus implies that the observed alteration of sperm characteristics may more likely be due to toxicity to cells in testicular milieu without interference with the hypothalamic-pituitary axis.

From the results, the effects of the tobacco products may be associated with increase in oxidative stress. Oxidative stress in the testis results from an imbalance of the production of free radicals and antioxidant activities. TS, ST, and nicotine caused significant elevations of the lipid peroxidation product, malondialdehyde (MDA), which is consistent with previous results [4, 49]. In addition, reduced glutathione (GSH), catalase, and superoxide dismutase (SOD) were altered. SOD and catalase are essential antioxidant defenses of the body; both catalyze the detoxification of $O_2{}^-$ reactive radicals and prevent generation of free radicals in the cell. GSH, which contains thiol group, readily interacts with free radicals and is considered to be one of the most important cellular antioxidants to maintain cellular redox state [50, 51]. Testicular tissue is rich in these antioxidants which form effective antioxidant barrier against environmental reactive oxygen species and those generated endogenously by inhaled toxicants [52]. In TS exposed prepubertal rats, SOD activity was not affected, catalase was reduced, and GSH was increased. In both ST and nicotine exposed prepubertal rats, there were no changes in SOD and catalase activities, but GSH was decreased in the former and elevated in the latter. In the exposed adult rats, TS caused no significant alteration

of antioxidants; ST increased GSH but did not alter SOD and catalase, while nicotine decreased SOD and did not affect the other antioxidants. Reduced antioxidant activity would increase generation or reactivity of ROS and cause oxidative stress. This compromises testicular function [52] and may contribute to the observed toxic testicular effects of TS, ST, and nicotine. The elevations of the antioxidant levels, observed mostly in exposed prepubertal rats, may reflect the testis adaptation to stress induced by the tobacco products. Similar observations have been reported in the female rat [53].

The results show that subacute exposure to tobacco smoke, smokeless tobacco, and nicotine does not affect sperm morphology but causes dose-related reductions in sperm motility, sperm count, and testosterone, occurring more in prepubertal rats than adult rats. These effects are most pronounced with smokeless tobacco and least pronounced with nicotine, and their mechanism of toxicity may be linked to increase in oxidative stress in the testis. It is, however, important to note that the data in the present study did not address whether or not these effects are reversible, so, there is need for further studies to evaluate the reversibility of these effects.

Conflict of Interests

The authors declare that there is no conflict of interests with respect to the research, authorship, and/or publication of this paper.

Acknowledgment

The authors thank the assistance of technical staff of the Departments of Pharmacology and Biochemistry, University of Port Harcourt, Nigeria, especially Mark Bam.

References

[1] I. B. Karaconji, "Facts about nicotine toxicity," *Archives of Industrial Hygiene & Toxicology*, vol. 56, pp. 363–371, 2005.

[2] B. O. Iranloye and A. F. Bolarinwa, "Effect of nicotine administration on weight and histology of some vital visceral organs in female albino rats," *Nigerian Journal of Physiological Sciences*, vol. 24, no. 1, pp. 7–12, 2009.

[3] B. Halliwell, "Cigarette smoking and health: a radical review," *Royal Society Journal of Social Heath*, vol. 113, no. 3, pp. 91–96, 1993.

[4] B. Halliwell and H. E. Poulsen, *Cigarette Smoke and Oxidative Stress*, Springer, New York, NY, USA, 2006.

[5] D. M. Fergusson, L. J. Horwood, F. T. Shannon, and B. Taylor, "Parental smoking and lower respiratory illness in the first three years of life," *Journal of Epidemiology and Community Health*, vol. 35, no. 3, pp. 180–184, 1981.

[6] G. W. Hunninghake and R. G. Crystal, "Cigarette smoking and lung destruction. Accumulation of neutrophils in the lungs of cigarette smokers," *American Review of Respiratory Disease*, vol. 128, no. 5, pp. 833–838, 1983.

[7] M. Weitzman, S. Gortmaker, D. Klein Walker, and A. Sobol, "Maternal smoking and childhood asthma," *Pediatrics*, vol. 85, no. 4, pp. 505–511, 1990.

[8] N. A. Rigotti and R. C. Pasternak, "Cigarette smoking and coronary heart disease: risks and management," *Cardiology Clinics*, vol. 14, no. 1, pp. 51–68, 1996.

[9] G. N. Connolly, P. Richter, A. Aleguas Jr., T. F. Pechacek, S. B. Stanfill, and H. R. Alpert, "Unintentional child poisonings through ingestion of conventional and novel tobacco products," *Pediatrics*, vol. 125, no. 5, pp. 896–899, 2010.

[10] M. Parascandola, E. Augustson, M. E. O'Connell, and S. Marcus, "Consumer awareness and attitudes related to new potential reduced-exposure tobacco product brands," *Nicotine & Tobacco Research*, vol. 11, no. 7, pp. 886–895, 2009.

[11] O. O. Desalu, K. R. Iseh, A. B. Olokoba, F. K. Salawu, and A. Danburam, "Smokeless tobacco use in adult nigerian population," *Nigerian Journal of Clinical Practice*, vol. 13, no. 4, pp. 382–387, 2010.

[12] Tobacco Products Scientific Advisory Committee (TPSAC), *The Nature and Impact of the Use of Dissolvable Tobacco Products on the Public Health: A Report from the Tobacco Products Scientific Advisory Committee*, Food and Drug Administration, 2012.

[13] C. Augood, K. Duckitt, and A. A. Templeton, "Smoking and female infertility: a systematic review and meta-analysis," *Human Reproduction*, vol. 13, no. 6, pp. 1532–1539, 1998.

[14] C. Ward, S. Lewis, and T. Coleman, "Prevalence of maternal smoking and environmental tobacco smoke exposure during pregnancy and impact on birth weight: retrospective study using Millennium Cohort," *BMC Public Health*, vol. 7, article 81, 2007.

[15] D. P. Misra and R. H. N. Nguyen, "Environmental tobacco smoke and low birth weight: a hazard in the workplace?" *Environmental Health Perspectives*, vol. 107, no. 6, pp. 897–904, 1999.

[16] R. A. Walsh, "Effects of maternal smoking on adverse pregnancy outcomes: examination of the criteria of causation," *Human Biology*, vol. 66, no. 6, pp. 1059–1092, 1994.

[17] S. C. Birnbaum, N. Kien, R. W. Martucci et al., "Nicotine- or epinephrine-induced uteroplacental vasoconstriction and fetal growth in the rat," *Toxicology*, vol. 94, no. 1–3, pp. 69–80, 1994.

[18] D. Economides and J. Braithwaite, "Smoking, pregnancy and the fetus," *Journal of the Royal Society of Health*, vol. 114, no. 4, pp. 198–201, 1994.

[19] I. P. Oyeyipo, Y. Raji, B. O. Emikpe, and A. F. Bolarinwa, "Effects of nicotine on sperm characteristics and fertility profile in adult male rats: a possible role of cessation," *Journal of Reproduction and Infertility*, vol. 12, no. 3, pp. 201–207, 2011.

[20] I. P. Oyeyipo, Y. Raji, and A. F. Bolarinwa, "Nicotine alters male reproductive hormones in male albino rats: the role of cessation," *Journal of Human Reproductive Sciences*, vol. 6, no. 1, pp. 40–44, 2013.

[21] M. F. Vine, C.-K. J. Tse, P.-C. Hu, and K. Y. Truong, "Cigarette smoking and semen quality," *Fertility & Sterility*, vol. 65, no. 4, pp. 835–842, 1996.

[22] H. Trummer, H. Habermann, J. Haas, and K. Pummer, "The impact of cigarette smoking on human semen parameters and hormones," *Human Reproduction*, vol. 17, no. 6, pp. 1554–1559, 2002.

[23] B. A. Hanadi, A. M. Kelany, F. M. ElQudsi, H. A. Ameen, and S. A. El Karium, "The possible protective role of antioxidants (selenium, vitamin E) in reducing smoking effects on testes

of albino rats," *Assiut University Bulletin for Environmental Researches*, vol. 14, no. 1, 2011.

[24] R. Abdul-Ghani, M. Qazzaz, N. Dabdoub, R. Muhammad, and A.-S. Abdul-Ghani, "Studies on cigarette smoke induced oxidative DNA damage and reduced spermatogenesis in rats," *Journal of Environmental Biology*, vol. 35, no. 5, pp. 943–947, 2014.

[25] H. Ozyurt, H. Pekmez, B. S. Parlaktas, I. Kus, B. Ozyurt, and M. Sarsilmaz, "Oxidative stress in testicular tissues of rats exposed to cigarette smoke and protective effects of caffeic acid phenethyl ester," *Asian Journal of Andrology*, vol. 8, no. 2, pp. 189–193, 2006.

[26] J. B. Dai, Z. X. Wang, and Z. D. Qiao, "The hazardous effects of tobacco smoking on male fertility," *Asian Journal of Andrology*, 2015.

[27] L. Samanta, A. Sahoo, and G. B. N. Chainy, "Age-related changes in rat testicular oxidative stress parameters by hexachlorocyclohexane," *Archives of Toxicology*, vol. 73, no. 2, pp. 96–107, 1999.

[28] K. N. Chandrashekar and Muralidhara, "Evidence of oxidative stress and mitochondrial dysfunctions in the testis of prepubertal diabetic rats," *International Journal of Impotence Research*, vol. 21, no. 3, pp. 198–206, 2009.

[29] Canadian Council on Animal Care (CCAC), *The Care and Use of Farm Animals in Research, Teaching and Testing*, Canadian Council on Animal Care (CCAC), Ottawa, Canada, 2009.

[30] D. C. Dorman, B. A. Wong, M. F. Struve et al., "Development of a mouse whole-body exposure system from a directed-flow, rat nose-only system," *Inhalation Toxicology*, vol. 8, no. 1, pp. 107–120, 1996.

[31] B. A. Wong, "Inhalation exposure systems: design, methods and operation," *Toxicologic Pathology*, vol. 35, no. 1, pp. 3–14, 2007.

[32] D. Vitarella, R. A. James, K. L. Miller, M. F. Struve, B. A. Wong, and D. C. Dorman, "Development of an inhalation system for the simultaneous exposure of rat dams and pups during developmental neurotoxicity studies," *Inhalation Toxicology*, vol. 10, no. 12, pp. 1095–1117, 1998.

[33] D. J. Baker, "Semen analysis," *Clinical Laboratory Science*, vol. 20, no. 3, pp. 172–187, 2007.

[34] O. Ochei and A. Kolhatker, *Medical Laboratory Science, Theory and Practice*, Tata McGraw-Hill Publishing Company Limited, New Delhi, India, 5th edition, 2002.

[35] M. Sun and S. Zigman, "An improved spectrophotometric assay for superoxide dismutase based on epinephrine autoxidation," *Analytical Biochemistry*, vol. 90, no. 1, pp. 81–89, 1978.

[36] H. Aebi, "Catalase *in vitro*," in *Method in Enzymology*, S. P. Colowick and N. O. Kaplane, Eds., Academic Press, New York, NY, USA, 1984.

[37] J. Sedlak and R. H. Lindsay, "Estimation of total, protein-bound, and nonprotein sulfhydryl groups in tissue with Ellman's reagent," *Analytical Biochemistry*, vol. 25, pp. 192–205, 1968.

[38] J. A. Buege and S. D. Aust, "Microsomal lipid peroxidation," *Methods in Enzymology*, vol. 52, pp. 302–310, 1978.

[39] M. O. Araoye, "Epidemiology of infertility: social problems of the infertile couples," *West African Journal of Medicine*, vol. 22, no. 2, pp. 190–196, 2003.

[40] T. Bushnik, J. L. Cook, A. A. Yuzpe, S. Tough, and J. Collins, "Estimating the prevalence of infertility in Canada," *Human Reproduction*, vol. 27, no. 3, pp. 738–746, 2012.

[41] E. Jauniaux and G. J. Burton, "Morphological and biological effects of maternal exposure to tobacco smoke on the feto-placental unit," *Early Human Development*, vol. 83, no. 11, pp. 699–706, 2007.

[42] G. Holzki, H. Gall, and J. Hermann, "Cigarette smoking and sperm quality," *Andrologia*, vol. 23, no. 2, pp. 141–144, 1991.

[43] R. Künzle, M. D. Mueller, W. Hänggi, M. H. Birkhäuser, H. Drescher, and N. A. Bersinger, "Semen quality of male smokers and nonsmokers in infertile couples," *Fertility & Sterility*, vol. 79, no. 2, pp. 287–291, 2003.

[44] A. M. E. de Jong, R. Menkveld, J. W. Lens, S. E. Nienhuis, and J. P. T. Rhemrev, "Effect of alcohol intake and cigarette smoking on sperm parameters and pregnancy," *Andrologia*, vol. 46, no. 2, pp. 112–117, 2014.

[45] O. E. Orisakwe, Z. N. Igweze, K. O. Okolo, and G. C. Ajaezi, "Heavy metal hazards of Nigerian smokeless tobacco," *Tobacco Control*, vol. 23, no. 6, pp. 513–517, 2014.

[46] J. S. Aprioku and A. W. Obianime, "Evaluation of the effects of *Citrus aurantifolia* (lime) juice in lead-induced hematological and testicular toxicity in rats," *Pharmacologia*, vol. 5, no. 1, pp. 36–41, 2014.

[47] C. H. Ramlau-Hansen, A. M. Thulstrup, A. S. Aggerholm, M. S. Jensen, G. Toft, and J. P. Bonde, "Is smoking a risk factor for decreased semen quality? A cross-sectional analysis," *Human Reproduction*, vol. 22, no. 1, pp. 188–196, 2007.

[48] F. F. Pasqualotto, B. P. Sobreiro, J. Hallak, E. B. Pasqualotto, and A. M. Lucon, "Cigarette smoking is related to a decrease in semen volume in a population of fertile men," *BJU International*, vol. 97, no. 2, pp. 324–326, 2006.

[49] A. R. Kiziler, B. Aydemir, I. Onaran et al., "High levels of cadmium and lead in seminal fluid and blood of smoking men are associated with high oxidative stress and damage in infertile subjects," *Biological Trace Element Research*, vol. 120, no. 1–3, pp. 82–91, 2007.

[50] A. Pastore, G. Federici, E. Bertini, and F. Piemonte, "Analysis of glutathione: implication in redox and detoxification," *Clinica Chimica Acta*, vol. 333, no. 1, pp. 19–39, 2003.

[51] E. Nozik-Grayck, H. B. Suliman, and C. A. Piantadosi, "Extra-cellular superoxide dismutase," *International Journal of Biochemistry & Cell Biology*, vol. 37, no. 12, pp. 2466–2471, 2005.

[52] J. S. Aprioku, "Pharmacology of free radicals and the impact of reactive oxygen species on the testis," *Journal of Reproduction and Infertility*, vol. 14, no. 4, pp. 158–172, 2013.

[53] E. Florek and A. Marszalek, "An experimental study of the influences of tobacco smoke on fertility and reproduction," *Human & Experimental Toxicology*, vol. 18, no. 4, pp. 272–278, 1999.

23

Selenium Attenuates HPV-18 Associated Apoptosis in Embryo-Derived Trophoblastic Cells but Not Inner Cell Mass In Vitro

Jennifer A. Tolen,[1] **Penelope Duerksen-Hughes,**[2] **Kathleen Lau,**[1] **and Philip J. Chan**[1]

[1]*Department of Gynecology and Obstetrics, 11370 Anderson Street, Suite 3950, Loma Linda University School of Medicine, Loma Linda, CA 92354, USA*
[2]*Department of Basic Sciences, Center for Health Disparities and Molecular Medicine, 11021 Campus Street, Loma Linda University School of Medicine, Loma Linda, CA 92350, USA*

Correspondence should be addressed to Philip J. Chan; pjchan@llu.edu

Academic Editor: Kai-Fai Lee

Objectives. Human papillomaviruses (HPV) are associated with cell cycle arrest. This study focused on antioxidant selenomethionine (SeMet) inhibition of HPV-mediated necrosis. The objectives were to determine HPV-18 effects on embryonic cells and to evaluate SeMet in blocking HPV-18 effects. *Methods.* Fertilized mouse embryos were cultured for 5 days to implanted trophoblasts and exposed to either control medium (group 1), HPV-18 (group 2), combined HPV-18 and 0.5 μM SeMet (group 3), or combined HPV-18 and 5.0 μM SeMet (group 4). After 48 hrs, trophoblast integrity and, apoptosis/necrosis were assessed using morphometric and dual-stain fluorescence assays, respectively. *Results.* HPV-18 exposed trophoblasts nuclei (253.8 ± 28.5 sq·μ) were 29% smaller than controls (355.6 ± 35.9 sq·μ). Supplementation with 0.5 and 5.0 μM SeMet prevented nuclear shrinkage after HPV-18 exposure. HPV-18 infected trophoblasts remained larger with SeMet supplementation. HPV-18 decreased cell viability by 44% but SeMet supplementation sustained cell viability. Apoptosis was lower when SeMet was present. HPV-18 decreased inner cell mass (ICM) viability by over 60%. *Conclusions.* HPV-18 decreased nuclear size and trophoblast viability but these effects were attenuated by the antioxidant SeMet. SeMet blocked HPV-18 associated apoptosis process in trophoblasts but not ICM cells suggesting involvement of different oxidative stress pathways.

1. Introduction

Human papillomaviruses (HPV) are classified group 1 human carcinogens (IARC, International Agency for Research on Cancer) extensively studied for their role in cervical cancer [1]. HPV are double-stranded DNA viruses with a well-defined affinity for epithelial cells. The high risk HPV serotypes 16 and 18 are responsible for 50–70% of all cases. HPV has been recovered more frequently in placentas obtained from patients with spontaneous preterm labor and spontaneous abortions than from term or elective abortions [2–6]. Gomez et al. [2] showed that HPV infection of trophoblasts induces cell death and reduces cell invasion, possibly placental invasion into the uterine wall. Preterm birth is the single largest direct cause of neonatal deaths,

directly resulting in 35% of the world's 3.1 million deaths a year [7]. Recently, HPV has been shown to increase oxidative stress [8] that is associated with pregnancy complications, premature rupture of membrane, and preterm birth [9–11]. However, treatment modalities for HPV-mediated placental pathogenesis are lacking and studies are warranted.

The trace element selenium is a component of antioxidative selenoenzymes, Glutathione Peroxidase (GPx) and Thioredoxin Reductase (ThxRed), that decrease oxidative stress. Studies in BeWo and JEG-3 trophoblast cell lines provided evidence that inorganic sodium selenite and organic selenomethionine (SeMet) protected cells from oxidative stress [12, 13]. SeMet is a selenium-containing amino acid that upregulates the 2 selenoenzymes GPx and ThxRed responsible for depleting reactive oxygen species (ROS) and reactive nitrogen species (RNS) thereby reducing oxidative stress [13, 14]. The role of selenium compounds as anticancer agents has been reviewed [15, 16].

We hypothesized that treatment with antioxidant promoting SeMet would inhibit HPV-mediated embryonic cell necrosis. Recently, cultured trophoblast cells from implanted embryos were used as a model for HPV infectivity studies [17, 18]. In this study, the objectives were (1) to determine the effects of HPV-18 exposure on cultured cells from the trophoblast and inner cell mass (ICM) layers and (2) to evaluate the role of SeMet in preventing the damaging effects of HPV-18 on the ICM and trophoblast cells.

2. Materials and Methods

2.1. HeLa Cell Lysate Procedure. The preparation of HeLa cell lysates was as previously reported [17, 18]. HeLa cells (ATCC, American Type Culture Collection, Manassas, VA) derived from human cervical cell carcinoma contained multiple copies of HPV-18 integrated at chromosome 8, band q24 [19, 20]. The HeLa cells were cultured in Eagle Minimal Essential Medium (MEM, Invitrogen, Carlsbad, CA), supplemented with 10% fetal bovine serum (Invitrogen), 100 U/mL penicillin, 0.1 mg/mL streptomycin, and 0.25 μg/mL amphotericin B (Sigma Aldrich Chemical Co., St. Louis, MO). The cells were passaged and processed after reaching 80% confluence [21]. The HeLa cells were centrifuge-washed at 300 ×g for 10 mins and the pellets of cells combined in a microfuge tube containing 0.4 mL of G-2 plus version 5 medium (G-2 v5, VitroLife, Englewood, CO). HPV-18 gene fragments were extracted from cells lysed using a sterile rod and pestle apparatus. The cell extract was stored frozen in cryovials at −23°C. The lysates were warmed to 37°C prior to their use in the mouse embryo experiments.

2.2. Culture of Pronuclear Mouse Embryo to the Implanted Stage. The procedure for culturing embryos to the implanted stage was as previously reported [22, 23]. Briefly, cryopreserved 1-cell mouse fertilized oocytes in cryostraws (Embryotech Laboratories Inc., Haverhill, MA) were thawed into a droplet of G-1 v5 medium (G-1 v5, VitroLife, Englewood, CO) in a Petri dish. The 1-cell fertilized embryos were washed through 2 additional droplets of G-1 v5 medium. The embryos were pooled at the center well of a double-well culture dish (Falcon 3037, Becton Dickinson, Franklin Lakes, NJ) containing 1 mL of G-1 v5 medium. Water was placed on the outer moat for humidity and each dish was placed in an incubator at 37°C, 5% CO_2 in air mixture. After 3 days, the embryos were randomly divided into 4 groups and placed into 4 culture dishes containing G-2 v5 medium with more nutrients for blastocyst growth. Embryos that had not developed to the early blastocyst stage were not used. The embryos were further incubated for an additional 2 days until they reached the implanted stage.

A concentrated stock solution of the selenium-containing amino acid, selenomethionine (SeMet, Sigma Aldrich Chemical Co., St. Louis, MO), was dissolved in G-2 v5 medium and used in the preparation of the 0.5 and 5.0 μM SeMet culture media. The 0.5 μM concentration was based on a previous study in trophoblast cells [13]. Implanted embryos in each group were exposed to either control medium containing heat-inactivated HPV-18 HeLa lysate (10 μL) (group 1), thawed HeLa cell lysate (10 μL) containing active HPV-18 (group 2), combined HeLa lysate and 0.5 μM SeMet medium (group 3), or combined HeLa lysate and 5.0 μM SeMet medium (group 4). The cell cultures were further incubated for 48 hrs. Cell viability status, trophoblast nuclear size, and cell area were assessed as described below.

2.3. Dual Fluorescence Stain Analysis for Cell Status. The dual fluorescence stain method [18, 22] was used to distinguish viable, apoptotic, or necrotic trophoblast cells in each embryo. Briefly, a drop of bisbenzimide (5 μL of 10 μM, Hoechst 33342, Sigma Chemical Co., St. Louis, MO) was added to the implanted embryos and after 1 minute, 5 μL of propidium iodide (32 μM, Sigma Chemical Co., St. Louis, MO, dissolved in saline) was added to the embryos. After another minute, the culture medium with the stains was discarded and prewarmed culture medium (0.5 mL) was added to each dish. The culture dish was placed on the stage of an epifluorescence UV-microscope set at magnification of 500x (Nikon Optiphot, Nikon Instruments, Melville, NY) and images of the fluorescent colored cells in each embryo were captured on a digital camera. The percentages of viable, apoptotic, and necrotic cells of the ICM and trophoblast layers were determined for each embryo. In this study, a viable cell was defined as the capacity of the cell to exclude the fluorescent dyes and possessed a clear coloration. In contrast, an apoptotic (completely blue color) or necrotic (pink-red color) cell was identified by the cell capacity to absorb bisbenzimide or propidium iodide stain, respectively.

2.4. Trophoblast Morphology Stain Procedure. Trophoblast cells and inner cell mass nuclei and cytoplasm were stained using a sequential Fast Green FCF and Rose Bengal (Spermac Stain Enterprises Inc., Republic of South Africa) staining procedure [18, 23]. The procedure involved rinsing the implanted embryos with culture medium followed by fixation in 4% formalin (5 mins). The fixative was rinsed off with water and Spermac stain A (Rose Bengal mixture) was added (2 minutes). Stain A was rinsed off and stain B (Pyronin Y mixture) was added (1-minute staining) followed by rinsing and staining with stain C (Fast Green FCF-Janus Green mixture, 1 minute). The stained embryos were rinsed in water, air-dried, and stored in a dark drawer until the time of analyses.

2.5. Spectrophotodensitometry. Cell dimensions were measured using a spectrophotodensitometric method which facilitated the determination of embryo growth and migration [18]. The Spermac-stained inner cell mass and trophoblast cells were located on each slide using the Nikon Diaphot inverted microscope (400x magnification) and the images digitized and recorded. The preanalytical phase included using Adobe Photoshop software to standardize each image [24]. The image outline of each nucleus or

TABLE 1: Comparison of the area (mean ± S.E.M.) of each trophoblast nucleus or each trophoblast cell size after 24-hour exposure (at 37°C, 5% CO_2 in air) to either (1) control medium with heat-inactivated HPV-18 HeLa lysate, (2) HPV-18 HeLa lysate, (3) HPV-18 HeLa lysate and 0.5 μM selenomethionine (SeMet), or (4) HPV-18 HeLa lysate and 5.0 μM SeMet. The ICM cells were not analyzed due to limitations in stained compacted cells.

Treatment groups	Number of cells (n)	Size of nucleus (μ^2)	Size of trophoblast (μ^2)
(1) Control	23	355.6 ± 35.9	45,620.5 ± 10,440.3
(2) HPV-18 HeLa lysate	28	253.8 ± 28.5[a]	54,477.3 ± 10,352.0
(3) HPV-18 HeLa lysate and 0.5 μM SeMet	20	401.9 ± 47.8[b]	63,651.1 ± 16,106.9[a]
(4) HPV-18 HeLa lysate and 5.0 μM SeMet	26	275.5 ± 23.1	105,038.0 ± 8,802.0[a,b]

[a]Different from the control (1) group ($p < 0.05$).
[b]Different from the HPV-18 HeLa lysate (2) group ($p < 0.05$).

TABLE 2: Day 6 in vitro implanted mouse embryos were exposed (at 37°C, 5% CO_2 in air) for 48 hours to either (1) control medium with heat-inactivated HPV-18 HeLa lysate, (2) HPV-18 HeLa lysate, (3) HPV-18 HeLa lysate and 0.5 μM selenomethionine (SeMet), or (4) HPV-18 HeLa lysate and 5.0 μM SeMet. The percentages of live, apoptotic, and necrotic trophoblast cells were assessed using bisbenzimide and propidium iodide dual-stain epifluorescence analyses.

Trophoblast cells group	Total cells (n)	Number of viable cells (%)	Number of apoptotic cells (%)	Number of necrotic cells (%)	Number of total nonviable cells (%)
(1) Control group	64	17 (23.6)	47 (76.4)	0 (0)	47 (76.4)
(2) HPV-18 HeLa lysate	134	16 (13.3)[a]	109 (79.8)	9 (6.9)[a]	118 (86.7)[a]
(3) HPV-18 HeLa and 0.5 μM SeMet	187	51 (24.2)[b]	111 (62.2)[b]	25 (13.6)[a,b]	136 (75.8)[b]
(4) HPV-18 HeLa lysate and 5.0 μM SeMet	132	35 (24.0)[b]	74 (58.7)[b]	23 (17.4)[a,b]	97 (76.1)[a,b]

[a]Different from the control (1) group ($p < 0.05$).
[b]Different from the HPV-18 HeLa lysate (2) group ($p < 0.05$).

the entire trophoblast cell was traced onscreen and measurements were determined using the Adobe Photoshop histogram function. The recorded data was entered into Microsoft Excel spreadsheets and analyzed.

2.6. Statistical Analysis. Data from the morphometric analyses of cell dimensions were presented as mean ± standard error of the mean (S.E.M.). For each treatment group, the mean dimension of the ICM or trophoblast nucleus and entire cell area were calculated and tested using ANOVA and significance of means was compared using the two-tailed Student's t-test. The numbers of viable, apoptotic, or necrotic trophoblast cells for each treatment group were tested using the two-tailed Mantel-Haenszel chi-square test statistics (http://OpenEpi.com/, Open Source Epidemiologic Statistics for Public Health, Emory University, Atlanta, GA). A value of $p < 0.05$ was considered significant.

3. Results

The nuclear size (Table 1) of HPV-18 exposed trophoblasts (253.8 ± 28.5 sq·μ) was 29% smaller ($p < 0.03$) than control trophoblasts (355.6 ± 35.9 sq·μ). The supplementation with 0.5 μM SeMet significantly reversed ($p < 0.005$) the nuclear shrinkage in the HPV-18 exposed trophoblasts (401.9 ± 47.8 sq·μ). Interestingly, the addition of the higher concentration of SeMet (5.0 μM) also prevented nuclear shrinkage in the HPV-18 infected trophoblasts but the effect was less pronounced (275.5 ± 23.1 sq·μ). A shrunken reduced

nucleus in the trophoblast cell was indicative of inhibited endoreduplication [25]. Endoreduplication is required for rapid differentiation and intensive cell growth [26].

In terms of the entire cell size, the HPV-18 exposed trophoblast cells demonstrated cell growth and hypertrophy (Figure 1) in the presence of both low (63651.1 ± 16106.9 sq·μ) and high (105038.0 ± 8802.0 sq·μ) SeMet concentrations when compared with the control (45620.5 ± 10440.3 sq·μ). Exposure to HPV-18 alone (54477.3 ± 10352 sq·μ) did not affect overall trophoblast cell dimension ($p < 0.09$). Trophoblast cell hypertrophy has been reported to be associated with activating F-actin cytoskeleton assembly correlated with migratory or invasive activity [27]. Although the nuclear size of HPV-18 exposed trophoblasts treated with the higher 5 μM concentration SeMet remained unchanged, the mean cell dimension in this group was over 93% larger in size (Figure 1).

The presence of HPV-18 decreased ($p < 0.005$) trophoblast cell viability (13.3% live) when compared with the control (23.6%) after 48 hours of culture (Table 2). However, when SeMet was also present in the HPV-18 exposed groups, cell viability was sustained similar to the control group ($p > 0.49$). Furthermore, the percentages of apoptotic cells were lower when SeMet was present in the HPV-18 exposed groups. Although a small increase in necrosis was noted in the SeMet groups, the higher apoptosis in the HPV-18 only group yielded an overall higher cell viability in the groups with SeMet supplementation. There was no dose response observed based on the 2 concentrations of SeMet tested in this study.

TABLE 3: Day 6 in vitro implanted mouse embryos were exposed (at 37°C, 5% CO_2 in air) for 48 hours to either (1) control medium with heat-inactivated HPV-18 HeLa lysate, (2) HPV-18 HeLa lysate, (3) HPV-18 HeLa lysate and 0.5 μM selenomethionine (SeMet), or (4) HPV-18 HeLa lysate and 5.0 μM SeMet. The percentages of live, apoptotic, and necrotic inner cell mass (ICM) cells were assessed using bisbenzimide and propidium iodide dual-stain epifluorescence analyses.

Treated ICM cells groups	Total cells (n)	Number of viable cells (%)	Number of apoptotic cells (%)	Number of necrotic cells (%)	Number of total nonviable cells (%)
(1) Control group	71	32 (45.5)	38 (53.2)	1 (1.3)	39 (54.5)
(2) HPV-18 HeLa lysate	365	41 (17.5)[a]	236 (55.3)	88 (27.2)[a]	324 (82.5)[a]
(3) HPV-18 HeLa and 0.5 μM SeMet	236	44 (19.2)[a]	123 (50.6)	69 (30.1)[a]	192 (80.8)[a]
(4) HPV-18 HeLa lysate and 5.0 μM SeMet	210	36 (20.6)[a]	148 (68.0)	26 (11.4)[a,b]	174 (79.4)[a]

[a]Different from the control (1) group ($p < 0.05$).
[b]Different from the HPV-18 HeLa lysate (2) group ($p < 0.05$).

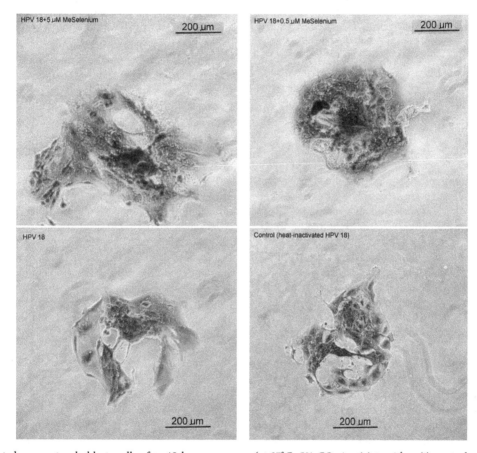

FIGURE 1: Implanted mouse trophoblasts cells after 48-hour exposure (at 37°C, 5% CO_2 in air) to either (1) control medium with heat-inactivated HPV-18 HeLa lysate, (2) HPV-18 HeLa lysate, (3) HPV-18 HeLa lysate and 0.5 μM selenomethionine (SeMet), or (4) HPV-18 HeLa lysate and 5.0 μM SeMet. The stain used was Rose Bengal and Fast Green-based Spermac staining kit and images were taken using the Nikon Diaphot inverted microscope (400x magnification). The cell sizes for the images were as follows: (1) control, 515 μ, (2) HPV-18 HeLa lysate, 609 μ, (3) HPV-18 HeLa lysate with 0.5 μM SeMet, 622 μ, and (4) HPV-18 HeLa lysate with 5.0 μM SeMet, 915 μ at the greatest width.

Using the dual fluorescence stains procedure, the status of each compacted cell of the ICM layer was readily assessed as a colored point of light. The results (Table 3) showed that HPV-18 decreased ICM cell viability by over 60% when compared with the control (17.5 versus control 45.5% live). The addition of SeMet to the HPV-18 exposed ICM cells did not prevent cell death resulting from HPV-18.

The percentages of apoptotic ICM cells were the highest in the HPV-18 with 5.0 μM SeMet group indicating a slower demise of ICM cells in the higher concentration of SeMet group. In contrast to trophoblast cells, the addition of SeMet to the ICM cells did not have a positive response in terms of sustaining viability when challenged with HPV-18 exposure.

4. Discussion

HPV infection rates in spontaneous abortions of the first and second trimesters have been reported to be in the 50–70% range [2, 3]. The presence of HPV has been detected in the placentas derived from spontaneous abortions and preterm deliveries cases [2]. The origin of the HPV found in the placental cells was postulated to be circulating cell-free HPV DNA in the blood. Indeed, using the sensitive QIAamp circulating nucleic acid kit procedure and TaqMan technology, Mazurek and colleagues provided evidence of the circulating cell-free HPV DNA in blood plasma [28]. Recent evidence suggested that one of the etiologies of placental pathology was impaired trophoblast cell adhesion and trophoblast cellular necrosis in the HPV-infected placenta [5, 6, 17, 29]. Trophoblast cells are placental cells that participate in embryonic implantation and form critical cellular layers to facilitate fetal and maternal blood interactions in the pregnant uterus. Another group of cells from the ICM layer gives rise to the fetus. During placental inflammation, the HPV expressed oncogenes E5, E6, and E7 correlated with increased reactive oxygen species (ROS) and oxidative stress in the trophoblasts [2–5, 30–33].

The trace element selenium is a component of antioxidative selenoenzymes, Glutathione Peroxidase (GPx) and Thioredoxin Reductase (ThxRed), that decrease oxidative stress. Recent studies provided evidence that inorganic sodium selenite and organic selenomethionine (SeMet) protected cells from oxidative stress caused by peroxides and metabolic inhibitors such as antimycin and rotenone [12, 13]. SeMet is a selenium-containing amino acid that upregulates the 2 selenoenzymes GPx and ThxRed responsible for depleting ROS and reactive nitrogen species (RNS) thereby reducing oxidative stress [13, 14]. Other studies have shown the involvement of SeMet in altered cell signaling and inhibited gene expression of the proinflammatory cytokine IL-1β [34]. However, for in vitro studies of isolated cultured cells, the SeMet effects would most likely involve only oxidative reactions.

In the present study, the results showed that the addition of SeMet prevented nuclear shrinkage in the HPV-18 exposed trophoblasts. A shrunken nucleus in the trophoblast cell would be indicative of inhibited endoreduplication [24, 25]. The mechanism of action likely involved SeMet upregulating GPx and ThxRed to enzymatically catalyze ROS into inert molecules such as water possibly through transference of energy away from the reactive peroxides [35]. In this manner, SeMet protected the trophoblast nucleus from damage. Furthermore, SeMet had a hypertrophic effect on the trophoblast cells in terms of expanded cell size, even in the presence of HPV-18. Previous reports in specific cell types such as mammary epithelial cells showed that SeMet increased cell proliferation and cell viability [36]. This suggested that SeMet supplementation blocked HPV-18 mediated damaging effects on structural aspect of the placental cell. An obvious issue to address was whether or not SeMet would sustain cell viability in the presence of HPV-18.

The results showed that when SeMet was present in the HPV-18 exposed trophoblast cells, viability was sustained similar to the control cells. Furthermore, the percentages of apoptotic cells were lower when SeMet was present in the HPV-18 exposed groups. In the absence of SeMet supplementation, HPV-18 decreased trophoblast cell viability by 44%. This confirmed the protective role of SeMet in placental trophoblast cells. However, more studies are still needed to address another important group of cells associated with the trophoblast, namely, the ICM or embryoblast cells.

Dual fluorescence stain analysis showed that HPV-18 decreased ICM cell viability by over 60% when compared with the control. The addition of SeMet to the HPV-18 exposed ICM cells had no effect on blocking cell death. Moreover, apoptosis of ICM cells was the highest in the HPV-18 with 5.0 μM SeMet group. This suggested that SeMet had a differential effect on cell viability that depended on the specific cell type. Previous studies have reported variable results of SeMet from cytotoxicity in lymphocytes and fibroblasts [37, 38] to protective effects in chondrocytes and BeWo trophoblasts [33, 39], hence reinforcing the need to study SeMet differential effects on placental cell types.

Limitations and precautions of the present study included the use of cultured cells which might generate a different response in the in vivo environment and the lack of pretreatment cell morphology assessment which would have required invasive cell fixing and staining procedures. Although studies showed SeMet upregulated selenoenzymes that reduced oxidative stress, a limitation here was that possible effects of SeMet affecting the stability of the HPV-18 gene fragments or cellular uptake were not evaluated as these effects were beyond the scope of the present study. It is recognized that the HPV oncogenes also affect other pathways involving p53 and Rb genes and these have been reviewed [40]. Nevertheless, the end result of HPV exposure was trophoblast cell death and SeMet could be a potential supplement for the prevention of HPV-related pregnancy losses. Further studies are needed to corroborate the present findings of SeMet treatment to abrogate HPV-related pathogenesis in the placenta.

Conflict of Interests

The authors declare that they have no conflict of interests regarding the publication of this paper.

Acknowledgments

The HeLa cells were kindly donated by Drs. Duerksen-Hughes and her laboratory team, the Department of Basic Sciences in the Division of Biochemistry at Loma Linda University, CA, USA.

References

[1] P. E. Castle, "The evolving definition of carcinogenic human papillomavirus," *Infectious Agents and Cancer*, vol. 4, article 7, 5 pages, 2009.

[2] L. M. Gomez, Y. Ma, C. Ho, C. M. McGrath, D. B. Nelson, and S. Parry, "Placental infection with human papillomavirus is associated with spontaneous preterm delivery," *Human Reproduction*, vol. 23, no. 3, pp. 709–715, 2008.

[3] M. E. Sarkola, S. E. Grénman, M. A. M. Rintala, K. J. Syrjänen, and S. M. Syrjänen, "Human papillomavirus in the placenta and umbilical cord blood," *Acta Obstetricia et Gynecologica Scandinavica*, vol. 87, no. 11, pp. 1181–1188, 2008.

[4] H. You, Y. Liu, N. Agrawal et al., "Multiple human papillomavirus types replicate in 3A trophoblasts," *Placenta*, vol. 29, pp. 30–38, 2008.

[5] M. Manavi, K. F. Czerwenka, B. Schurz, W. Knogler, E. Kubista, and E. Reinold, "Latent cervical virus infection as a possible cause of early abortion," *Gynakologisch-Geburtshilfliche Rundschau*, vol. 32, no. 2, pp. 84–87, 1992.

[6] P. L. Hermonat, L. Han, P. J. Wendel et al., "Human papillomavirus is more prevalent in first trimester spontaneously aborted products of conception compared to elective specimens," *Virus Genes*, vol. 14, no. 1, pp. 13–17, 1997.

[7] H. Blencowe, S. Cousens, D. Chou et al., "Born too Soon: the global epidemiology of 15 million preterm births," *Reproductive Health*, vol. 10, no. 1, article S2, 2013.

[8] C. Foppoli, F. De Marco, C. Cini, and M. Perluigi, "Redox control of viral carcinogenesis: the human papillomavirus paradigm," *Biochimica et Biophysica Acta*, vol. 1850, no. 8, pp. 1622–1632, 2015.

[9] Z. Zuo, S. Goel, and J. E. Carter, "Association of cervical cytology and HPV DNA status during pregnancy with placental abnormalities and preterm birth," *American Journal of Clinical Pathology*, vol. 136, no. 2, pp. 260–265, 2011.

[10] G. Cho, K.-J. Min, H.-R. Hong et al., "High-risk human papillomavirus infection is associated with premature rupture of membranes," *BMC Pregnancy and Childbirth*, vol. 13, article 173, 2013.

[11] M. McDonnold, H. Dunn, A. Hester et al., "High risk human papillomavirus at entry to prenatal care and risk of preeclampsia," *American Journal of Obstetrics and Gynecology*, vol. 210, no. 2, pp. 138.e1–138.e5, 2014.

[12] A. S. Rahmanto and M. J. Davies, "Catalytic activity of selenomethionine in removing amino acid, peptide, and protein hydroperoxides," *Free Radical Biology and Medicine*, vol. 51, no. 12, pp. 2288–2299, 2011.

[13] M. Watson, L. van Leer, J. J. Vanderlelie, and A. V. Perkins, "Selenium supplementation protects trophoblast cells from oxidative stress," *Placenta*, vol. 33, no. 12, pp. 1012–1019, 2012.

[14] R. Walter and J. Roy, "Selenomethionine, a potential catalytic antioxidant in biological systems," *Journal of Organic Chemistry*, vol. 36, no. 17, pp. 2561–2563, 1971.

[15] L. Novotny, P. Rauko, S. B. Kombian, and I. O. Edafiogho, "Selenium as a chemoprotective anti-cancer agent: reality or wishful thinking?" *Neoplasma*, vol. 57, no. 5, pp. 383–391, 2010.

[16] A. P. Fernandes and V. Gandin, "Selenium compounds as therapeutic agents in cancer," *Biochimica et Biophysica Acta—General Subjects*, vol. 1850, no. 8, pp. 1642–1660, 2015.

[17] L. J. Hong, B. T. Oshiro, and P. J. Chan, "HPV-16 exposed mouse embryos: a potential model for pregnancy wastage," *Archives of Gynecology and Obstetrics*, vol. 287, no. 6, pp. 1093–1097, 2013.

[18] S. S. Chen, B. S. Block, and P. J. Chan, "Pentoxifylline attenuates HPV-16 associated necrosis in placental trophoblasts," *Archives of Gynecology and Obstetrics*, vol. 291, no. 3, pp. 647–652, 2015.

[19] A. Mincheva, L. Gissmann, and H. zur Hausen, "Chromosomal integration sites of human papillomavirus DNA in three cervical cancer cell lines mapped by in situ hybridization," *Medical Microbiology and Immunology*, vol. 176, no. 5, pp. 245–256, 1987.

[20] J. D. Meissner, "Nucleotide sequences and further characterization of human papillomavirus DNA present in the CaSki, SiHa and HeLa cervical carcinoma cell lines," *Journal of General Virology*, vol. 80, no. 7, pp. 1725–1733, 1999.

[21] L. R. Gooding, L. Aquino, P. J. Duerksen-Hughes et al., "The E1B 19,000-molecular-weight protein of group C adenoviruses prevents tumor necrosis factor cytolysis of human cells but not of mouse cells," *Journal of Virology*, vol. 65, no. 6, pp. 3083–3094, 1991.

[22] S. C. Rowland, J. D. Jacobson, W. C. Patton, A. King, and P. J. Chan, "Dual fluorescence analysis of DNA apoptosis in sperm," *American Journal of Obstetrics & Gynecology*, vol. 188, no. 5, pp. 1156–1157, 2003.

[23] P. J. Chan, J. U. Corselli, J. D. Jacobson, W. C. Patton, and A. King, "Spermac stain analysis of human sperm acrosomes," *Fertility and Sterility*, vol. 72, no. 1, pp. 124–128, 1999.

[24] J. Tolivia, A. Navarro, E. del Valle, C. Perez, C. Ordoñez, and E. Martínez, "Application of photoshop and scion image analysis to quantification of signals in histochemistry, immunocytochemistry and hybridocytochemistry," *Analytical and Quantitative Cytology and Histology*, vol. 28, no. 1, pp. 43–53, 2006.

[25] L. Hinck, J. P. Thissen, S. Pampfer, and R. De Hertogh, "Effect of high concentrations of glucose on differentiation of rat trophoblast cells in vitro," *Diabetologia*, vol. 46, no. 2, pp. 276–283, 2003.

[26] V. S. Yang, S. A. Carter, Y. Ng et al., "Distinct activities of the anaphase-promoting complex/cyclosome (APC/C) in mouse embryonic cells," *Cell Cycle*, vol. 11, no. 5, pp. 846–855, 2012.

[27] J. Han, L. Li, J. Hu et al., "Epidermal growth factor stimulates human trophoblast cell migration through Rho A and rho C activation," *Endocrinology*, vol. 151, no. 4, pp. 1732–1742, 2010.

[28] A. M. Mazurek, A. Fiszer-Kierzkowska, T. Rutkowski et al., "Optimization of circulating cell-free DNA recovery for KRAS mutation and HPV detection in plasma," *Cancer Biomarkers*, vol. 13, no. 5, pp. 385–394, 2013.

[29] J. Wang, L. Mayernik, and D. R. Armant, "Trophoblast adhesion of the peri-implantation mouse blastocyst is regulated by integrin signaling that targets phospholipase C," *Developmental Biology*, vol. 302, no. 1, pp. 143–153, 2007.

[30] S. Boulenouar, C. Weyn, M. van Noppen et al., "Effects of HPV-16 E5, E6 and E7 proteins on survival, adhesion, migration and invasion of trophoblastic cells," *Carcinogenesis*, vol. 31, no. 3, pp. 473–480, 2010.

[31] H. You, Y. Liu, M. J. Carey, C. L. Lowery, and P. L. Hermonat, "Defective 3A trophoblast-endometrial cell adhesion and altered 3A growth and survival by human papillomavirus type 16 oncogenes," *Molecular Cancer Research*, vol. 1, no. 1, pp. 25–31, 2002.

[32] D. Lai, C. L. Tan, J. Gunaratne et al., "Localization of HPV-18 E2 at at mitochondrial membranes induces ROS release and modulates host cell metabolism," *PLoS ONE*, vol. 8, no. 9, Article ID e75625, 2013.

[33] M. A. Whiteside, E. M. Siegel, and E. R. Unger, "Human papillomavirus and molecular considerations for cancer risk," *Cancer*, vol. 113, no. 10, pp. 2981–2994, 2008.

[34] A. W. M. Cheng, T. V. Stabler, M. Bolognesi, and V. B. Kraus, "Selenomethionine inhibits IL-1β inducible nitric oxide synthase (iNOS) and cyclooxygenase 2 (COX2) expression in primary human chondrocytes," *Osteoarthritis and Cartilage*, vol. 19, no. 1, pp. 118–125, 2011.

[35] L. Flohé, "Glutathione peroxidase: fact and fiction," *Ciba Foundation Symposium*, no. 65, pp. 95–122, 1978.

[36] S. G. Miranda, N. Purdie, V. Osborne, B. L. Coomber, and J. P. Cant, "Selenomethionine increases proliferation and reduces apoptosis in bovine mammary epithelial cells under oxidative stress," *Journal of Dairy Science*, vol. 94, no. 1, pp. 165–173, 2011.

[37] J. Wu, G. H. Lyons, R. D. Graham, and M. F. Fenech, "The effect of selenium, as selenomethionine, on genome stability and cytotoxicity in human lymphocytes measured using the cytokinesis-block micronucleus cytome assay," *Mutagenesis*, vol. 24, no. 3, pp. 225–232, 2009.

[38] F. Hazane-Puch, P. Champelovier, J. Arnaud et al., "Six-day selenium supplementation led to either UVA-photoprotection or toxic effects in human fibroblasts depending on the chemical form and dose of Se," *Metallomics*, vol. 6, no. 9, pp. 1683–1692, 2014.

[39] A. Khera, J. J. Vanderlelie, and A. V. Perkins, "Selenium supplementation protects trophoblast cells from mitochondrial oxidative stress," *Placenta*, vol. 34, no. 7, pp. 594–598, 2013.

[40] K. K. Mighty and L. A. Laimins, "The role of human papillomaviruses in oncogenesis," *Recent Results in Cancer Research*, vol. 193, pp. 135–148, 2014.

24

Sexual and Reproductive Health: Knowledge, Attitude, and Perceptions among Young Unmarried Male Residents of Delhi

Jitendra Kumar Meena,[1] Anjana Verma,[1] Jugal Kishore,[2] and Gopal Krishan Ingle[1]

[1]Department of Community Medicine, Maulana Azad Medical College, New Delhi 110002, India
[2]Department of Community Medicine, Vardhman Mahavir Medical College, New Delhi 110029, India

Correspondence should be addressed to Jitendra Kumar Meena; zypexian@gmail.com

Academic Editor: Hind A. Beydoun

Context. Men play a significant role in all spheres of domestic life including reproduction. Youth is a period of critical development and ignoring sexual and reproductive health (SRH) needs of young men ought to have wider social and health consequences. *Aims and Objectives.* To assess the knowledge, attitude, and perceptions regarding SRH among young unmarried men (18–25 years). *Settings and Design.* A semiqualitative study conducted across four health centers (2 rural, 2 urban) across Delhi. *Materials and Methods.* Focus group discussions (FGDs) were held among sixty-four participants regarding various aspects of SRH. *Data Analysis.* The data generated were analyzed using free listing and thematic content analysis along with simple quantitative proportions for different variable groups. *Results.* Good knowledge regarding HIV/AIDS was observed though found poor regarding other STIs/RTIs. Inadequate knowledge and negative attitude towards SRH and condom use were observed among rural participants. Peer group and mass media were the commonest SRH information sources among rural and urban participants, respectively. *Conclusions.* Poor SRH knowledge, perceptions, and available nonformal, unreliable information sources expose young men to poor SRH outcomes. Early, comprehensive SRH information provision can have life-long protective benefits to them and their partners.

1. Introduction

Good reproductive health should include freedom from risk of sexually transmitted diseases, the right to regulate one's own fertility with full knowledge of contraceptive choices, and the ability to control sexuality without being discriminated against because of age, marital status, income, or similar considerations [1]. Male involvement in reproductive health issues had been poor in India and women often depend on husband and other family members for making decision in sexual and reproductive health matters [2]. Men are mutually indispensable partners in sexual and reproductive relationships, marriage, and family building and should be potential partners and advocate for good reproductive health rather than bystanders, barriers, or adversaries. The WHO (1998) emphasized that men should be empowered through the provision of information and services targeting boys, youth, and adults within home, community, and work settings.

With advent of HIV/AIDS pandemic, increasing prevalence of STIs, and the problem of unwanted pregnancies, need of male involvement has become important than ever before [3]. A study done in Bangladesh found significant association between husbands' fertility preferences, background and socioeconomic characteristics, and current use of any family planning method by the couple [4]. The problem is profound in rural areas where inadequate health services, lack of information, social stigma, and policy barriers combined with personal and cultural fears predispose young people to poor knowledge, attitude, and practices regarding SRH. In a study conducted on young unmarried rural Indian men it was seen that their sexual and reproductive health (SRH) knowledge is limited, although the majority were familiar with condoms (99%). Electronic mass media (67%) were the prime source of reproductive health information, yet they lacked detailed knowledge of various contraceptives and felt ignored by health providers, who, they felt, would be capable of providing SRH information through interpersonal communication [5].

A similar study among Khairwar tribe males reported that only 17% of respondents had ever heard of HIV/AIDS infection and STI/RTIs and most had no proper knowledge of its transmission [6]. Lack of correct knowledge regarding reproductive and sexual health among men could be detrimental to their SRH and of their sexual partners. Early sexual activity outside marriage exposes many young men to the risks of unwanted pregnancy and STI/RTIs. In a study done in Turkey, male university students who were sexually active lacked enough knowledge about family planning methods and were reported to engage in high risk behavior [7]. In a similar study in Mumbai, India, it was reported that most sexually active college students did not use condoms and a substantial number of them had sex with commercial sex workers (CSW) [8].

Young adulthood is a period of critical development involving physical, physiological, cognitive, and psychosocial changes. Increasing evidence exists that ignoring SRH needs of young men has wider social and health consequences. In a study done in two boys and two girls' senior secondary schools of rural Delhi, it was found that 25% students had premarital sexual experience [9]. In a study done among male college students of Mumbai it was observed that exposure to erotic materials, a liberal attitude towards sex combined with poor knowledge, and perceived peer norms regarding sexual behavior are some of the most important predictors of risky sexual behavior among male students [10].

Due to the sensitive nature of the subject, little is known about burden and factors associated with SRH problems among men and their knowledge, attitudes, and practices. A study carried out on 120 men attending a reproductive health checkup in a village in rural West Bengal, India, found that SRH issues prevalent and concerning men were sexual weakness, itching around genital areas, burning sensation during urination, early ejaculation, wounds on the genitals, white discharge, and so forth. Other issues raised by men included masturbation, nocturnal emission, consequences of loss of semen, menstruation, pregnancy, and AIDS [11]. Despite wide range of morbidities concerning SRH, treatment seeking behavior among people remains poor as shown in surveys conducted in Bangladesh and India where most people with STI symptoms seek care from unregulated (untrained) private practitioners. The National AIDS Control Organization in India estimates that only 5–10 percent of patients with STIs present to public sector health care. This is true not just for STIs, but for a wide range of curative services, and it is not only the economically wealthy who seek private medical care; the poor also choose private providers for a variety of reasons [12].

Young men are frequently more willing to consider alternative views about their roles in reproductive health and if brought into a wide range of reproductive health services, better SRH outcomes can be expected however; despite all the evidence, there remains a poor male involvement in SRH matters and keeping in view such deficiency the current study was planned and conducted.

2. Subjects and Methods

2.1. Study Locations. The present study was carried out at four different locations (health centers) affiliated to the Department of Community Medicine, Azad Medical College, New Delhi. These health centers were conveniently chosen as they were functioning under investigator's parent department and had well-maintained population records to facilitate community health action. Two of the health centers were located in rural areas (Pooth and Barwala village) and the other two were urban health centers (Balmiki basti slums and Gokulpuri resettlement colony).

2.2. Study Design. It was a semiqualitative study, conducted to assess young men's SRH information needs, perceptions. and preferences through focus group discussions (FGDs). Semiqualitative research involves systematic integration, or "mixing," of quantitative estimates within qualitative data therefore permitting a more complete understanding and synergistic utilization of data.

2.3. Sample Design and Implementation. A convenient sample size of sixty-four was predetermined by the authors based on availability of resources and time constraints. Therefore, to maintain uniformity sixteen participants were included from each health center by selecting first eight eligible men attending general outpatient clinic on two randomly selected days. In case of any refusal the next eligible person was asked to participate in the study. Nonpermanent residents, those not falling in age bracket (18–25 years), and participants with SRH complaints were excluded from the study.

2.4. Study Methodology. Selected participants were informed regarding the subject and objectives of the study and informed verbal consent was obtained. The majority of participants were participating for the first time in similar discussion. Prior approval for conducting the study was taken from designated officials at the health centers and community members. A total of eight FGDs consisting of eight participants in each session were held at selected health centres. The study participants were grouped on the basis of their place of residence (rural/urban) during data collection. However, during data analysis stage they were grouped on the basis of residence, education, and age for differential comparisons. The FGDs were carried out at designated health facilities in separate rooms with adequate facilities and privacy. Due to confidentiality of the study participants proper care was taken during data analysis and publication. Study participants were not paid any incentives for participating in the study.

Discussions were held in Hindi language which is the vernacular language of the region and was easily understood by participants. With participants' permission, audio tapes were used to record proceedings from the FGDs. Two male researchers, one investigator and the other recorder/facilitator, conducted the sessions ranging in length from one to one and half hours. To facilitate equal participation, ground rules were communicated to the participants at the outset of discussions. Group members were asked to respect other participants' confidentiality and privacy, wait for their turn to sign or speak, and respect the right of everyone to freely express their views.

Sexual and reproductive health (SRH) is defined as "a state of complete physical, mental and social well-being and not merely the absence of disease or infirmity, in all matters relating to the sexuality and reproductive system. Sexual and Reproductive health therefore implies that people are able to have a satisfying and safe sex life and that they have the capability to reproduce and the freedom to decide if, when and how often to do so" [13]. Good SRH knowledge indicates sufficient knowledge of key sexual and reproductive health (SRH) topics and issues. The topics should reflect those of primary importance for protecting and promoting SRH. In the present study participants were asked to express their views on similar topics such as SRH and its importance, knowledge regarding various SRH problems, prevention, and treatment of reproductive diseases, and high risk behavior; SRH problems and issues refer to multiple disorders which afflict sexual and reproductive functions in men, for example, testicular swelling, loss of libido, urinary symptoms, erectile difficulty, RTI/STI, HIV, infertility, and genital cancers.

A structured vignette about two fictional people from either gender was used to contextualize and simplify the discussions and to provide an acceptable means of exploring potentially sensitive issues when needed. During each focus group session, the investigator led the discussions while the recorder summarized and noted down important points that were made for each of the questions which were used to back up the audio recordings. After each session, the participants were provided with basic SRH information package based on the feedback received.

2.5. Data Analysis. The data collected in form of audio recordings and notes was translated into English by three authors and after cross-checking a consensus final report was made. Transcribed data were organized into categories and content thematic approach was used for analyzing data using categories from the dataset. Relevant quotes were also mentioned in the text to illustrate these categories. Simple quantitative proportions for different variable groups were also used to analyze the data.

3. Results

A total of seventy-eight people were offered participation in the study with a response rate of 82.1% ($n = 64$). The median age of participants was 23 years and half of them were residing in rural areas of Delhi. The majority of participants had completed high school education (10th std.) and almost half of them were pursuing higher education at the time of data collection. The following themes were identified in the data: (a) knowledge of sexual and reproductive health, (b) importance of sexual and reproductive health, (c) sexual and reproductive health problems and their causation, (d) prevention of sexual and reproductive health problems, (e) treatment of sexual and reproductive health problems, and (f) sexual and reproductive health information and sources.

3.1. Knowledge of Sexual and Reproductive Health. The study participants had variable understanding of good SRH, and more than half of them identified it as the ability of a person to perform sexual activity and procreate. However, some younger rural men believed that it is the absence of any disease or symptoms in reproductive organs. One of the rural participant said "*Ghar mein jitney jyada baccche matlab baap utna hi swasthya hai*" (the more the number of offsprings, the better the SRH of the father). Two-thirds of participants had correct knowledge about the male reproductive organs and functions especially among urban residents. Most of the rural participants felt the need of better knowledge regarding SRH and were willing to acquire the same. The majority of participants reiterated the deficiency of correct and easily accessible SRH information sources.

3.2. Importance of Sexual and Reproductive Health. Most participants felt the importance of SRH and believed that privilege of mobility and freedom of decision making in sexual matters make men more vulnerable and responsible for unfavorable SRH outcomes, for example, STIs/RTIs and unwanted pregnancy. Most rural participants were afraid of such outcomes as they carried social stigma and blame. Nearly all participants agreed that good SRH is important for better fertility outcomes. Around half of the participants said SRH is important matter of concern only for sexually active people and nonindulgence in premarital or high risk sex ensures good SRH. One rural participant said "*Allah ki marzi ke bina sex karne se bimari ho jati hai jisse napunsak ban sakte hain*" (indulging in sex without almighty's wish can lead to disease which can manifest as infertility).

3.3. Sexual and Reproductive Health Problems and Their Causation. Around three-fourths of participants had ever heard of one or more SRH problems. It was observed that urban participants enrolled in college had comparatively better knowledge regarding SRH problems, risk factors, and their modes of transmission. Most of the participants felt that male gender role denies them the space to express fears and anxieties regarding personal SRH problems. Participants with higher age were more concerned of sexual performance related issues like sexual weakness or loss of desire (Kamjori, icchanahona), early dysfunction or ejaculation (Jaldi Girna), penile bent (Ling ka tedhapan), infertility or impotency (Napunsakta), and so forth, while younger participants perceived nocturnal emission (Swapnadosh), excess sexual desire (Garmi), and masturbation (Hasthmaithun) as major SRH problems. Most participants felt that SRH problems are caused by highly frequent or risky sexual behavior with some rural participants' quoting "*sex ke side effects*" (side effects of sex).

The majority of participants except few rural residents knew about HIV/AIDS linkage to sexual activity. Urban participants had better knowledge regarding other transmission modes of HIV/AIDS. Awareness regarding other SRH issues, for example, STI/RTI, functional problems, and fertility, was found particularly low among younger rural participants. Frequently mentioned general symptoms of SRH problems were ulcer/sore on private parts, genital discharge, itching around genital areas, burning or pain on urination, and so forth.

Most of the urban and around half of rural participants felt that unhealthy life style (alcohol, tobacco, and drug addiction) and high risk sexual behavior (unprotected sex, visiting CSW, multiple sex partners, etc.) are detrimental to SRH. Few urban participants also mentioned that poor genital hygiene can also increase risk of SRH problems. Knowledge regarding modes of transmission of SRH problems was fair but some rural participants mentioned dirty water, infected blood transfusion, insect bite, and so forth. Rural participants perceived themselves to be at risk of STIs/RTIs due to their lack of SRH knowledge

Most urban participants were able to identify truck/carriage drivers, single men, CSW, widowers, homosexuals, transgender and drug addicts, and so forth as high risk groups for SRH problems. However, rural participants mostly felt that people visiting CSW, indulging in pornography or unnatural sex (homosexuals), and the ones who are not faithful to their partners are at a higher risk of SRH problems. Some rural participants mentioned that sexual activity is meant for procreation and not for recreation quoting "*sex bhagwan ka tohfa hai ek nayi zindagi lane ke liye naaki beja istemaal maze ke liye*" (sex is a gift of God to bring new life to this world not just to misuse it for pleasure) and some rural participants strongly believed that immoral sexual indulgence paves the way to SRH problems.

3.4. Prevention of Sexual and Reproductive Health Problems. The majority of participants were aware of the preventive role of condoms in transmission of HIV and AIDS and their contraceptive role but knowledge regarding their preventive role in other STIs was low. Half of the participants felt that being faithful to single partner, avoiding commercial sex workers, and regular medical checkup are important preventive strategies. It was seen that urban participants mostly emphasized role of condoms and proper genital hygiene in prevention of SRH problems while rural participants mentioned reduced high risk behavior. One urban participant said "*jannang ki safai evam nirodh ka istemaal humein aise rogon se bachate hain*" (genital hygiene and use of condoms protect us from such diseases). Negative perceptions regarding condom use were widely observed among rural participants. Some rural participants said condom use promotes promiscuous behavior; that is, it is unnatural and not sanctified religiously and hence should be discouraged, while urban participants had different issues regarding condom use and some felt that condoms are difficult to wear and significantly reduce sexual pleasure. Most participants especially rural participants said that condoms are not socially acceptable and it is an embarrassing experience to purchase them. Few participants mentioned the need of premarital SRH screening because of increasing burden of HIV/AIDS. One of the urban participant said "*shadi se pehle yaun rogon ki jaanch jaroor honi chahiye jisse ki dusre ki zindagi barbad na ho*" (it is essential to check for SRH problems before marriage so that health of the other partner can be protected).

3.5. Treatment of Sexual and Reproductive Health Problems. Most of the participants said that only few people seek treatment of SRH problems from qualified medical practitioners, primarily due to social stigma and privacy concerns. More than half of participants believed that public health facilities cater only to female SRH problems. While most participants said they had faith and prefer treatment available at public health facilities, some rural participants preferred private doctors, traditional healers (Bengali doctor, vaidyas, hakims, etc.), and home remedies (eating groundnuts, herbs mixed in drinks like milk or buttermilk). Reasons established for alternative treatment seeking behavior were poor knowledge, privacy concern, and callous attitude of doctors and lack of specialists. One rural participant said "*Keval padhe likhe samajhdar log hi sarkari ilaj samajhte hain, baki sabko vaidya ka ilaj chahiye*" (only educated wise people understand treatment at public health facilities and others want treatment by local healers).

3.6. Sexual and Reproductive Health Information and Sources. Peer group (friends, colleagues, etc.) and mass media (television, internet, newspaper, books, etc.) were the most important sources for SRH information among rural and urban participants, respectively. SRH information was common regarding HIV/AIDS and condom use as they were the most widely discussed subjects. Peers were the most common sources for SRH information related to personal sexual matters and anxieties. The participants especially the urban felt that SRH information from peer sources might be wrong and could lead to further confusion and increased vulnerability. SRH information received from peers and mass media was most often not fully understood and was frequently ignored by most of the participants. Some rural participants believed that SRH information received through mass media encourages young people to indulge in risky sexual activity. Paucity of correct SRH information was reiterated by participants and some mentioned that SRH chapters in school textbooks were intentionally skipped by teachers. Very few participants received SRH information from health care personnel or dispensary boards or notices in health facilities.

3.7. Feedbacks. The majority of participants felt the need for correct and adequate information regarding SRH, especially among urban participants. Information sought was mostly regarding safe ways to have sex, "right time" to start having sex, best practices, prevention of STI, facts regarding sexual physiological issues (night fall, masturbation), and so forth. Half of the participants advocated that SRH is a very important subject and should be formally taught during schooling. Some urban participants said that wide scale dissemination of SRH information will lead to higher societal acceptance and hence better prevention of SRH problems.

4. Discussion

Analysis of the FGDs reflects poor SRH knowledge among study participants especially among rural residents. Lack and poor quality of health services were major constraints in adoption of healthy SRH practices. Substantial felt need regarding correct SRH information was observed reflecting lacunae and missed opportunities in public SRH services.

Most participants agreed to the importance of SRH but related it to sexual activity and its outcomes. Importance of SRH was felt but not realized in rural participants mostly due to fear of social stigma, isolation, and blame. Similar findings were observed in rural Nepal where young people rarely visited health posts to seek sexual health services [14]. In our study, SRH problems reported by elder participants were mostly sexual dysfunctions and related anxieties, while younger participants were concerned regarding physiological SRH issues, for example, nocturnal emission, masturbation, and so forth. The majority of participants had good knowledge about HIV/AIDS, but knowledge regarding other STIs/RTIs was poor especially among rural participants. Predictors for better SRH knowledge were higher age, urban residence, postschool education, and so forth among study participants. The findings of our study do not conform to a study conducted at health camp attendees in rural West Bengal, where no statistically significant difference was found in age, monthly income, days of absence from home, or marital status between men reporting SRH problems [11]. Some rural participants perceived themselves to be at higher risk of contracting SRH problems owing to the lack of SRH information. Misconceptions regarding transmission of STIs and immorality ascribed to sexual activity were commonly observed among rural participants similar to the findings of a Nigerian study [15]. The majority of participants held rejective perceptions regarding condom because of difficulty in its use, reduction in sexual pleasure, unnaturality, and religious unacceptance. Most of the participants in our study were doubtful of contraceptive role of condoms and had poor knowledge regarding their use in preventing STIs other than HIV/AIDS. Similar findings were documented in a study among young unmarried men in rural districts of central India where only 68% young men were aware of condoms and their HIV/AIDS preventive role, and 40% participants knew of their role in preventing unwanted pregnancies [5]. In a Nepalese study it was seen that condoms were not easily available in rural markets and their use was often stigmatized; similar findings were seen in the current study [14].

Poor utilization of trained doctors or public health facilities regarding SRH complaints was seen among rural participants due to social stigma, dissatisfaction, callous attitude of staff, lack of specialists, and privacy concerns. Almost half of the participants felt that public health facilities mostly serve women clients in SRH matters. Important SRH knowledge sources were peer group and mass media among rural and urban study participants, respectively. Similar findings were seen in a study conducted in Nepal, where friends and the media, such as newspapers, radios, and television, were the main reported sources of information about sexual matters [14]. However, in our study SRH information received was inadequate and unreliable and mostly related to HIV/AIDS and condom use only.

Strengths. Semiqualitative research gives us a broader and in-depth understanding of the sociomedical subject like SRH along with proportional estimates. Inclusion of participants from both rural and urban backgrounds is enabling to understand sociocultural determinants of SRH. It is one of the very few studies conducted to assess young men's perception regarding SRH in North India.

Limitations. Data were collected from specified age group of men and may not be representative of the whole range of SRH perceptions among males. The study groups were non-homogenous in terms of characteristics like age, education, socioeconomic status, and so forth which could have affected the quality of data generated.

5. Conclusions

Men have their own SRH concerns and needs which are not always met mostly due to their ascribed gender role and lack of access to specialized health care and information sources. Little knowledge about their own reproductive physiology and SRH problems exposes young men to unsafe behaviors and practices. Young males especially those belonging to rural areas remain disadvantaged in access to correct SRH information compared to urban counterparts, therefore remaining at higher risk of developing SRH problems. Conventional nonformal SRH information sources like peers, mass media, and so forth remain the only source of information to young men and are unreliable and there is a scope of subjective misinterpretations. Providing young men with formal early, correct, comprehensive SRH information can have life-long protective benefits to them along with their partners. IEC activities targeted at this group can prove instrumental in allaying various societal misconceptions about SRH. Peer education programs and increasing access and effective utilization of electronic media especially in rural areas offer potential scope of improvement.

Abbreviations

FGD: Focus group discussion
SRH: Sexual and reproductive health
STI: Sexually transmitted infection
RTI: Reproductive tract infections
CSW: Commercial sex worker
IEC: Information, education, and counseling.

Conflict of Interests

The authors declare that there is no conflict of interests regarding the publication of this paper.

References

[1] United Nations, *Fourth World Conference on Women, Action for Equity, Development and Peace*, United Nations, Beijing, China, 1995.

[2] M. S. Jayalakshmi, K. Ambwani, P. K. Prabhakar, and P. Swain, "A study of male involvement in family planning," *Health and Population: Perspectives and Issues*, vol. 25, no. 3, pp. 113–123, 2002.

[3] World Health Organization, *Reproductive Health Strategy for the African Region 1998–2007*, WHO Regional Office for Africa, Harare, Zimbabwe, 1998.

[4] M. B. Hossain, J. F. Phillips, and A. B. M. K. A. Mozumder, "The effect of husbands' fertility preferences on couples' reproductive behaviour in rural Bangladesh," *Journal of Biosocial Science*, vol. 39, no. 5, pp. 745–757, 2007.

[5] A. Char, M. Saavala, and T. Kulmala, "Assessing young unmarried men's access to reproductive health information and services in rural India," *BMC Public Health*, vol. 11, article 476, 2011.

[6] K. B. Saha, N. Singh, U. Chatterjee Saha, and J. Roy, "Male involvement in reproductive health among scheduled tribe: experience from Khairwars of central India," *Rural and Remote Health*, vol. 7, no. 2, p. 605, 2007.

[7] N. H. Sahin, "Male university students' views, attitudes and behaviors towards family planning and emergency contraception in Turkey," *Journal of Obstetrics and Gynaecology Research*, vol. 34, no. 3, pp. 392–398, 2008.

[8] G. Rangaiyan, *Sexuality & sexual behaviour in the age of AIDS: a study among college youth in Mumbai [Ph.D. dissertation]*, International Institute for Population Sciences (IIPS), Mumbai, India, 1996.

[9] A. K. Sharma and V. N. Sehgal, "Knowledge, attitude, belief and practice (K.A.B.P) study on AIDS among senior secondary students," *Indian Journal of Dermatology, Venereology and Leprology*, vol. 64, no. 6, pp. 266–269, 1998.

[10] R. K. Verma, J. Pulerwitz, V. Mahendra et al., "Challenging and changing gender attitudes among young men in Mumbai, India," *Reproductive Health Matters*, vol. 14, no. 28, pp. 135–143, 2006.

[11] K. M. Dunn, S. Das, and R. Das, "Male reproductive health: a village based study of camp attenders in rural India," *Reproductive Health*, vol. 1, pp. 7–12, 2004.

[12] S. Hawkes and K. G. Santhya, "Diverse realities: understanding HIV and STIs in India," *Sexually Transmitted Infections*, vol. 78, no. 1, pp. 531–539, 2002.

[13] United Nations, *Programme of Action. Adopted at the International Conference on Population and Development, Cairo, 5–13 September 1994*, Paragraph 7.2, United Nations, New York, NY, USA, 1994.

[14] P. R. Regmi, E. van Teijlingen, P. Simkhada, and D. R. Acharya, "Barriers to sexual health services for young people in Nepal," *Journal of Health, Population and Nutrition*, vol. 28, no. 6, pp. 619–627, 2010.

[15] N. Orobaton, "Strategies for increasing male involvement in family planning in Nigeria: a concept paper," 1993.

25

Women's Satisfaction of Maternity Care in Nepal and Its Correlation with Intended Future Utilization

Yuba Raj Paudel,[1] **Suresh Mehata,**[1] **Deepak Paudel,**[2] **Maureen Dariang,**[1] **Krishna Kumar Aryal,**[3] **Pradeep Poudel,**[1] **Stuart King,**[1] **and Sarah Barnett**[4]

[1]*Nepal Health Sector Support Program, Ministry of Health and Population, Kathmandu 44600, Nepal*
[2]*Department for International Development in Nepal, Country Office, Ekantakuna Road, Lalitpur 44600, Nepal*
[3]*Nepal Health Research Council, Ministry of Health and Population, Kathmandu 44600, Nepal*
[4]*Options Consultancy Services Limited, Devon House, 58 St. Katharine's Way, London E1W1LB, UK*

Correspondence should be addressed to Suresh Mehata; sureshmehata@nhssp.org.np

Academic Editor: Robert Gaspar

The impact of rapid increase in institutional birth rate in Nepal on women's satisfaction and planned future utilization of services is less well known. This study aimed to measure women's satisfaction with maternity care and its correlation with intended future utilisation. Data came from a nationally representative facility-based survey conducted across 13 districts in Nepal and included client exit interviews with 447 women who had either recently delivered or had experienced complications. An eight-item quality of care instrument was used to measure client satisfaction. Multivariate probit model was used to assess the attribution of different elements of client satisfaction with intended future utilization of services. Respondents were most likely to suggest maintaining clean/hygienic health facilities (42%), increased bed provision (26%), free services (24%), more helpful behaviour by health workers (18%), and better privacy (9%). Satisfaction with the information received showed a strong correlation with the politeness of staff, involvement in decision making, and overall satisfaction with the care received. Satisfaction with waiting time ($p = 0.035$), information received ($p = 0.02$), and overall care in the maternity care (<0.001) showed strong associations with willingness to return to facility. The findings suggest improving physical environment and interpersonal communication skills of service providers and reducing waiting time for improving client satisfaction and intention to return to the health facility.

1. Introduction

The Government of Nepal has promoted institutional births through the expansion of birthing centers in existing peripheral health institutions and the availability of 24-hour comprehensive emergency obstetric care at hospitals [1]. In addition, the Ministry of Health and Population (MoHP) introduced maternity incentives to reduce financial barriers to accessing institutional births in 2005, which evolved into free maternity care and transport incentives (the Aama program) in 2009 [2]. As a result of this demand generation and service expansion, the institutional birth rate tripled from 18% in 2006 to 55% in 2014 [3–6]. However, increasing the access and utilization of health services is unlikely to bring improved health outcomes unless services meet benchmarks for good quality [7]. The midterm review of current Nepal Health

Sector Program (NHSP II) acknowledged that attention to date has focused on improving access to care, and, although this needs to continue, more attention on quality of care is required as a matter of priority [8]. Furthermore, quality of care is also a central focus in the National Health Policy 2014 [9].

Women's experience and satisfaction are an important element of quality of maternity care [10, 11]. Satisfaction is a complex and multidimensional concept embracing structure, process, and outcome of care [12, 13]. The literature suggests that factors such as women's participation in decision making during pregnancy and childbirth [14, 15], women's sense of control, both internal and external, over the whole process [13, 14], client-provider relationships [16], respectful care [7], and the physical environment of the maternity ward [15] are significant factors associated with women's satisfaction and future utilization of health services. A systematic review highlights the importance of staff attitude and respectful behaviour over pain management or sociodemographic factors on maternity client satisfaction [17]. Hence, to understand service user's perception of quality service, and interaction among different elements of quality of care, it is necessary to study correlation of satisfaction with these elements. Administrators and managers can use such information to improve quality score in a cost-effective way.

Client satisfaction measures the ability of services to meet consumers' expectations [18], and is an important determinant of the choice of health facility and of future utilization of services [19–22]. Satisfied clients will be more likely to return in the future and recommend the institution to their relatives/friends [23, 24]. A study conducted in outpatient setting to investigate association of patient satisfaction with return behaviour concluded that many of the standard elements of quality of care have a very less effect on return behaviour, whereas time and attention paid to health care users were the strongest predictor of returning to a health institution [24]. However, to our knowledge, no studies have examined the association between the likelihood of returning to facility with maternity clients' satisfaction in Nepal.

Increased institutional births are being successfully promoted in Nepal; however, the impact of rapid increases in utilisation on quality of care, women's experience, and client satisfaction is less well known. This paper aims to measure client satisfaction with key elements of quality of care and study the correlation between key quality measures and future utilisation. Understanding women's views and experiences provides an important insight for managers and policy makers to change practices to effectively address their needs and expectations and benefit future clients [25].

2. Methods

2.1. Data Source and Sampling. This paper used data from a nationally representative cross-sectional facility-based survey conducted by some of the authors: Service Tracking Survey (STS) 2013 [26]. Three questionnaires were administered in the survey: facility assessment, exit interviews with maternity clients, and exit interviews with outpatients. The survey provided national estimates for key reproductive, maternal, neonatal, and child health indicators related to availability, readiness, and quality of care. The detailed methodology is presented in the STS 2013 final report [26]. Briefly, a two-stage sampling design was adopted to select health facilities. In the first stage, five districts from Terai, five districts from hill, and 3 districts from mountain were selected considering one district (primary sampling unit) that was randomly selected from 13 subregions of Nepal. In the second stage, all district hospitals and Primary Health Care Centres (PHCCs) from selected districts were included, and sub/health posts (S/HPs) were selected using equal probability selection method (EPSEM). The selected health facilities included 17 public hospitals, 39 PHCCs, 100 HPs, and 86 SHPs. A total of 447 exit interviews were conducted with women who had either delivered recently or had experienced obstetric complications

(87% in hospitals, 8% in PHCCs, 4% in HPs, and less than 1% in SHPs). Due to low caseload and the short data collection time period, fewer clients were interviewed in HPs and SHPs.

2.2. Data Collection and Quality Assurance. Data collection was carried out between July and August 2013. Training Manual, Survey Field Manual, and Data Entry Manual were produced and used throughout the training, data collection, and data entry to ensure quality and consistency. Enumerators had a five-day training, focusing on objectives, approach, survey instruments, ethical issues, reporting, and other operational issues. Supervision and monitoring visits to the survey sites were made soon after survey started to identify and rectify any problems early on. Completed questionnaires were checked by the supervisors in the district before sending them to the central office for data entry. Feedback was provided to the enumerators during data collection.

2.3. Data Cleaning, Coding, and Entry. Completed questionnaires were checked for completeness, consistency of data, and the presence of outliers before data entry. Any suspect data were cross-checked against hard copies of completed questionnaires. The databases were developed in CSPro 5.0. The databases were pretested before data entry start and any errors were eliminated.

2.4. Measures

2.4.1. Client Satisfaction. Client satisfaction was measured using an eight-item instrument. The items covered several key dimensions of client satisfaction: accessibility (one question), interpersonal communication (two questions), physical environment (two questions), clinical care (two questions), and decision making (one question). The 8 items of quality of care showed a high internal consistency (Cronbach's alpha = 0.74) to measure client satisfaction. The responses were marked using a five-point Likert scale [27]: (1) fully dissatisfied, (2) unsatisfied, (3) neutral, (4) satisfied, and (5) fully satisfied. The survey measured the likelihood of visiting the facility again with the question "if you are willing to have another baby, would you like to visit this facility for childbirth?"

2.4.2. Data Analysis. We acknowledged the weighing of the data, the approximate stratification, and the two-level clustering while computing statistical tests, using the survey functions of STATA 12 SE Version.

The sample weight was used during the descriptive bivariate and multivariate analysis. Descriptive analysis was carried out for all dimensions of clients' satisfaction (Table 3). Pearson's correlation was calculated between levels of satisfaction with waiting time, information received, provider competency, politeness of staff, involvement in decision making, cleanliness of facility, privacy, overall care received at the facility, and intended future use of services (Table 2). A correlation coefficient of ≥ 0.3 is considered to be a strong correlation for this analysis. A multivariate probit regression model was used to investigate factors associated

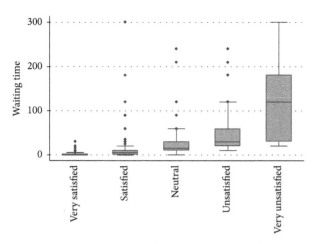

FIGURE 1: Waiting time (minutes) according to level of satisfaction with waiting time ($N = 447$).

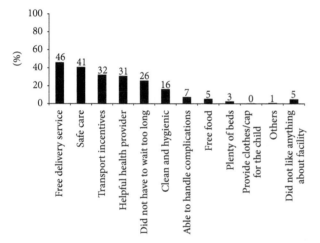

FIGURE 2: Maternity clients' likes about delivery care ($N = 447$).

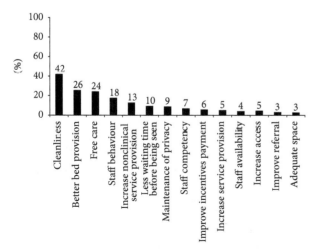

FIGURE 3: Maternity clients' recommendations ($N = 447$).

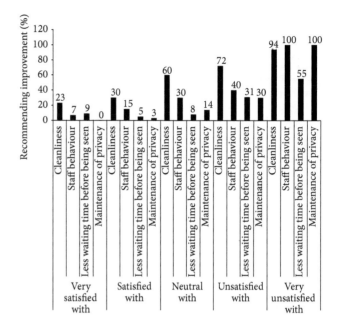

FIGURE 4: Maternity clients' recommendations according to level of satisfaction ($N = 447$).

with intention of future use of services (Table 4). The multivariate model included 8 items of client satisfaction. Level of satisfaction according to waiting time was investigated and presented in a box plot (Figure 1). Maternity clients' likes and recommendations to physical environment, staff behaviour, and facilities were calculated as percentage of total respondents (Figures 2 and 3). Furthermore, client's recommendations to improve various attributes (waiting time, cleanliness, privacy, and staff behaviour) according to their level of satisfaction to each item were also investigated (Figure 4).

3. Results

Table 1 depicts sociodemographic characteristics and accessibility factors for maternity clients. Among 447 respondents, nearly two-thirds were 20–29 years old (67%) and more than one-third were Brahmin/Chhetri (37%). Nearly half (46%) of the total sample had completed secondary education. It took less than 30 minutes for around one-third of the respondents (37%) to reach the health facility, while it took more than an hour to reach health facility for more than a quarter (26%) of respondents.

The percentages of clients satisfied with individual elements of quality of care are presented in Table 2. Most of them were satisfied with (very satisfied and satisfied) care received at the facility (86%), provider's skills (85%), politeness of staff (83%), waiting time (80%), involvement in decision making (77%), cleanliness (70%), information received (69%), and assured confidentiality (67%). Mean satisfaction score was the highest for level of skill of service provider (4.0) and was the lowest for cleanliness of the facilities (3.4).

Table 3 shows the correlation between the various elements of client satisfaction. Satisfaction with information

TABLE 1: Sociodemographic characteristics and geographical/accessibility factors of maternity clients ($N = 447$).

Variables	N	%
Sociodemographic characteristics		
Age (years)		
<20	109	24.38
20–29	300	67.11
≥30	38	8.50
Parity		
Primigravida	263	58.84
Multigravida	184	41.16
Education status		
Never attended school	92	20.58
Primary education	57	12.75
Secondary education	204	45.64
Further education	94	21.03
Caste/ethnicity		
Brahmin/Chhetri	164	36.69
Terai/Madhesi other castes	91	20.36
Dalits	68	15.21
Newar	15	3.36
Janajati	96	21.48
Muslim	13	2.91
Geographic/assessable factors		
Ecological zone		
Mountain	38	8.50
Hill	136	30.43
Terai	273	61.07
Place of residence		
Urban	346	77.40
Rural	101	22.60
Reaching time (minutes)		
<30	167	37.36
30–59	160	35.79
≥60	120	26.85

received showed a strong correlation with politeness of staff, involvement in decision making, and satisfaction about care at facility. Likewise, satisfaction with skill of service provider also showed a strong correlation with politeness of staff and satisfaction with care received. Furthermore, a strong correlation was observed between future use of services and the overall care received at the facility.

Determinants for willingness to visit the facility again are shown in Table 4. Just more than half of the respondents (56%) reported that they were willing to visit the facility again (data not shown). Multivariate analysis revealed that satisfaction with waiting time (coef.: 0.47; 95% CI: 0.03–0.90), information received at the facility (coef.: 0.64; 95% CI: 0.09–1.19), and satisfaction with overall care at facility (coef.: 1.03; 95% CI: 0.55–1.50) were positively associated with willingness to visit the facility again. No significant association was observed with willingness to visit the facility

again and politeness of staff, involvement in decision making, cleanliness of facility, and privacy at facility.

Figure 1 describes satisfaction with waiting time versus waiting time duration at the facility, and study revealed that the likelihood of dissatisfaction with waiting time is increased with increase in waiting time at the facility. The significant difference in waiting time was observed by level of satisfaction; the lowest waiting time was observed for those who were very satisfied (mean: 2 minutes and median = 0 minutes) compared to those who were very unsatisfied (mean: 144 minutes and median: 120 minutes).

Maternity clients were asked what they liked or disliked about the childbirth care they had received. Most commonly, clients liked the provision of free delivery services (46%); safe care (41%); transportation incentives (36%); the helpful attitude of health workers; short waiting times; and the clean and hygienic conditions of health facilities (Figure 2). The most common dislikes reported by maternity clients were a lack of cleanliness (22%), a scarcity of beds and bed linen (21%), and a lack of privacy (9%).

Figure 3 presents major recommendations made by maternity clients to improve services. Most of them suggested maintaining clean/hygienic health facilities (42%), better bed provision (26%), improvement/continuity of free services (24%), more helpful behaviour from health workers (18%), less waiting time (10%), and better privacy at the health facilities (9%). About 17% of maternity clients responded that everything was good in the facility and required no improvement.

Figure 4 shows recommendations of maternity clients by level of satisfaction to cleanliness, staff behavior, waiting time, and privacy. More than 9 in 10 (94%) of clients who were very unsatisfied with cleanliness recommended improving the cleanliness of the facility. More than half of clients who were satisfied or very satisfied with cleanliness also recommended improving cleanliness of the facilities. All of the clients who were very unsatisfied with staff behavior and privacy recommended improving staff behaviour, and privacy, respectively, in the facility. More than half of the clients (55%) who were very unsatisfied with waiting time made recommendation to reduce waiting time between arriving at the facility and being seen by service provider.

4. Discussion

This study measured client satisfaction using 8 items of quality of care. Mean satisfaction score was the highest for level of skill of service providers. On one hand, clients may not be able to differentiate dimensions of competence and incompetence. On the other hand, clients may relate provider skill with politeness and good communication skill of service providers as shown by correlation matrix (Table 2). Previous studies have also found that frequency of explanations [15], skillful interactions, and responsiveness of service provider to client's need [28, 29] were strongly associated with satisfaction with maternity care received. Furthermore, quality of care might have different meaning to different individuals [10]. Relational component could be more important to

TABLE 2: Percentage of the mothers by level of satisfaction with perinatal care ($N = 447$).

Dimension	Very satisfied	Satisfied	Mean satisfaction score[*]	Standard deviation
Accessibility				
Waiting time	27.9	52.5	3.9	0.95
Interpersonal communication aspects				
Information received	11.2	57.7	3.7	0.70
Politeness of staff	12.8	69.9	3.9	0.64
Physical environment				
Assurance of confidentiality	4.0	62.7	3.6	0.73
Cleanliness of facility	7.2	62.4	3.4	0.99
Decision making				
Involvement in decision making	8.9	68.3	3.8	0.65
Technical aspect				
Level of skill of provider	17.3	67.6	4.0	0.62
Care at facility	12.9	72.8	3.9	0.60

[*]The satisfaction score was constructed by giving scores: fully satisfied = 5; satisfied = 4; neutral = 3; dissatisfied = 2; and fully dissatisfied = 1.

some clients compared to technical competency of service providers [7].

Cleanliness of the facility was a major concern among both satisfied and unsatisfied clients. Just more than two-thirds of the clients were satisfied or very satisfied with cleanliness. While a similar proportion of clients were satisfied or very satisfied with cleanliness in service tracking survey of 2012 [30], higher dissatisfaction with cleanliness of maternity facilities was shown in studies conducted in Malawi [21] and Kenya [20] in comparison to current study. Since cleanliness is easily discernible to clients in comparison to other aspects of quality of care, this could have resulted in lower satisfaction with cleanliness. However, poor cleanliness in maternity wards has been reported in previous studies conducted in Nepal and elsewhere [20, 21, 31]. A study that used pattern approach to studying satisfaction to maternity care showed that women who were unsatisfied with physical environment were more likely to be educated [29]; since more than two-thirds of clients in current study had secondary or higher education, cleanliness could have been pointed out clearly. It is interesting to note that almost a quarter of clients who were very satisfied with cleanliness also expressed recommendation to improve cleanliness of the facilities (Figure 4).

Satisfaction with information received showed a strong correlation with politeness of service provider, skill of service provider, and satisfaction toward the care received. This finding suggests that women want to be well informed about the process and outcome of childbirth and most likely relate it to competency of service provider. A good communication between provider and clients is highly valued by maternity clients [25]. Although research has shown that cognitive and emotional support for women during labour is beneficial for well-being of women and newborn by reducing duration of labour and possibility of postpartum depression [32], many studies have highlighted that maternity experience in medical setting has been dominated by professionals. Health workers share very less information with mothers about childbirth process, let alone participating them in decision making about childbirth [25, 33]. Furthermore, although clients expect service providers to have knowledge and technical competency, their satisfaction is mainly determined by behaviour, communication skill of service providers, and amount of time spent in interaction [17, 34]. Hence, maternity health care need to be restructured in a way to cater to the multidimensional needs of women during childbirth.

Only two-thirds of clients were satisfied or very satisfied with privacy in the facility. A study conducted in a maternity health centre from Malawi found that, despite being treated politely, lack of auditory and visual privacy led women to not using a maternity facility [21]. Hence provisions to ensure privacy in health facilities are warranted.

Similar to the findings from other studies [18, 34, 35], the current study found that client satisfaction decreased with higher waiting time. Being seen only after 2 hours of arriving at facility could have brought feeling of being ignored at the health facility and brought dissatisfaction. Another possible explanation for dissatisfaction with longer waiting time could be due to less time to talk with service providers owing to overcrowded facility, despite having to wait for long time. Furthermore, a study conducted in Ethiopia found that delay in receiving care once women had reached the maternity hospital was mainly due to operational issues such as "shortage of medicines, blood, equipment, or to the absence of qualified/competent staff, poor organization of care or combination of all" [36]. Although current study could not investigate what caused longer waiting time, it is likely that poor organization and readiness of care could have resulted in longer waiting time since Jahn et al. found that conduction of caesarean section took an average of 4.5 hours (range of 40 minutes to 11 hours) in rural Nepal once the decision to operate has been made [37]. Longer waiting time was reported to be associated with the worst outcomes among women who experienced similar childbirth complications [36]. Increased demand with staff shortage is likely to result in overcrowded facilities, longer waiting time, poor behaviour from overburdened staff, and shortage of supplies [38], which

TABLE 3: Correlation matrix ($N = 447$).

	Waiting time	Information received	Level of skill of provider	Politeness of staff	Involvement in decision making	Cleanliness of facility	Level of privacy	Care received at facility	Intention for future use of services
Satisfaction with									
Waiting time	1.00								
Information received	0.23	1.00							
Level of skill of provider	0.28	0.41	1.00						
Politeness of staff	0.31	0.36	0.49	1.00					
Involvement in decision making	0.19	0.43	0.30	0.38	1.00				
Cleanliness of facility	0.19	0.25	0.20	0.15	0.19	1.00			
Level of privacy	0.11	0.33	0.23	0.26	0.24	0.27	1.00		
Care received at facility	0.24	0.40	0.43	0.43	0.31	0.32	0.38	1.00	
Intention for future use of services	0.19	0.14	0.13	0.23	0.15	0.08	0.09	0.38	1.00

TABLE 4: Determinants of willingness to return to facility (N = 447).

		Linearized			95% confidence interval	
	Coef.	Std. err.	z	p	Lower	Upper
Waiting time	0.47	0.22	2.11	0.035	0.03	0.90
Information received	0.64	0.28	2.29	0.022	0.09	1.19
Politeness of staff	0.00	0.26	−0.02	0.986	−0.51	0.50
Privacy at facility	−0.39	0.24	−1.64	0.100	−0.86	0.08
Cleanliness of facility	−0.18	0.20	−0.91	0.365	−0.56	0.21
Involvement in decision making	0.15	0.22	0.68	0.500	−0.29	0.59
Level of skill of provider	−0.28	0.27	−1.05	0.292	−0.81	0.24
Overall care at facility	1.03	0.24	4.24	<0.001	0.55	1.50

are often interrelated. Since childbirth is a stressful event, women want quick response when they need a support, while a longer waiting time causes frustration/dissatisfaction [34].

Current study found an association of willingness to return to the facility with satisfaction to waiting time, information received, and overall care in the facility. These results are in concert with findings from other recent studies [23, 34, 39–41]. A study from the US also showed that reducing waiting-room wait time in a primary-care practice significantly improved patient satisfaction and willingness to refer relatives/friends to the facility [41]. Willingness to refer friends/relatives was treated as a proxy measure for overall satisfaction and willingness to return to the primary care. A previous study concluded that service providers need to assess expectation of clients regarding realistic waiting time in order to meet their expectations and improve satisfaction [34]. Reduced intention to return to health facility among those who had to wait for long time could be attributed to poor outcomes among mothers having to wait longer before being seen [36].

Consistent with findings from previous studies [23, 40], information received from service providers, and patient satisfaction have been shown to be a strong correlate of return behaviour in the current study. Garman et al. showed that satisfied clients were more likely to return to the hospital [24]. The clients who returned for subsequent health care were more likely to have received adequate information and attention from service providers. The time and attention provided to the patients and their families counted a lot in increasing likelihood for subsequent visit to the same institution. Hence, high quality patient-clinician relationship is instrumental for client satisfaction. Similarly, Al-Mailam studied satisfaction of hospital care and found that satisfaction to overall care was significantly associated with satisfaction to nursing care. And satisfaction to nursing care showed a strong correlation with intention to return to the hospital [23]. Studies show that if nurses are satisfied with their own jobs, they will behave with clients in a respectful manner [23, 42]. Since most of the care in maternity care is associated with nursing care, behaviour of nurses is likely to determine overall satisfaction and probability of returning in the future.

The findings of this study need to be interpreted in the light of some limitations. Since the majority of women were interviewed within 24 hours of birth in institution, there is a possibility of women being less critical due to the joy of childbirth and overlooking negative experiences due to a phenomenon called halo effect [43]. Further, women of early postnatal period feel difficulty to report negative experiences of childbirth if the child is healthy [44]. In addition, being interviewed within institutional setting might have caused women to response in a positive way. Although other studies have used willingness to recommend the facility as a measure of satisfaction, this study only examined willingness to return to facility. However, researchers have treated willingness to recommend the health facility to friends/relatives as a proxy measure for willingness to return to health facility [41]. Since only few maternity clients (5% of total sample) could be interviewed from sub/health posts, the findings from this study might be closer to the scenario of PHCCs and hospitals of Nepal. We measured intention to return to the health facility for next childbirth which could be different to their actual behaviour. First-time mothers, less educated [29] ones, or who gave childbirth at institutions for the first time might have different perception of quality of care compared to mothers who are educated and who have a previous experience of giving birth at institution.

The findings of this study have implications for policy, maternity care practice, and future research. With increasing focus on institutional birth with skilled birth attendants there is a fear that biomedical interventions overshadow the psychosocial model of care for women [33, 45]. Hence women's expectations need to be understood and addressed upon. Being treated with kindness and meeting their expectations increase women's satisfaction of childbirth experience [25, 46]. Cleanliness of maternity facilities and adequate beds and bed linens need to be ensured and privacy needs to be maintained. Reducing waiting time and providing adequate information are critical for increasing the likelihood to return in the future. Altogether, a renewed focus needs to be given to provide women with full information without having to wait for too long. They need to be provided with opportunity to ask questions and allowed to be involved in decision making. Further qualitative studies examining expectation of clients and satisfaction with self (internal control) need to be undertaken to better understand women's experiences. Response time (duration between calling for service and receiving service) need to be included as measures of satisfaction in future studies.

5. Conclusion

Mean satisfaction score was the highest for skill of service providers and the lowest for cleanliness of facilities. Satisfaction with information received was strongly correlated with politeness of staff, involvement in decision making, and satisfaction with overall care at facility. Willingness to return to facility showed a strong association with information received, waiting time, and overall care at facility. Hence, the measures to improve client experience of maternity care in Nepal should focus on improvement in physical environment along with improving attitude and communication skill of service providers with prompt response.

Conflict of Interests

The authors have no conflict of interests.

Authors' Contribution

Sarah Barnett, Deepak Paudel, Suresh Mehata, and Yuba Raj Paudel had the concept of the paper. Yuba Raj Paudel and Suresh Mehata conducted literature review, carried out the data analysis, and prepared the first draft. Stuart King, Sarah Barnett, Deepak Paudel, Maureen Dariang, and Krishna Kumar Aryal suggested the methodology and reviewed the paper. All authors read and agreed on the final version of paper.

Acknowledgments

The authors would like to thank all of the advisors of NHSSP. The STS 2013 was funded by UK Department for International Development (DFID).

References

[1] Department of Health Services, *Annual Report—2012/13*, Department of Health Services, Kathmandu, Nepal, 2014.

[2] Family Health Division, *Aama Program Guideline*, Second Revision 2069, Family Health Division, DoHS, Kathmandu, Nepal, 2012.

[3] Ministry of Health, New Era, and Macro International, *Nepal Demographic and Health Survey 2006*, Ministry of Health, New Era, Macro International, Calverton, Md, USA, 2007.

[4] Ministry of Health, New Era, and Macro International, *Nepal Demographic and Health Survey 2011*, Ministry of Health, New Era, Macro International, Calverton, Md, USA, 2012.

[5] Central Bureau of Statistics, *Nepal Living Standard Survey-2010/2011. Statistical Report*, vol. 1, Central Bureau of Statistics, Kathmandu, Nepal, 2011.

[6] CBS, *Nepal Multiple Indicator Cluster Surevy 2014: Key Findings*, Central Bureau of Statistics, 2015.

[7] L. Hulton, Z. Matthews, and R. W. Stones, *A Framework for the Evaluation of Quality of Care in Maternity Services*, University of Southampton, Southampton, UK, 2000.

[8] D. Daniels, K. Ghimire, P. Thapa et al., *The Mid Term Review of Nepal Health Sector Programme II (2010–2015)*, 2013, http://www.nhssp.org.np/jar/NHSP%20II%20-%20MTR%20Report.pdf.

[9] Ministry of Health and Population, *National Health Policy 2071*, Ministry of Health and Population, Kathmandu, Nepal, 2014.

[10] R. Pittrof, O. M. R. Campbell, and V. G. A. Filippi, "What is quality in maternity care? An international perspective," *Acta Obstetricia et Gynecologica Scandinavica*, vol. 81, no. 4, pp. 277–283, 2002.

[11] L. A. Hulton, Z. Matthews, and R. W. Stones, "Applying a framework for assessing the quality of maternal health services in urban India," *Social Science and Medicine*, vol. 64, no. 10, pp. 2083–2095, 2007.

[12] M. Redshaw, "Women as consumers of maternity care: measuring 'satisfaction' or 'dissatisfaction'?" *Birth*, vol. 35, no. 1, pp. 73–76, 2008.

[13] J. M. Green and H. A. Baston, "Feeling in control during labor: concepts, correlates, and consequences," *Birth*, vol. 30, no. 4, pp. 235–247, 2003.

[14] M. Morgan, N. Fenwick, C. McKenzie, and C. D. A. Wolfe, "Quality of midwifery led care: assessing the effects of different models of continuity for women's satisfaction," *Quality in Health Care*, vol. 7, no. 2, pp. 77–82, 1998.

[15] L. Séguin, R. Therrien, F. Champagne, and D. Larouche, "The components of women's satisfaction with maternity care," *Birth*, vol. 16, no. 3, pp. 109–113, 1989.

[16] S. R. Baker, P. Y. L. Choi, C. A. Henshaw, and J. Tree, "'I felt as though I'd been in Jail': women's experiences of maternity care during labour, delivery and the immediate postpartum," *Feminism & Psychology*, vol. 15, no. 3, pp. 315–342, 2005.

[17] E. D. Hodnett, "Pain and women's satisfaction with the experience of childbirth: a systematic review," *American Journal of Obstetrics & Gynecology*, vol. 186, no. 5, supplement, pp. S160–S172, 2002.

[18] R. Amdemichael, M. Tafa, and H. Fekadu, "Maternal satisfaction with the delivery services in Assela Hospital, Arsi Zone, Oromia Region, Ethiopia, 2013," *Obstetrics & Gynecology (Sunnyvale)*, vol. 4, article 257, 2014.

[19] S. Agha, A. M. Karim, A. Balal, and S. Sosler, "The impact of a reproductive health franchise on client satisfaction in rural Nepal," *Health Policy and Planning*, vol. 22, no. 5, pp. 320–328, 2007.

[20] M. O. Audo, A. Ferguson, and P. K. Njoroge, "Quality of health care and its effects in the utilisation of maternal and child health services in Kenya," *East African Medical Journal*, vol. 82, no. 11, pp. 547–553, 2005.

[21] G. S. Lule, J. Tugumisirize, and M. Ndekha, "Quality of care and its effects on utilisation of maternity services at health centre level," *East African Medical Journal*, vol. 77, no. 5, pp. 250–255, 2000.

[22] A. Tayelgn, D. T. Zegeye, and Y. Kebede, "Mothers' satisfaction with referral hospital delivery service in Amhara Region, Ethiopia," *BMC Pregnancy and Childbirth*, vol. 11, no. 1, article 78, 2011.

[23] F. F. Al-Mailam, "The effect of nursing care on overall patient satisfaction and its predictive value on return-to-provider behavior: a survey study," *Quality Management in Healthcare*, vol. 14, no. 2, pp. 116–120, 2005.

[24] A. N. Garman, J. Garcia, and M. Hargreaves, "Patient satisfaction as a predictor of return-to-provider behavior: analysis and assessment of financial implications," *Quality Management in Health Care*, vol. 13, no. 1, pp. 75–80, 2004.

[25] R. Hatamleh, I. A. Shaban, and C. Homer, "Evaluating the experience of Jordanian women with maternity care services," *Health Care for Women International*, vol. 34, no. 6, pp. 499–512, 2013.

[26] Ministry of Health and Population (MOHP), Health Research and Social Development Forum (HERD), and Nepal Health Sector Support Programme (NHSSP), *Service Tracking Survey 2013*, MOHP, HERD, NHSSP, Kathmandu, Nepal, 2014.

[27] R. Likert, "A technique for the measurement of attitudes," *Archives of Psychology*, vol. 22, no. 140, pp. 5–53, 1932.

[28] P. Goodman, M. C. Mackey, and A. S. Tavakoli, "Factors related to childbirth satisfaction," *Journal of Advanced Nursing*, vol. 46, no. 2, pp. 212–219, 2004.

[29] A. Rudman, B. El-Khouri, and U. Waldenström, "Women's satisfaction with intrapartum care—a pattern approach," *Journal of Advanced Nursing*, vol. 59, no. 5, pp. 474–487, 2007.

[30] S. Mehata, S. Lekhak, P. Chand, D. Singh, P. Poudel, and S. Barnett, *Service Tracking Survey 2012*, Ministry of Health and Population, Kathmandu, Nepal, 2013.

[31] Family Health Division and NHSSP, *Responding to Increased Demand for Institutional Childbirths at Referral Hospitals in Nepal: Situational Analysis and Emerging Options*, NHSSP, 2013.

[32] M. Klaus, J. Kennell, G. Berkowitz, and P. Klaus, "Maternal assistance and support in labor: father, nurse, midwife, or doula," *Clinical Consultations in Obstetrics and Gynecology*, vol. 4, no. 4, pp. 211–217, 1992.

[33] T. Kabakian-Khasholian, O. Campbell, M. Shediac-Rizkallah, and F. Ghorayeb, "Women's experiences of maternity care: satisfaction or passivity?" *Social Science & Medicine*, vol. 51, no. 1, pp. 103–113, 2000.

[34] J. Senti and S. D. LeMire, "Patient satisfaction with birthing center nursing care and factors associated with likelihood to recommend institution," *Journal of Nursing Care Quality*, vol. 26, no. 2, pp. 178–185, 2011.

[35] J. K. Obamiro, "Effects of waiting time on patient satisfaction: Nigerian hospitals experience," *The International Journal of Economic Behavior*, vol. 3, no. 1, pp. 117–126, 2013.

[36] E. Kabali, C. Gourbin, and V. De Brouwere, "Complications of childbirth and maternal deaths in Kinshasa hospitals: testimonies from women and their families," *BMC Pregnancy and Childbirth*, vol. 11, no. 1, article 29, 2011.

[37] A. Jahn, M. D. Iang, U. Shah, and H. J. Diesfeld, "Maternity care in rural Nepal: a health service analysis," *Tropical Medicine & International Health*, vol. 5, no. 9, pp. 657–665, 2000.

[38] S. Ng'anjo Phiri, K. Fylkesnes, A. L. Ruano, and K. M. Moland, "'Born before arrival': user and provider perspectives on health facility childbirths in Kapiri Mposhi district, Zambia," *BMC Pregnancy and Childbirth*, vol. 14, no. 1, article 323, 2014.

[39] W. D. Klinkenberg, S. Boslaugh, B. M. Waterman et al., "Inpatients' willingness to recommend: a multilevel analysis," *Health Care Management Review*, vol. 36, no. 4, pp. 349–358, 2011.

[40] H. R. Rubin, B. Gandek, W. H. Rogers, M. Kosinski, C. A. McHorney, and J. E. Ware Jr., "Patients' ratings of outpatient visits in different practice settings: results from the medical outcomes study," *The Journal of the American Medical Association*, vol. 270, no. 7, pp. 835–840, 1993.

[41] M. Michael, S. D. Schaffer, P. L. Egan, B. B. Little, and P. S. Pritchard, "Improving wait times and patient satisfaction in primary care," *Journal for Healthcare Quality*, vol. 35, no. 2, pp. 50–60, 2013.

[42] N. A. Khan, S. K. Aslam, A. U. Rehman et al., "Satisfaction level and its predictors among out patients at public sector hospital in Karachi," *Journal of Dow University of Health Sciences*, vol. 8, no. 3, 2014.

[43] D. Polit and C. Beck, *Nursing Research: Principles and Methods*, Lippincott Williams & Wilkins, Philadelphia, Pa, USA, 2004.

[44] J. E. Soet, G. A. Brack, and C. DiIorio, "Prevalence and predictors of women's experience of psychological trauma during childbirth," *Birth*, vol. 30, no. 1, pp. 36–46, 2003.

[45] P. Larkin, C. M. Begley, and D. Devane, "Women's experiences of labour and birth: an evolutionary concept analysis," *Midwifery*, vol. 25, no. 2, pp. e49–e59, 2009.

[46] S. Hassan-Bitar and L. Wick, "Evoking the guardian angel: childbirth care in a palestinian hospital," *Reproductive Health Matters*, vol. 15, no. 30, pp. 103–113, 2007.

Permissions

All chapters in this book were first published in IJRMED, by Hindawi Publishing Corporation; hereby published with permission under the Creative Commons Attribution License or equivalent. Every chapter published in this book has been scrutinized by our experts. Their significance has been extensively debated. The topics covered herein carry significant findings which will fuel the growth of the discipline. They may even be implemented as practical applications or may be referred to as a beginning point for another development.

The contributors of this book come from diverse backgrounds, making this book a truly international effort. This book will bring forth new frontiers with its revolutionizing research information and detailed analysis of the nascent developments around the world.

We would like to thank all the contributing authors for lending their expertise to make the book truly unique. They have played a crucial role in the development of this book. Without their invaluable contributions this book wouldn't have been possible. They have made vital efforts to compile up to date information on the varied aspects of this subject to make this book a valuable addition to the collection of many professionals and students.

This book was conceptualized with the vision of imparting up-to-date information and advanced data in this field. To ensure the same, a matchless editorial board was set up. Every individual on the board went through rigorous rounds of assessment to prove their worth. After which they invested a large part of their time researching and compiling the most relevant data for our readers.

The editorial board has been involved in producing this book since its inception. They have spent rigorous hours researching and exploring the diverse topics which have resulted in the successful publishing of this book. They have passed on their knowledge of decades through this book. To expedite this challenging task, the publisher supported the team at every step. A small team of assistant editors was also appointed to further simplify the editing procedure and attain best results for the readers.

Apart from the editorial board, the designing team has also invested a significant amount of their time in understanding the subject and creating the most relevant covers. They scrutinized every image to scout for the most suitable representation of the subject and create an appropriate cover for the book.

The publishing team has been an ardent support to the editorial, designing and production team. Their endless efforts to recruit the best for this project, has resulted in the accomplishment of this book. They are a veteran in the field of academics and their pool of knowledge is as vast as their experience in printing. Their expertise and guidance has proved useful at every step. Their uncompromising quality standards have made this book an exceptional effort. Their encouragement from time to time has been an inspiration for everyone.

The publisher and the editorial board hope that this book will prove to be a valuable piece of knowledge for researchers, students, practitioners and scholars across the globe.

List of Contributors

Kavita Agarwal, Achla Batra and Aruna Batra
Department of Obstetrics & Gynaecology, Safdarjung Hospital, G-14, 92 Vrindavan Apartment, Gali No. 4, Krishna Nagar, Safdarjung Enclave, New Delhi 110029, India

Abha Aggarwal
NIMS, Delhi 110029, India

N. Ellissa Baskind and Vinay Sharma
The Leeds Centre for Reproductive Medicine, Leeds Teaching Hospitals NHS Trust, Seacroft Hospital, York Road, LS14 6UH Leeds, UK

Nicolas M. Orsi
Women's Health Research Group, Leeds Institute of Cancer & Pathology, St James's University Hospital, Well come Trust Brenner Building, Beckett Street, LS9 7TF Leeds, UK

F. Coelho, L. F. Aguiar, G. S. P. Cunha and N. Cardinot
Centro de Infertilidade e Medicina Fetal do Norte Fluminense, Hospital Escola Álvaro Alvim, Rua Barão da Lagoa Dourada, 409-2° pavimento, Centro, 28035-210 Campos dos Goytacazes, RJ, Brazil

E. Lucena
Centro Colombiano de Fertilidad y Esterilidad (CECOLFES) S.A.S., Calle 102 No. 14A-15, 56769 Bogota, Colombia

Ghulam Mustafa, Waqas Hameed, Safdar Ali, Muhammad Ishaque, Wajahat Hussain and Aftab Ahmed
Marie Stopes Society, Research, Monitoring and Evaluation, Technical Services Department, 21-C, Commercial Area, Old Sunset Boulevard, DHA-II, Karachi, Sindh 75500, Pakistan

Syed Khurram Azmat
Marie Stopes Society, Research, Monitoring and Evaluation, Technical Services Department, 21-C, Commercial Area, Old Sunset Boulevard, DHA-II, Karachi, Sindh 75500, Pakistan
Department of Urogynecology, Faculty of Medicine and Health Sciences, University of Gent, Sint-Pietersnieuwstraat 25, 9000 Gent, Belgium

Erik Munroe
Marie Stopes International, Research, Monitoring and Evaluation Department, 1 Conway Street, Fitzroy Square, London W1T 6LP, UK

Tal Lazer, Shir Dar, Ekaterina Shlush and Basheer S. Al Kudmani
CReATe Fertility Centre, 790 Bay Street, Suite 1100, Toronto, ON, Canada M5G 1N8
Department of Obstetrics & Gynecology, University of Toronto, Toronto, ON, Canada M5S 2J7

Kevin Quach and Agata Sojecki
CReATe Fertility Centre, 790 Bay Street, Suite 1100, Toronto, ON, Canada M5G 1N8

Karen Glass, Prati Sharma, Ari Baratz and Clifford L. Librach
CReATe Fertility Centre, 790 Bay Street, Suite 1100, Toronto, ON, Canada M5G 1N8
Department of Obstetrics & Gynecology, University of Toronto, Toronto, ON, Canada M5S 2J7
Division of Reproductive Endocrinology and Infertility, Department of Obstetrics and Gynecology, Women's College Hospital, Toronto, ON, Canada M5S 1B2

Anjana Verma, Jitendra Kumar Meena and Bratati Banerjee
Department of Community Medicine, Maulana Azad Medical College, New Delhi 110002, India

Bernd Rosenbusch
Department of Gynaecology and Obstetrics, University of Ulm, Prittwitzstraße 43, 89075 Ulm, Germany

Ignace Habimana-Kabano
Demography and Statistics, University of Rwanda, P.O. Box 117, Huye, Rwanda
Utrecht University, P.O. Box 80115, 3508 TC Utrecht, Netherlands

Annelet Broekhuis and Pieter Hooimeijer
Utrecht University, P.O. Box 80115, 3508 TC Utrecht, Netherlands

Prashanth Adiga, Indumathi Kantharaja, Shripad Hebbar, Lavanya Rai, Shyamala Guruvare and Anjali Mundkur
Department of Obstetrics and Gynaecology, Kasturba Medical College, Manipal University, Manipal 576104, India

Abdul Quaiyum
Centre for Reproductive Health, icddr,b, Bangladesh

Rukhsana Gazi and Shahed Hossain
Centre for Equity and Health Systems, icddr,b, Mohakhali C/A, Dhaka 1212, Bangladesh

Andrea Wirtz
Department of Epidemiology, The Centre for Public
Health and Human Rights, Johns Hopkins Bloomberg
School of Public Health, 615 North Wolfe Street/E7144,
Baltimore, MD 21205, USA

Nirod Chandra Saha
Health Systems and Infectious Diseases Division, icddr,b,
Bangladesh

Abdulsalam Saliu and Babatunde Akintunde
Department of Community Medicine, Ladoke Akintola
University of Technology Teaching Hospital, Ogbomoso
201, Oyo State, Nigeria

**Waqas Hameed, Wajahat Hussain, Ghulam Mustafa,
Muhammad Ishaque, Safdar Ali and Aftab Ahmed**
Marie Stopes Society, Research, Monitoring & Evaluation
Department-Technical Services, Karachi, Sindh 75500,
Pakistan

Syed Khurram Azmat
Marie Stopes Society, Research, Monitoring & Evaluation
Department-Technical Services, Karachi, Sindh 75500,
Pakistan
Department of Uro-Gynecology, University of Ghent,
9000 East Flanders, Belgium

Moazzam Ali
Department of Reproductive Health and Research, World
Health Organization, 1211 Geneva, Switzerland

Marleen Temmerman
Department of Uro-Gynecology, University of Ghent,
9000 East Flanders, Belgium
Department of Reproductive Health and Research, World
Health Organization, 1211 Geneva, Switzerland

**Nasreen Noor, Mehkat Ansari, S. Manazir Ali and
Shazia Parveen**
Department of Obstetrics and Gynaecology and
Department of Pediatrics, JNMCH, AMU, L-Block 107
Safina Apartment, Medical Road, Aligarh 202002, India

**Joselyn Rojas, Mervin Chávez-Castillo and Valmore
Bermúdez**
Endocrine and Metabolic Diseases Research Center,
School of Medicine, University of Zulia, 20th Avenue,
Maracaibo 4004, Venezuela

Tayebeh Naderi and Samaneh Omidi
Research Center for Health Services Management,
Institute of Futures Studies in Health, Kerman University
of Medical Sciences, Kerman 76175-113, Iran

Shohreh Foroodnia and Faezeh Samadani
Research Center for Social Determinants of Health,
Institute of Futures Studies in Health, Kerman University
of Medical Sciences, Kerman 76175-113, Iran

Nouzar Nakhaee
Neuroscience Research Center, Institute of
Neuropharmacology, Kerman University of Medical
Sciences, Kerman 76175-113, Iran

Samer Sourial
Department of Women's and Children's Health, Institute
of Translational Medicine, University of Liverpool,
Liverpool L69 3BX, UK

Nicola Tempest and Dharani K. Hapangama
Department of Women's and Children's Health, Institute
of Translational Medicine, University of Liverpool,
Liverpool L69 3BX, UK
Centre for Women's Health Research, Liverpool Women's
Hospital NHS Foundation Trust, Liverpool L8 7SS, UK

**Juan Torrado, Yanina Zócalo, Ignacio Farro, Federico
Farro and Daniel Bia**
Centro Universitario de Investigación, Innovación
y Diagnóstico Arterial (CUiiDARTE), Physiology
Department, Faculty of Medicine, Republic University,
General Flores 2125, 11800 Montevideo, Uruguay

Claudio Sosa, Santiago Scasso and Justo Alonso
Department of Obstetrics and Gynecology "C", Pereira-
Rossell Hospital, Faculty of Medicine, Republic University,
Br. Artigas 1550, 11600 Montevideo, Uruguay

Ida Lilywaty Md Latar and Nuguelis Razali
Department of Obstetrics & Gynaecology, Universiti
Malaya, 59100 Kuala Lumpur, Malaysia

Vidyashree Ganesh Poojari and Vidya Vishwanath Bhat
Department of OBG, Radhakrishna Multispeciality
Hospital, Bangalore, Karnataka, India

Ravishankar Bhat
Department of General Surgery, Radhakrishna
Multispeciality Hospital, Bangalore, Karnataka, India

Khaled Kasim
Department of Public Health and Community Medicine,
Faculty of Medicine, Al-Azhar University, Nasr City,
Cairo, Egypt

Ahmed Roshdy
Assisted Reproductive Technology (ART) Unit,
International Islamic Centre for Population Studies and
Research (IICPSR), Al-Azhar University, Cairo, Egypt

Jila Amirkhani
Medical Science Research Center, Medical Department,
Islamic Azad University, Tehran Medical Sciences Branch,
Tehran, Iran

Soheila Yadollah-Damavandi and Yekta Parsa
Young Researchers Club, Islamic Azad University,
Tehran Medical Sciences Branch, Tehran, Iran

Seyed Mohammad-Javad Mirlohi and Seyede Mahnaz Nasiri
Student Research Committee, Islamic Azad University, Tehran Medical Sciences Branch, Tehran, Iran

Mohammad Gharehbeglou
Department of Medicine, Islamic Azad University, Qom Branch, Qom, Iran

Jonah Sydney Aprioku and Theresa Chioma Ugwu
Department of Pharmacology, Faculty of Basic Medical Sciences, University of Port Harcourt, PMB 5323, Port Harcourt, Nigeria

Jennifer A. Tolen, Kathleen Lau and Philip J. Chan
Department of Gynecology and Obstetrics, 11370 Anderson Street, Suite 3950, Loma Linda University School of Medicine, Loma Linda, CA 92354, USA

Penelope Duerksen-Hughes
Department of Basic Sciences, Center for Health Disparities and Molecular Medicine, 11021 Campus Street, Loma Linda University School of Medicine, Loma Linda, CA 92350, USA

Jitendra Kumar Meena, Anjana Verma and Gopal Krishan Ingle
Department of Community Medicine, Maulana Azad Medical College, New Delhi 110002, India

Jugal Kishore
Department of Community Medicine, Vardhman Mahavir Medical College, New Delhi 110029, India

Yuba Raj Paudel, Suresh Mehata, Maureen Dariang, Pradeep Poudel and Stuart King
Nepal Health Sector Support Program, Ministry of Health and Population, Kathmandu 44600, Nepal

Deepak Paudel
Department for International Development in Nepal, Country Office, Ekantakuna Road, Lalitpur 44600, Nepal

Krishna Kumar Aryal
Nepal Health Research Council, Ministry of Health and Population, Kathmandu 44600, Nepal

Sarah Barnett
Options Consultancy Services Limited, Devon House, 58 St. Katharine's Way, London E1W1LB, UK

Printed in the USA
CPSIA information can be obtained
at www.ICGtesting.com
JSHW051444221024
72173JS00006B/1578